Geometric Dynamics

Mathematics and Its Applications

Volume 513

Geometric Dynamics

by

Constantin Udrişte

Department of Mathematics and Physics,
University Politehnica of Bucharest,
Bucharest, Romania

SPRINGER-SCIENCE+BUSINESS MEDIA, B.V.

A C.I.P. Catalogue record for this book is available from the Library of Congress.

DOI 10.1007/978-94-011-4187-1

Printed on acid-free paper

To my parents,
DUMITRA and NICOLAE

CONTENTS

PREFACE

Geometric dynamics is a tool for developing a mathematical representation of real world phenomena, based on the notion of a field line described in two ways:

-as the solution of any Cauchy problem associated to a first-order autonomous differential system;

-as the solution of a certain Cauchy problem associated to a second-order conservative prolongation of the initial system.

The basic novelty of our book is the discovery that a field line is a geodesic of a suitable geometrical structure on a given space (Lorentz-Udrişte world-force law). In other words, we create a wider class of Riemann-Jacobi, Riemann-Jacobi-Lagrange, or Finsler-Jacobi manifolds, ensuring that all trajectories of a given vector field are geodesics. This is our contribution to an old open problem studied by H. Poincaré, S. Sasaki and others.

From the kinematic viewpoint of corpuscular intuition, a field line shows the trajectory followed by a particle at a point of the definition domain of a vector field, if the particle is sensitive to the related type of field. Therefore, field lines appear in a natural way in problems of theoretical mechanics, fluid mechanics, physics, thermodynamics, biology, chemistry, etc.

This book concentrates on the modern concepts that are necessary to state the properties of flows and of geometric dynamics. Therefore, the order and coverage of topics where chosen for maximum efficiency, effectiveness, and balance. The key words of the summary of the book are: scalar fields, vector fields, differential operators, geometrical and physical vector fields (potential, irrotational, solenoidal, Killing, conformal, linear, affine, projective, torse-forming, Hamiltonian, biscalar, electric, magnetic etc.), field lines, flows, stability of equilibrium points, potential systems and catastrophe theory, field hypersurfaces, bifurcation in the equilibrium set, flow bifurcation, distribution orthogonal to a vector field, extrema with nonholonomic constraints, thermodynamic systems, energies, geometric dynamics induced by a vector field, Lorentz-Udrişte world-force law, magnetic fields around piecewise rectilinear electric circuits, nonclassical magnetic dynamics, hypoelastic materials, granular materials, stability domains, constitutive equations, Cauchy stress tensor, deformation tensor, stress history, accessible stress path, volume stress power, total stress power.

From the viewpoint of mathematical expression, we appreciate that accessible calculations are much more useful than exposition of hermetic mathematical language. In this sense, we prefer examples furnished by the applied sciences, promoting especially those that do not bury the mathematical concepts in unessential data, and we have carefully balanced theory with applications and geometric intuition. Also, at the beginning of each chapter is given a short description of the contents, of the applications and of the examples, all suggesting the theoretical and practical meaning of the respective chapter. These short introductions supplement titles of some chapters which refer only to the mathematical contents and not to applications.

The book is addressed to graduate students, scientists and researchers whose work involves mathematics, mechanics, physics, engineering, biology, chemistry, economics, etc, being based on didactic and scientific experience accumulated by the author at the Department of Mathematics of the University Politehnica of Bucharest. Here the ideas of the book "*C. Udrişte, Field Lines (in Romanian), Technical Editorial House, Bucharest, 1988*" are developed further using the tools of dynamical systems and differential geometry. Completely new and original are Chapter 9 - Dynamics Induced by a Vector Field, Chapter 10 - Magnetic Dynamical Systems and Sabba Ştefănescu Conjectures, and Chapter 11 - Bifurcations in the Mechanics of Hypoelastic Granular Materials. Chapter 11 was competently realized by Prof. Dr. Lucia Drăguşin, a famous specialist in the mathematical theory of materials.

We would like to express our appreciation to all people and institutions who helped us while this book was being prepared. Special thanks go to Prof. Dr. Ionel Ţevy for scientific discussions, to Prof. Magdalena Toda for translating a part of the original manuscript from Romanian into English, to Mr. Edwin Beschler for valuable suggestions regarding the English language and the style of the book, and to my wife Eng. Aneta Udrişte, Prof. Dr. Constantin Drăguşin, Student Andrei Soeanu for their WP assistance. I gratefully aknowledge the Ministry of Education, Ministry of Research and Technology, and the Romanian Academy for financial support of our research during the past ten years. A part of this research is strongly reflected by the topics in Chapters 9 and 10.

I am deeply obliged to Kluwer Academic Publishers for accepting my offer and for their valuable technical assistance.

June 10, 1999 Prof. Dr. Constantin Udrişte
BUCHAREST

1. VECTOR FIELDS

Scalar fields (see 1.1) and vector fields (see 1.2 and 1.5) are mathematical models derived from laws of nature, among which we cite the following examples:

1) the law of molecular sublimation speed and the law of the pressure that is necessary for producing this phenomenon, the equilibrium condition and the volume after dilatation while creating some spherical products in the universe;

2) the velocity of local evolution of a biological system made up from a predator species and a prey species, the gravitational field, the electrostatic field, the field of velocities in the mass of a fluid and the gradient of a scalar field.

The Inverse Function Theorem and the Implicit Function Theorem are the basis of Differential Geometry. The elementary part of this geometry refers to the submanifolds of R^n *(see 1.3).*

Some quantitative and qualitative properties of scalar and vector fields arise from the derivative with respect to a vector or to a vector field, explained in 1.4, or from the gradient, Hessian, curl, divergence and Laplacian operators presented in 1.6.

In 1.5 and in problems 2 and 3 from 1.7, we describe some alternatives for defining tangent vectors and, consequently, vector fields, imposed by the necessity of abstraction, namely passing from R^n *to finite or infinite-dimensional differentiable manifolds. In 1.7 we give some problems that we consider to be useful in rationalizing and completing the theory.*

1.1. SCALAR FIELDS

Let R be the set of real numbers and R^n the canonical Euclidean space of dimension n.

A function $f: R^n \to R$ is called a *scalar field* on R^n. Abbreviating, the scalar field is denoted by f, while its value at the point $x = (x_1, \ldots, x_n)$ is denoted by $f(x)$.

A continuous scalar field is called *of class* C^0. A scalar field that has continuous partial derivatives up to the order p inclusively $(p = 1, 2, \ldots)$ is called *of class* C^p. A scalar field that admits an expansion in a Taylor series in a neighborhood of any point $x \in R^n$ is called *of class* C^∞ or *analytic*.

Notice. Let S be any subset of R^n. The scalar field $f: S \to R$ is called *of class* C^p, $p \geq 1$, if there exists an open set $D \subset R^n$ that includes also S and a scalar field $F: D \to R$ of class C^p, $p \geq 1$, such that $f = F|_S$.

Let $f: R^n \to R$ be a scalar field of class C^1. The solutions of the system

$$\frac{\partial f}{\partial x_1}(x_1,\ldots,x_n)=0\,,\ldots,\frac{\partial f}{\partial x_n}(x_1,\ldots,x_n)=0$$

are called *critical points* of the scalar field f. The points in which at least one partial derivative $\frac{\partial f}{\partial x_1},\ldots,\frac{\partial f}{\partial x_n}$ does not vanish are called *regular points* of f.

Let c be a real number. The set

$$M_c=f^{-1}(c)=\{(x_1,\ldots,x_n)\,|\,(x_1,\ldots,x_n)\in R^n, f(x_1,\ldots,x_n)=c\}$$

is called *the set of constant level* c or *the set of Cartesian implicit equation* $f(x_1,\ldots,x_n)=c$. For brevity, we write $M_c: f(x_1,\ldots,x_n)=c$. Obviously, if $c\notin f(R^n)$, then $M_c=\varnothing$.

The names of *constant level points, constant level curves* and *constant level surfaces* are given to certain sets of constant level in the cases $n=1$, $n=2$, respectively $n=3$ (see 1.3).

If we consider arbitrarily c in R, then the equations $f(x_1,\ldots,x_n)=c$ represent a family of sets of constant level. This family has the following properties:

1) through each point passes a set of constant level, mainly through $x_0=(x_{10},\ldots,x_{n0})\in R^n$ passes the set for which $c=f(x_0)$;

2) two sets of constant level have no common point. If there were any, the sets would coincide because each value of a function is unique.

The sets of constant level associated to the function f are strongly related to the graph of f, serving together to describe some qualitative properties of the scalar field. The graph of the scalar field $f: R^n\to R$ is the subset of R^{n+1} defined by

$$G(f)=\{(x_1,\ldots,x_n,x_{n+1})\,|\,(x_1,\ldots,x_n)\in R^n,\ x_{n+1}=f(x_1,\ldots,x_n)\}.$$

Thus it can be seen that M_c is precisely the projection on R^n of the intersection of the graph of f and the hyperplane $x_{n+1}=c$. On the other hand, $G(f)$ is the set of constant zero level attached to the function

$$F: R^{n+1}\to R,\ F(x_1,\ldots,x_{n+1})=f(x_1,\ldots,x_n)-x_{n+1}.$$

M_c contains both regular and critical points of f. Those critical points which belong to M_c are called *critical* or *singular points* of M_c.

If f is a polynomial of degree n, then M_c is called an n-th *order algebraic hypersurface*. In particular, we have the following names: *first-order algebraic hypersurfaces (hyperplanes), second-order algebraic hypersurfaces (hyperquadrics)* etc.

Examples. Let us consider the scalar fields defined on R^2 respectively by

$$x^2+y^2 (or\ -x^2-y^2),\ x^2-y^2,\ x^3-3xy^2,\ x^2,\ x^2y^2.$$

These fields are visualized either by corresponding graphs which respectively have shapes from Figs.1-5, a, or by the constant level curves which are drawn in Figs.1-5, b.

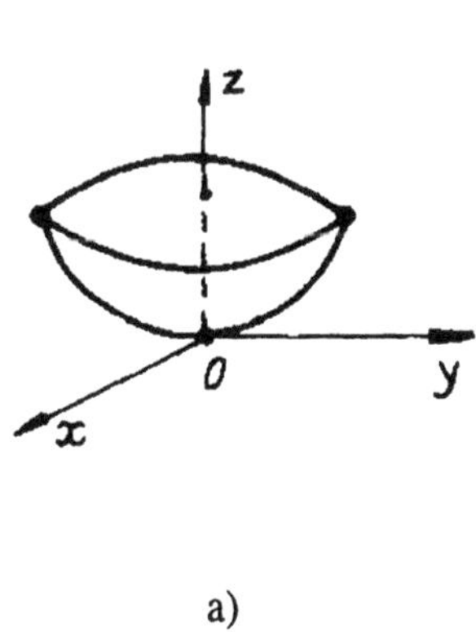

a)

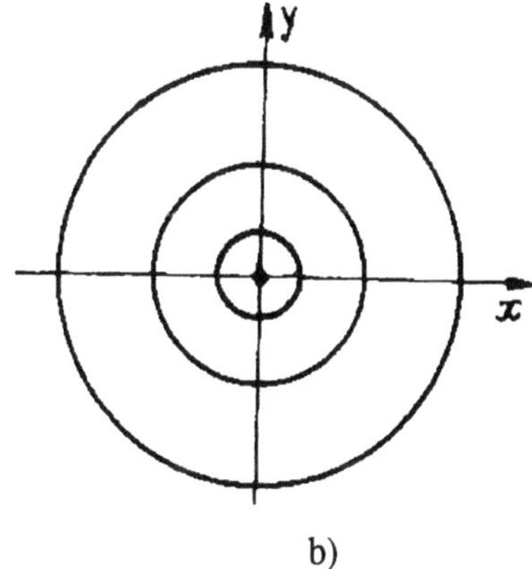

b)

Fig. 1

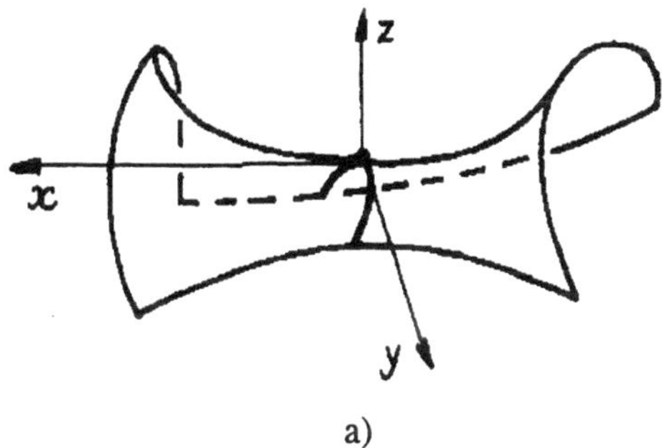

a)

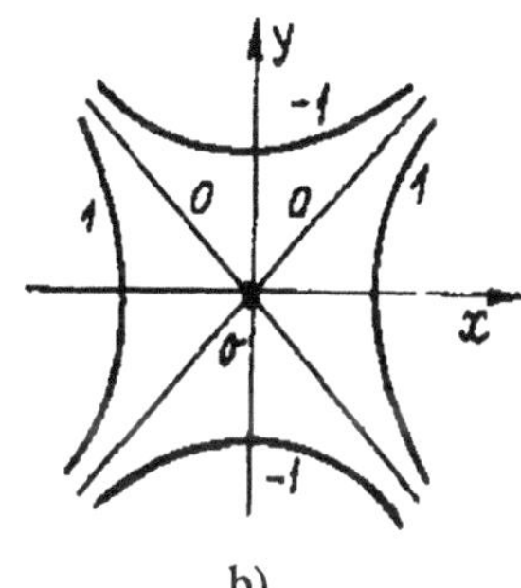

b)

Fig. 2

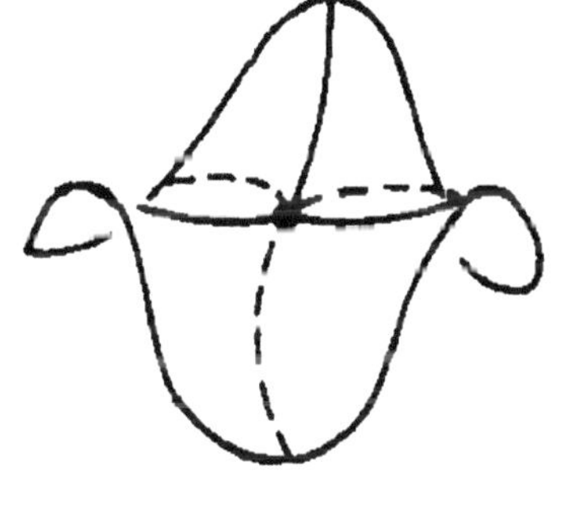

a)

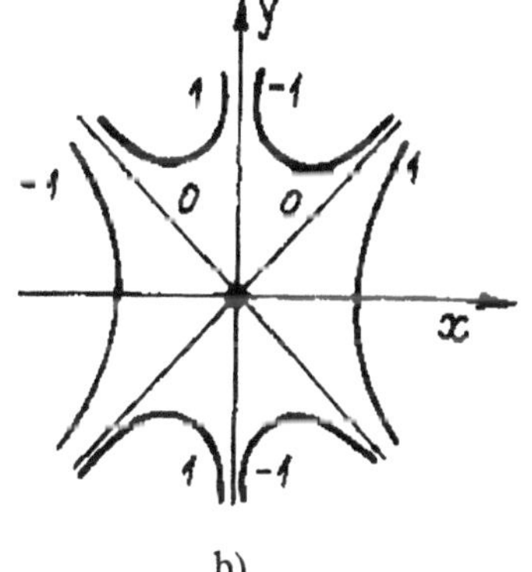

b)

Fig. 3

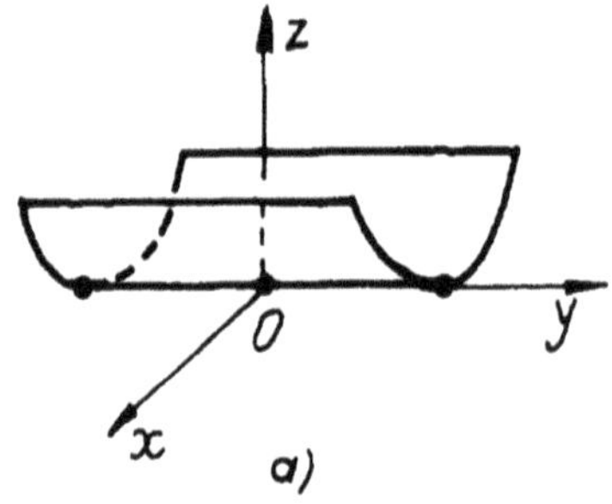

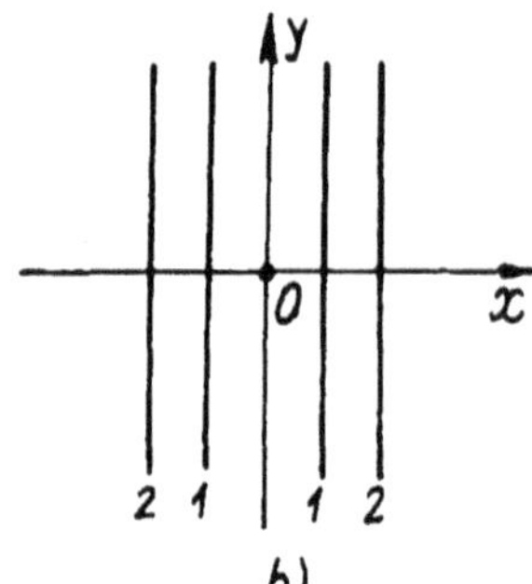

Fig. 4

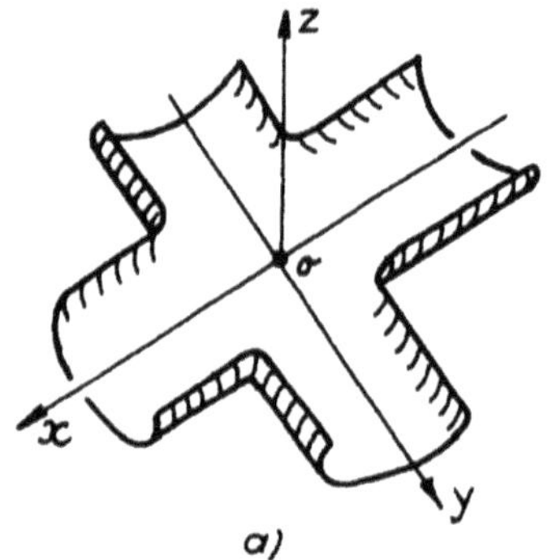

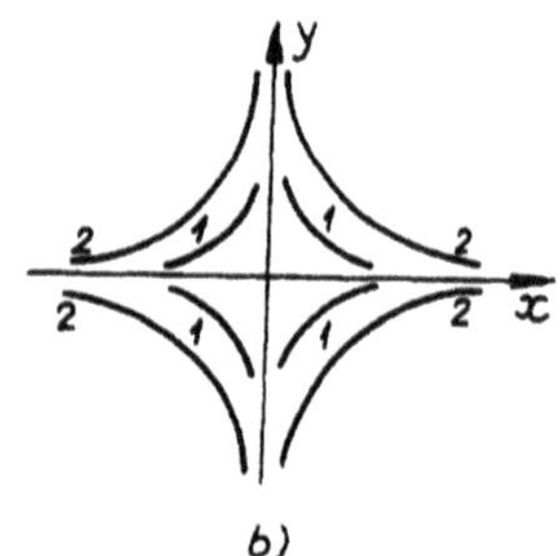

Fig. 5

Applications. 1) A vacuum-like cosmic medium produces the sublimation of metals. The sublimation speed of the molecules on the surface of the bodies made of inorganic substances is given by the relation [33]

$$V = \frac{p}{2320}\sqrt{\frac{M}{T}}\,, \tag{1}$$

where V is the sublimation speed, p is the pressure of the steam, M is the molecular mass of the steam, while T is the absolute temperature. The relation which determines the pressure necessary for producing the sublimation phenomenon is

$$lg\, p = A - \frac{B}{T}, \quad A, B = \text{constants} > 0. \tag{2}$$

A mathematical model of the physical law (1) is the scalar field $f: D \to R$, $D = R \times (-\infty, 0] \times (-\infty, 0) \cup R \times [0, \infty) \times (0, \infty) \subset R^3$,

$$f(x,y,z) = \frac{x}{2320}\sqrt{\frac{y}{z}}$$

(or a restriction of this function).

The sets of constant level attached to the function f are subsets of D characterized by Cartesian implicit equations, $c^2 z = x^2 y$. These are ruled surfaces, since their intersections with the planes $x = k$ are portions of straight lines, $x = k$, $a^2 z = k^2 y$. The graph of f is a hypersurface of R^4.

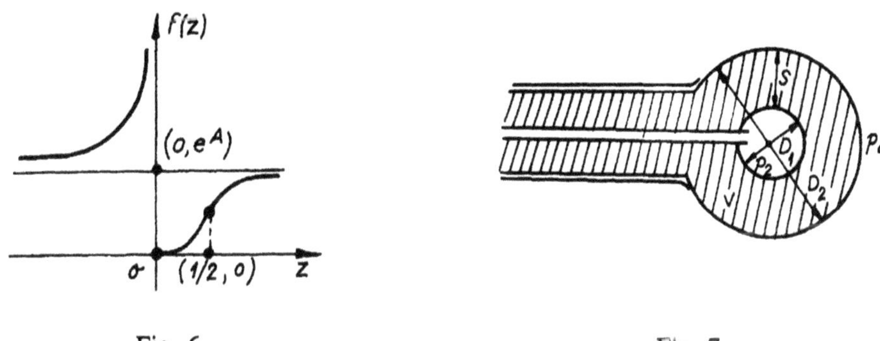

Fig. 6 Fig. 7

The physical relation (2) is strongly related to the function

$$f : R \setminus \{0\} \to R,\ f(z) = \exp\left(A - \frac{B}{z}\right),\ A, B = \text{const} > 0$$

or to the restriction $f|_{(0,T_0]}$. The table of variation of f is (Fig.6)

z	$-\infty$			0		1/2		∞
$f'(z)$	0	+	∞	0		+		0
$f''(z)$		+			+	0	-	
$f(z)$	e^A	↗	∞	0		↗		e^A

2) Creation of spherical products in the universe starts with dilation of balls (in liquid state) by injection of gas under pressure into their interior. The interior diameter D_1 of the cavity which contains gas is determined by the pressure of gas p_2 and by the stress σ of the surrounding liquid. On the other hand, the stress σ is determined by the diameter of the

ball D_2 and by the external pressure p_0. The equilibrium condition for each point on the spherical surface is given by the relation

$$p_2 - p_0 = 4\sigma\left(\frac{1}{D_1} - \frac{1}{D_2}\right), \tag{3}$$

where D_1 is the interior diameter and D_2 is the exterior diameter of the spherical ring (Fig.7). The single constant quantity of the process is the volume V of the material, initially established in order to obtain the final thickness S of the walls and the external diameter D_2. The dependence between the internal pressure p_2, the external diameter D_2 and the volume V of the material is given by the relation [33]

$$V = \frac{\pi}{6}\left[D_2^3 - \left(\frac{4}{p_2}\frac{\sigma D_2}{D_2 - 4\sigma}\right)^3\right]. \tag{4}$$

The law (3) suggests the scalar field

$$f: E \to R,\ E = R^3 \setminus (yOz \cup xOz),\ f(x,y,z) = 4z\left(\frac{1}{x} - \frac{1}{y}\right).$$

The constant level sets of f are the portions inside E of the cones of equations $cxy = zy - zx$. The graph of f is a hypersurface of R^4.

The scalar field with the largest possible domain of definition (from a mathematical point of view) that models the law (4) is

$$f: E \to R,\ E = R^3 \setminus (yOz \cup \{(x,y,z) \in R^3, y - 4z = 0\}),$$

$$f(x,y,z) = \frac{\pi}{6}\left[y^3 - \frac{64y^3z^3}{x^3(y-4z)^3}\right].$$

Related to this, the law (4) represents the sets of positive constant level of a restriction of the function f.

1.2. VECTOR FIELDS

Let R^n be the (real) canonical Euclidean vector space with dimension n. Like any Euclidean vector space, R^n is implicitly a Euclidean point space.

Let x and y be two arbitrary points of R^n. The ordered pair (x,y) is called a *tangent vector* to R^n at the point x (oriented segment, vector applied to the point x) and is graphically represented by an arrow starting from the point x and ending at the point y.

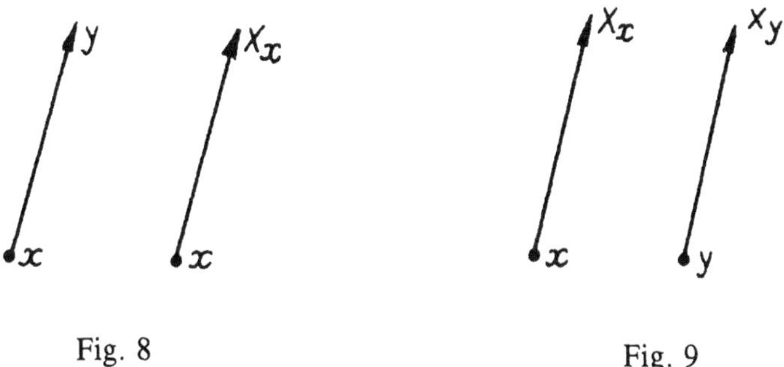

Fig. 8 Fig. 9

The point x is called the *origin* or the *point of application* of the tangent vector, while y is called its *extremity (end point)*. If $x = (0, 0, \ldots, 0)$ is the origin of R^n, then (x, y) is called the *position vector* (Fig. 8) of the point y.

The point $\boldsymbol{X} = y - x$ is called the *vector part* of the tangent vector and, instead of (x, y), we can write $\boldsymbol{X}_x$ or even $\boldsymbol{X}$ if the point of application is clear from the context.

From the definition of the tangent vector to R^n at a point it follows that the tangent vectors $\boldsymbol{X}_x$ and $\boldsymbol{Y}_y$ coincide (are equal) if and only if they have the same vector part, $\boldsymbol{X} = \boldsymbol{Y}$, and the same point of application, $x = y$.

Two vectors $\boldsymbol{X}_x$ and $\boldsymbol{Y}_y$ which have the same vector part $\boldsymbol{X} = \boldsymbol{Y}$, but different points of application, $x \neq y$, are said to be *parallel* (Fig.9).

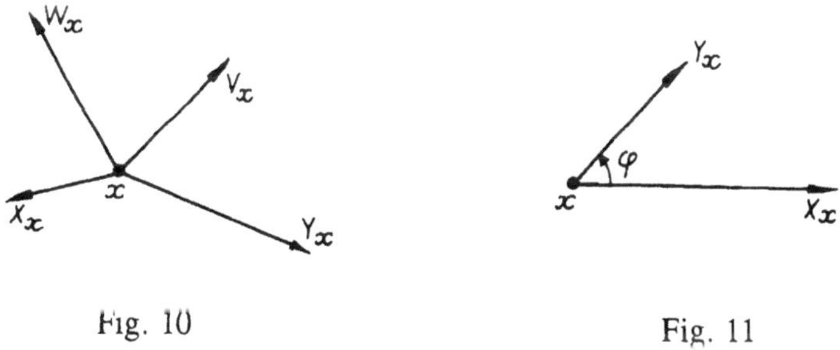

Fig. 10 Fig. 11

We fix a point $x \in R^n$ and consider all the tangent vectors to R^n at x. The set of all the tangent vectors to R^n at x is called the *tangent space* to R^n at the point x, denoted by $T_x R^n$ (Fig.10). The tangent space is organized as a vector space with the laws

$$\boldsymbol{X}_x + \boldsymbol{Y}_x = (\boldsymbol{X} + \boldsymbol{Y})_x, \quad r\boldsymbol{X}_x = (r\boldsymbol{X})_x .$$

In fact the vector space $T_x R^n$ is isomorphic to R^n, the isomorphism being given by the correspondence $\boldsymbol{X} \to \boldsymbol{X}_x$.

The *scalar product* in $T_x R^n$ is defined by

$$(X_x, Y_x) = (X, Y),$$

where the right side represents the scalar product on R^n. In particular, the *norm (length)* of the vector X_x is the number $\|X_x\| = \|X\|$. A vector of length 1 is called a *unit vector* or a *versor*. If $(X, Y) = 0$, then the tangent vectors X_x, Y_x are called *orthogonal*.

From the Cauchy-Schwarz inequality it follows that

$$-1 \leq \frac{(X, Y)}{\|X\|\,\|Y\|} \leq 1.$$

Therefore the formula

$$\cos\varphi = \frac{(X, Y)}{\|X\|\,\|Y\|}, \quad \varphi \in [0, \pi],$$

defines the angle between two nonzero tangent vectors X_x and Y_x (Fig.11).

An ordered system of n unit vectors, mutually orthogonal, tangent to R^n at x, is called a *frame* at the point x. If $\{E_1, E_2, \dots, E_n\}$ is a frame at $x \in R^n$, then for any $X \in T_x R^n$ we may write

$$X = (X, E_1)E_1 + (X, E_2)E_2 + \cdots + (X, E_n)E_n.$$

The real numbers $r_i = (X, E_i)$, $i = 1, 2, \dots, n$, are called the *components* of X with respect to the fixed frame and are algebraic measures of some projections.

The frame $(1, 0, \dots, 0)_x, (0, 1, \dots, 0)_x, \dots, (0, 0, \dots, 1)_x$ is called the *natural frame* and the components of a vector with respect to this frame are called *Euclidean components*.

Let

$$X_2 = r_{21}E_1 + r_{22}E_2 + \cdots + r_{2n}E_n,$$
$$\dots\dots\dots\dots\dots\dots\dots\dots\dots\dots$$
$$X_n = r_{n1}E_1 + r_{n2}E_2 + \cdots + r_{nn}E_n$$

be $n - 1$ vectors from $T_x R^n$ related to the frame $\{E_1, E_2, \dots, E_n\}$.

The vector

$$X_2 \times \cdots \times X_n = \begin{vmatrix} E_1 & E_2 & \dots & E_n \\ r_{21} & r_{22} & \dots & r_{2n} \\ \dots & \dots & \dots & \dots \\ r_{n1} & r_{n2} & \dots & r_{nn} \end{vmatrix} \in T_x R^n,$$

where the right side is a symbolic determinant developed upon the first row, is called the *vector product* between $X_2, \dots, X_n$. Obviously, $X_2 \times \cdots \times X_n$ is orthogonal to each vector $X_2, \dots, X_n$.

Let us consider n vectors $X_i \in T_x R^n$. The number $(X_1, X_2 \times \cdots \times X_n)$ is called the *mixed product* of the n vectors. If

$$X_1 = (r_{11}, \dots, r_{1n}), X_2 = (r_{21}, \dots, r_{2n}), \dots, X = (r_{n1}, \dots, r_{nn}),$$

then

$$(X_1, X_2 \times \cdots \times X_n) = \begin{vmatrix} r_{11} & r_{12} & \cdots & r_{1n} \\ r_{21} & r_{22} & \cdots & r_{2n} \\ \cdots & \cdots & \cdots & \cdots \\ r_{n1} & r_{n2} & \cdots & r_{nn} \end{vmatrix}.$$

The modulus of this number represents the volume of the n-parallelepiped constructed on the vectors $X_1, X_2, \dots, X_n$.

In R^3, the natural frame is $i_x = (1,0,0)_x$, $j_x = (0,1,0)_x$, $k_x = (0,0,1)_x$ and one may talk about the *vector product* of two tangent vectors (Fig.12),

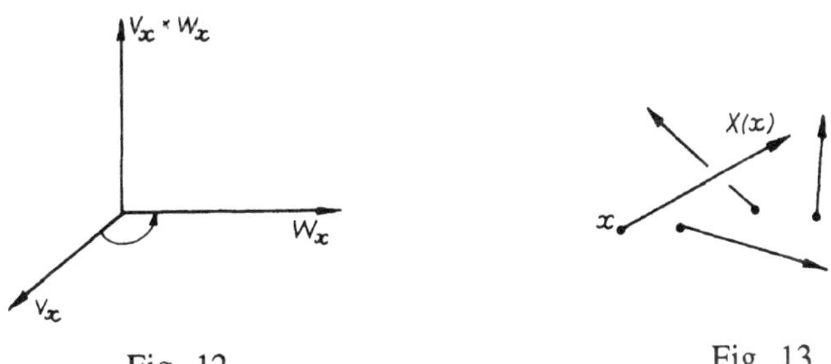

Fig. 12

Fig. 13

$$V_x = ai_x + bj_x + ck_x, \quad W_x = ei_x + fj_x + gk_x, \quad V_x \times W_x = \begin{vmatrix} i_x & j_x & k_x \\ a & b & c \\ e & f & g \end{vmatrix}.$$

A function X that associates to each point x of R^n a vector $X(x)$ tangent to R^n at x is called a *vector field* on R^n (Fig.13).

A vector field X for which $X(x)$ is parallel to $X(y)$, for any $x, y \in R^n$, is called a *parallel* or *constant vector field*. The set of values of a parallel field identifies with a free vector.

The parallel fields $U_1, U_2, \dots, U_n$ defined by

$$U_1(x) = (1,0,\dots,0)_x, U_2(x) = (0,1,\dots,0)_x, \dots, U_n(x) = (0,0,\dots,1)_x,$$

are called *fundamental fields* and their ensemble is called the field of the *natural frame*.

Theorem. *If X is a vector field on R^n, then there exist n real functions $f_i : R^n \to R$, $i = 1, 2, \dots, n$, such that*

$$X = f_1 U_1 + f_2 U_2 + \cdots + f_n U_n.$$

The scalar fields f_i are called the *Euclidean components* of the vector field X.

Proof. By definition, X associates to x a vector $X(x)$ tangent to R^n at x. Since the vector part of $X(x)$ depends on x, it can be written in the form $(f_1(x), f_2(x), \dots, f_n(x))$ and thus we obtain the functions $f_i : R^n \to R$, $i = 1, 2, \dots, n$. Moreover, for any $x \in R^n$, we have

$$X(x) = (f_1(x), f_2(x), \dots, f_n(x))_x = f_1(x)(1, 0, \dots, 0)_x + f_2(x)(0, 1, \dots, 0)_x + \cdots + f_n(x)(0, 0, \dots, 1)_x$$
$$= f_1(x) U_1(x) + f_2(x) U_2(x) + \cdots + f_n(x) U_n(x).$$

Obviously the functions f_i are uniquely determined. In particular, any tangent vector X_x can be written in the form $X_x = \sum_{i=1}^{n} r_i U_i(x)$.

The algebra of the vector fields is constructed on the basis of the following pointwise laws

$$(X + Y)(x) = X(x) + Y(x), \quad (fX)(x) = f(x) X(x).$$

Define the *scalar product* of the vector fields X and Y as

$$(X, Y)(x) = (X(x), Y(x));$$

define the *vector product* of the vector fields $X_2, \dots, X_n$ as

$$(X_2 \times \cdots \times X_n)(x) = X_2(x) \times \cdots \times X_n(x);$$

define the *mixed product* of the vector fields $X_1, X_2, \dots, X_n$ as

$$(X_1, X_2 \times \cdots \times X_n)(x) = (X_1(x), X_2(x) \times \cdots \times X_n(x)).$$

The above defined laws, in a pointwise manner, can be expressed by operations on the components of the respective fields. We also notice that, basing on the foregoing theorem, any vector field X on R^n is equivalent with a function of type

$$F : R^n \to R^n, \quad F(x) = (f_1(x), f_2(x), \dots, f_n(x)).$$

Therefore it is natural to say that X is called a *vector field of class C^p* if its components are of class C^p (as real functions). On the hypothesis that X is of class C^p, $p \geq 1$, the distribution of the vectors $X(x)$ follows some precise additional rules, at least in the neighborhood of a point, rules imposed by the existence of field lines and of field hypersurfaces (see Chapters 3 and 6).

Let us assume that we refer to R^3. Here the field of the natural frame $\{i, j, k\}$ is defined by (Fig.14)

$$i(x) = i_x = (1, 0, 0)_x, \quad j(x) = j_x = (0, 1, 0)_x, \quad k(x) = k_x = (0, 0, 1)_x.$$

Any vector field on R^3 is written in the form (Fig.15)

$$X = f(x, y, z) i + g(x, y, z) j + h(x, y, z) k.$$

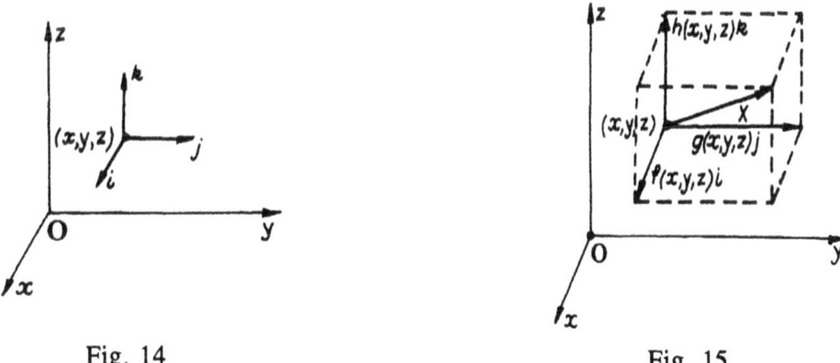

Fig. 14 Fig. 15

In the case of the space R^3, we can define the vector product of two vector fields X and Y, namely

$$(X \times Y)(x) = X(x) \times Y(x).$$

Remarks. 1) The domains of definition of the scalar or vector fields that we shall use from now on will generally be subsets D of R^n.

2) The vector fields $X_1, \dots, X_m$, $m \le n$, are called *linearly independent* on $D \subset R^n$ if $X_1(x), \dots, X_m(x)$ are linearly independent vectors, for any $x \in D$. This sort of "linear independence," used in elementary problems, does not have the same meaning as a linear independence defined on the real vector space of vector fields (space of functions that is infinite-dimensional, see 1.5).

3) Two vector fields X and Y are called *collinear* on D if there is a scalar field $f: D \to R$ such that $Y = fX$.

Three vector fields X, Y and Z are called *coplanar* on D if there exist two scalar fields $f, g: D \to R$ such that $Z = fX + gY$.

Examples. 1) In Fig.16 we present three specific vector fields on R^2.

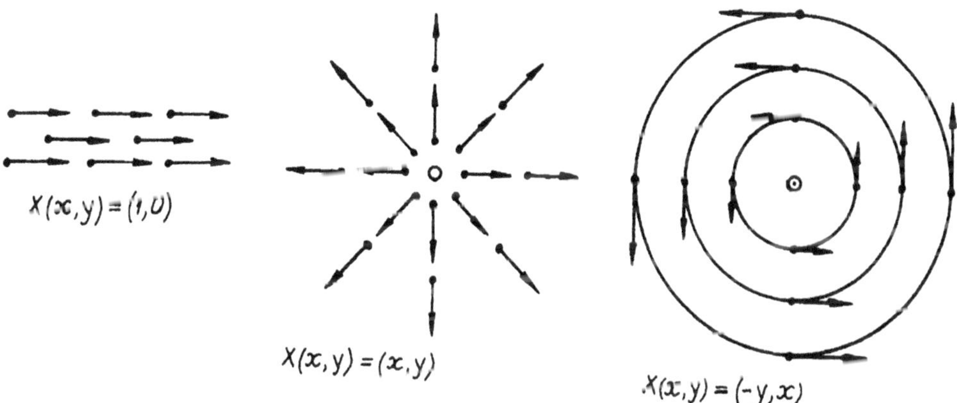

Fig. 16

2) An important problem for ecology is the "oscillation of populations" phenomenon. Studying this phenomenon on fish species in the Adriatic Sea, Volterra and Lotka concluded that the speed of local evolution of a biological system consisting of a "predator" species and a "prey" species has the expression

$$X(x,y) = (x(a-by), y(cx-d)),\ (x,y) \in R^2,$$

where a, b, c, d are constants.

3) **Gravitational field** (Fig.17). Let R^3 be a mathematical model of the tridimensional physical space and m a certain mass at the origin. The universal attraction force by which the mass m acts on the unit mass at the arbitrary point (x,y,z) is (see 2.2)

$$F(x,y,z) = -\frac{m}{(x^2+y^2+z^2)^{\frac{3}{2}}}(xi+yj+zk).$$

The function $(x,y,z) \to F(x,y,z)$ is called a *Newtonian* or *gravitational field* produced by the mass m on $R^3 \setminus \{(0,0,0)\}$.

4) **Electrostatic field** (Fig.17, 18). Let R^3 be a mathematical model of the tridimensional physical space and q_0 an electric charge at the origin. The force E by which the charge q_0 acts on the charge $q = +1$ (unit of charge in SI, 1 Coulomb = 1 As) at the arbitrary point (x,y,z) is (see 2.2)

$$E(x,y,z) = \frac{1}{4\pi\varepsilon}\frac{q_0}{(x^2+y^2+z^2)^{\frac{3}{2}}}(xi+yj+zk),$$

where ε is the permitivity of the medium in which the charges are placed.

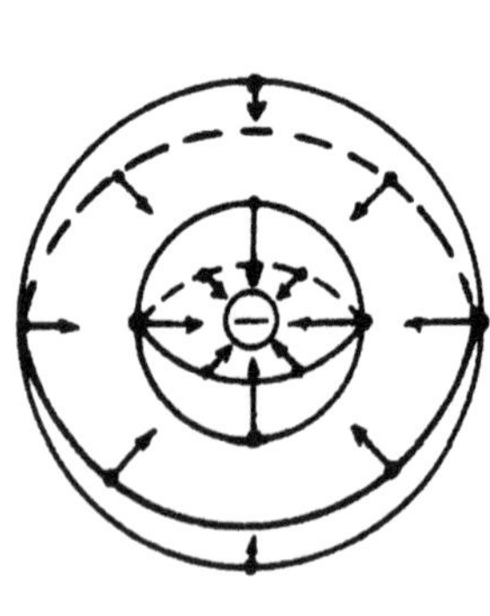

Fig. 17

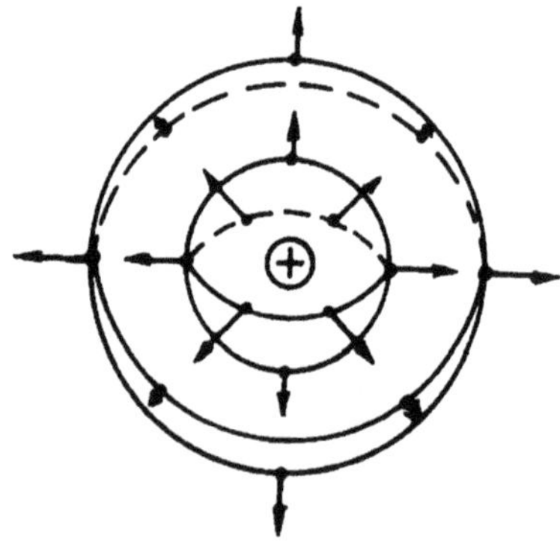

Fig. 18

The function $(x,y,z) \to E(x,y,z)$ is called the *electrostatic field* produced by the charge q_0 on $R^3 \setminus \{(0,0,0)\}$.

5) **The field of velocities inside a fluid**. Let R^3 be a mathematical model of the

tridimensional physical space and a source q located at the origin. When passing through the point (x,y,z), a particle of fluid springing from the origin has the velocity (see 2.3)

$$V(x,y,z) = \frac{1}{4\pi} \frac{q}{(x^2+y^2+z^2)^{\frac{3}{2}}}(x\boldsymbol{i}+y\boldsymbol{j}+z\boldsymbol{k}).$$

The function $(x,y,z) \to V(x,y,z)$ is called the *field of velocities* inside the fluid.

6) **The gradient.** Let D be an open set of R^n and $f: D \to R$ a scalar field of class C^1. To this scalar field we can associate the vector field

$$\text{grad} f = \frac{\partial f}{\partial x_1} \boldsymbol{U}_1 + \cdots + \frac{\partial f}{\partial x_n} \boldsymbol{U}_n$$

called *the gradient* of f.

Let $M_c : f(x_1, \ldots, x_n) = c$ be the set of constant level c attached to f and $x_0 \in M_c$. Let us show that $\text{grad} f(x_0)$ is orthogonal on every curve of M_c that passes through x_0 with the speed $\alpha'(t_0)$. In order to prove this fact, let $I \subset R$ and $\alpha = (x_1, \ldots, x_n) : I \to R^n$ be a curve of class C^1 with the properties $\alpha(t_0) = x_0$ and $\alpha(I) \subset M_c$. Differentiating the identity $f(x_1(t), \ldots, x_n(t)) = c$, $t \in I$, with respect to t, we get

$$\frac{\partial f}{\partial x_1}\frac{dx_1}{dt} + \cdots + \frac{\partial f}{\partial x_n}\frac{dx_n}{dt} = 0.$$

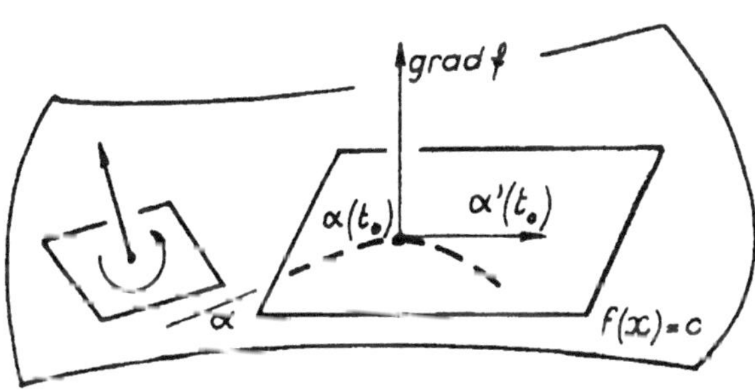

Fig. 19

In particular $(\text{grad} f(x_0), \alpha'(t_0)) = 0$, that is $\text{grad} f(x_0) \perp \alpha'(t_0)$. Based on this property, the gradient is a normal vector field to any of the sets of constant level M_c (Fig. 19).

1.3. SUBMANIFOLDS OF R^n

Let us consider a function of type $F: R^n \to R^m$. The functions $f_i = y_i \circ F: R^n \to R$, where y_i are the coordinate functions of R^m, are called the *Euclidean components* of F, and we write $F = (f_1, \dots, f_m)$. The set

$$G(F) = \{(x_1, \dots, x_n, f_1(x_1, \dots, x_n), \dots, f_m(x_1, \dots, x_n))\}$$

is called the *graph* of the function $F = (f_1, \dots, f_m)$. Obviously $G(F)$ coincides with the set of values of the function

$$(x_1, \dots, x_n) \to (x_1, \dots, x_n, f_1(x_1, \dots, x_n), \dots, f_m(x_1, \dots, x_n)).$$

The function F is of class C^p if and only if the components f_i, $i = 1, \dots, m$, are functions of class C^p. To a function F of class C^1 we attach the Jacobi matrix

$$J(F) = \begin{bmatrix} \frac{\partial f_1}{\partial x_1} & \dots & \frac{\partial f_1}{\partial x_n} \\ \dots & \dots & \dots \\ \frac{\partial f_m}{\partial x_1} & \dots & \frac{\partial f_m}{\partial x_n} \end{bmatrix}.$$

If $n = m$, then the determinant of the matrix $J(F)$ is called the *Jacobian* of f and it is denoted by $\frac{D(f_1, \dots, f_n)}{D(x_1, \dots, x_n)}$.

The function $F: R^n \to R^m$ is called:

1) *injective* if the relations $x, y \in R^n$, $F(x) = F(y) \in R^m$ imply $x = y$;
2) *surjective* if for any $z \in R^m$, there exists $x \in R^n$ such that $F(x) = z$;
3) *bijective* if it is both injective and surjective;
4) *immersion* if it is of class C^1 and $\operatorname{rank} J(F)(x) = n$, for any $x \in R^n (n \le m)$;
5) *submersion* if it is of class C^1 and $\operatorname{rank} J(F)(x) = m$, for any $x \in R^n (m \le n)$;
6) *regular* if it is either an immersion or a submersion;
7) *diffeomorphism* for $n = m$, if it is of class C^1 and possesses an inverse of class C^1.

If the function F is not regular at a point x, then x is called a *critical point* or *singular point*, while $F(x)$ is called *critical value* or *singular value*.

Inverse Function Theorem. *Let $F: R^n \to R^n$ be a function of class C^1. If $x_0 \in R^n$ is a point for which $\det J(F)(x_0) \neq 0$, then there exists a neighborhood D of x_0 such that the restriction of F to D is a diffeomorphism.*

Implicit Function Theorem. *Let* $F = (f_1, \ldots, f_m) : R^{n+m} \to R^m$ *be a function of class* C^1. *If at* $(a,b) \in R^{n+m}$ *we have* $F(a,b) = 0$ *and* $\dfrac{D(f_1, \ldots, f_m)}{D(y_1, \ldots, y_m)}(a,b) \neq 0$, *then there exists a neighborhood* D *of* a *and a function of class* C^1 *(a unique one)* $g : D \to R^m$ *such that* $g(a) = b$ *and* $f(x, g(x)) = 0$, *for any* $x \in D$.

Following the model of surfaces in R^3 defined by means of equations (implicit, explicit or parametric) attached to some functions at least of class C^1, which fulfil some conditions of smoothness and non self-intersection, we introduce the submanifolds of R^n.

A subset M of R^n is called a *submanifold of dimension* $m (\leq n)$ if for any point $x \in M$ there exists an open set D of R^n that contains x and a submersion $F : D \to R^{n-m}$ such that

$$M \cap D = \{x \mid x \in D, F(x) = 0\}.$$

Theorem. *Let* M *be a subset of* R^n. *The following properties are equivalent:*

1) M *is a submanifold of dimension* m *of* R^n;

2) for each point $x \in M$ *there exists an open set* D *of* R^n *which contains* x *and* $n - m$ *functions* $f_i : D \to R$, $i = 1, \ldots, n-m$, *of class* C^1 *such that the vectors* $\operatorname{grad} f_i(x)$ *are linearly independent and* $M \cap D = \{x \mid x \in D, f_1(x) = 0, \ldots, f_{n-m}(x) = 0\}$;

3) for each point $x \in M$ *there exists an open set* D *of* R^n *which contains* $x = (x_1, \ldots, x_n)$, *an open set* E *of* R^n *which contains* $(x_1, \ldots, x_m)$ *and* $n - m$ *functions* $h_i : E \to R$, $i = 1, \ldots, n-m$, *of class* C^1 *such that, modulo a permutation of coordinates (if need be),* $M \cap D$ *is the graph of the application* $(h_1, \ldots, h_{n-m}) : E \to R^{n-m}$;

4) for each point $x \in M$ *there exists an open set* D *of* R^n *which contains* x, *an open set* E *of* R^m *and an injective immersion* $g : E \to R^n$ *with image* $M \cap D$ *and with continuous inverse* $g^{-1} : M \cap D \to E$.

Proof. $1) \Leftrightarrow 2) \Rightarrow 3) \Rightarrow 4) \Rightarrow 2)$. The property 2) is a transcription of 1) that uses the components $f_1, \ldots, f_{n-m}$ of the submersion F. Conversely, if 2) is true, then

$$F = (f_1, \ldots, f_{n-m}) : D \to R^{n-m}$$

is a submersion at the point x. Since the determinants are continuous functions, the function F remains a submersion on an open set that contains x, and hence $2) \Rightarrow 1)$.

The property 3) follows from 2) based on the Implicit Function Theorem.

$3) \Rightarrow 4)$: the function

$$g : E \to R^n,\ g(u) = (u_1, \ldots, u_m, h_1(u), \ldots, h_{n-m}(u)),\ u = (u_1, \ldots, u_m),$$

is an injective immersion with image $M \cap D$ and with continuous inverse $g^{-1} : M \cap D \to E$.

$4) \Rightarrow 2)$: we represent the immersion g by its components

$$x_1 = g_1(u_1, \ldots, u_m), \ldots, x_n = g_n(u_1, \ldots, u_m).$$

If $\dfrac{D(g_1,\ldots,g_m)}{D(u_1,\ldots,u_m)}(u_0) \neq 0$, then by the Inverse Function Theorem

$$u_1 = \varphi_1(x_1,\ldots,x_m)\,,\ \ldots\ ,\ u_m = \varphi_m(x_1,\ldots,x_m)\,,$$

with the conditions

$$x_{m+1} = g_{m+1}(\varphi_1(x_1,\ldots,x_m)\,,\ \ldots\ ,\ \varphi_m(x_1,\ldots,x_m)),$$
$$\ldots\ldots\ldots\ldots\ldots\ldots\ldots\ldots\ldots\ldots\ldots\ldots\ldots\ldots\ldots\ldots\ldots$$
$$x_n = g_n(\varphi_1(x_1,\ldots,x_m)\,,\ \ldots\ ,\ \varphi_m(x_1,\ldots,x_m)).$$

The functions defined by

$$f_1(x) = x_{m+1} - g_{m+1}(\varphi_1(x_1,\ldots,x_m)\,,\ \ldots\ ,\ \varphi_m(x_1,\ldots,x_m)),$$
$$\ldots\ldots\ldots\ldots\ldots\ldots\ldots\ldots\ldots\ldots\ldots\ldots\ldots\ldots\ldots\ldots\ldots$$
$$f_{n-m}(x) = x_n - g_n(\varphi_1(x_1,\ldots,x_m)\,,\ \ldots\ ,\ \varphi_m(x_1,\ldots,x_m))$$

satisfy the conditions of 2).

Example. We consider an electric power RLC circuit having distributed resistance, inductance and capacity (Fig.20). On each branch the current intensity is i and the voltage v. At a certain moment, we associate two triples of real numbers (i_R, i_L, i_C), (v_R, v_L, v_C). These are linked by Kirchhoff's laws $i_R = i_L = -i_C$, $v_R + v_L = v_C$ and the generalized Ohm's law $v_R = \Phi(i_R)$, with Φ function of class C^1.

Changing the notations, we associate with this RLC circuit the set

$$M = \{(x_1,\ldots,x_6) \mid x_1 - x_2 = 0,\ x_2 + x_3 = 0,\ x_4 + x_5 - x_6 = 0,\ \Phi(x_1) - x_4 = 0\}\,,$$

which is a submanifold of dimension 2 of R^6.

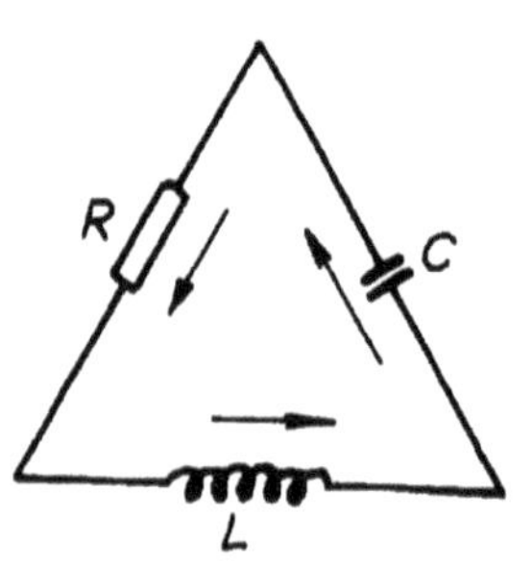

Fig. 20

If in each definition of a submanifold we use functions of class C^p, $p \geq 1$, then M is called a *submanifold* of class C^p.

The submanifold of dimension 0 are sets of isolated points of R^n. The submanifolds of dimension 1 are *curves*, while the submanifolds of dimension 2 are called *surfaces*. The submanifolds of dimension n are open sets of R^n, while the submanifolds of dimension $n-1$ are called *hypersurfaces*.

The image of an injective immersion is not always a submanifold (the inverse is not necessarily continuous). The image of a function of class C^1 can be a submanifold even if that function is not an immersion. Also, being given a submersion $F: R^n \to R^m$, the set $F^{-1}(z)$ is either void or a submanifold of dimension $n-m$ of R^n. Generally, being given two functions $G: R^n \to R^m$, $H: R^p \to R^n$ of class C^1 that do not satisfy everywhere the definition conditions for a submanifold, we can obtain submanifolds from $G^{-1}(z)$ or $H(R^p)$ eliminating the unsuitable points. These are either points at which the rank condition is not satisfied, or points of self-intersection.

Let M be a submanifold of R^n with dimension m and D an open set of R^m. A function $h : D \to R^n$ of class C^1 with the properties

1) $h(D) \subset M$,

2) h is an injective immersion,

is called a *chart* in M.

If h is only an immersion, then h is called a *parametrization* of the region $h(D)$ of M. According to the foregoing theorem, any point $x \in M$ admits some charts $h : D \to M$ such that $x \in h(D)$.

Let M be a submanifold of R^n and I an interval from R. A continuous function $\alpha : I \to M$ is called a *curve* in M. If $I = [a, b]$ and $\alpha(a) = \alpha(b)$, then the curve α is said to be *closed*. A closed curve $\alpha : [a, b] \to M$ is called a *closed and simple curve* if the restriction $\alpha : [a, b) \to M$ is injective.

A vector v of R^n is said to be *tangent* to the submanifold M at the point x if there exists a curve $\alpha : [a, b] \to M$ of class C^1 for which $\alpha(t_0) = x$, $\alpha'(t_0) = v$, $t_0 \in I$. The set of vectors of R^n tangent to M at x is a vector subspace of R^n of dimension m called *the tangent space* to M at x and denoted by $T_x M$. The set $TM = \bigcup_{x \in M} T_x M$ is called the *tangent bundle* of M (submanifold of R^{2n} of dimension $2m$).

A vector w of R^n is said to be *normal* to M at x if it is orthogonal to the tangent space $T_x M$. The set of all vectors normal to M at the point x is a vector space of dimension $n - m$ called the *normal space* to M at the point x and denoted by $N_x M$.

Let M be a submanifold of R^n. A function X that associates to every point $x \in M$ a vector $X(x)$ tangent to R^n at x is called a *vector field* on M. If $X(x) \in T_x M$, for any $x \in M$, then X is called a *tangent vector field* to M, while if $X(x) \in N_x M$, for any $x \in M$, then X is called a *normal vector field* to M.

A submanifold M is said to be *simply connected* if for any point $x_0 \in M$ and any closed curve $\alpha : [a, b] \to M$, $\alpha(a) = \alpha(b) = x_0$ there exists a continuous function $H : [a, b] \times [0, 1] \to M$ such that

$$H(t, 0) = \alpha(t), \; H(t, 1) = x_0, \quad \text{for any} \quad t \in [a, b],$$
$$H(a, s) = H(b, s) = x_0, \quad \text{for any } s \in [0, 1].$$

This definition contains the intuitive fact that α can be continuously deformed up to the point x_0.

A submanifold M is said to be *connected* if for any $x, y \in M$ there exists a curve $\alpha : [a, b] \to M$, piecewise of class C^1, which joins x and y, that is $\alpha(a) = x$, $\alpha(b) = y$.

A subset M of R^n is called a *submanifold of dimension* $m (\leq n)$, *with boundary*, if for each point $x \in M$ there exists an open set D of R^n that contains x and $n - m + 1$ functions $f_i : D \to R$, $i = 1, \dots, n - m + 1$, of class C^1 such that the vectors $\operatorname{grad} f_i(x)$ are linearly independent and

$$M \cap D = \{x \mid x \in D, f_1(x) = 0, \dots, f_{n-m}(x) = 0, f_{n-m+1}(x) \geq 0\}.$$

The set $\partial M = \{x \in M \text{ and } f_{n-m+1}(x) = 0\}$, called the *boundary* of M, is a submanifold of dimension $m - 1$. The set $M - \partial M$, called the *interior* of M, is a submanifold of dimension m.

1.4. DERIVATIVE WITH RESPECT TO A VECTOR

Let D be an open set of R^n, let $f, g : D \to R$ be two scalar fields of class C^1 and let c be a real number. The scalar fields $f + g$, cf, fg, $\frac{f}{g}$ are of class C^1 and the following relations are satisfied:

$$\operatorname{grad}(f+g) = \operatorname{grad} f + \operatorname{grad} g, \quad \operatorname{grad}(cf) = c \operatorname{grad} f,$$

$$\operatorname{grad}(fg) = g \operatorname{grad} f + f \operatorname{grad} g, \quad \operatorname{grad} \frac{f}{g} = \frac{g \operatorname{grad} f - f \operatorname{grad} g}{g^2}.$$

Remarks. 1) Since $df(x)(h) = (\operatorname{grad} f(x), h)$, to determine $\operatorname{grad} f(x)$ we can use the differential $df(x)(h)$.

2) Instead of "grad" we often write the symbol nabla, ∇.

Let D be an open set of R^n and $f : D \to R$ a scalar field of class C^1. Let $x = (x_1, \dots, x_n) \in D$ and X_x a tangent vector to D at the point x. We fix the interval I and $t \in I$ such that $x + tX \in D$, where X is the point corresponding to the vector X_x. Obviously $t \to x + tX$ represents the restriction of a straight line, and if f is of class C^1, then the composed function $t \to f(x + tX)$ is also of class C^1.

The number

$$D_{X_x} f = \frac{d}{dt} f(x + tX)\big|_{t=0}$$

is called the *derivative of f with respect to the vector X_x*.

The derivative of f with respect to the vector X_x represents the action of the vector X_x on the function f, indicating qualitatively the modification of $f(x)$ while x is moving in the sense of X_x. If X_x is a unit vector, then $D_{X_x} f$ is also called the *derivative of f along the direction X_x*.

Lemma. *If $X_x = (a_1, \dots, a_n)$, then*

$$D_{X_x} f = a_1 \frac{\partial f}{\partial x_1} + \cdots + a_n \frac{\partial f}{\partial x_n}(x) = (X_x, \nabla f(x)) = df(x)(X),$$

where ∇f is the gradient of f and df is the differential of the function f.

If $D_{X_x} f = (X_x, \nabla f(x)) = 0$, for any $X_x \in T_x D$, then x is a critical point of f, that is $\nabla f(x) = 0$.

Let $\nabla f(x) \neq 0$. Using the Cauchy-Schwarz inequality,

$$|D_{X_x} f| = |(X_x, \nabla f(x))| \le \|X_x\| \|\nabla f(x)\|,$$

in which the equality takes place if and only if X_x and $\nabla f(x)$ are collinear, it follows that the function $X_x \to D_{X_x} f$, $\|X_x\| = 1$ attains its minimum $- \|\nabla f(x)\|$ for $X_x = -\dfrac{\nabla f(x)}{\|\nabla f(x)\|}$ and its maximum $\|\nabla f(x)\|$ for $X_x = \dfrac{\nabla f(x)}{\|\nabla f(x)\|}$. Thus $-\nabla f(x)$ [respectively, $\nabla f(x)$] locally shows the direction and the sense in which f decreases (increases) in the steepest manner. Therefore, the gradient is often used in the Theory of Extrema.

In the hypothesis $\nabla f(x) \neq 0$, the relation $D_{X_x} f = 0$ is equivalent to the fact that X_x is tangent, at the point x, to the constant level hypersurface of f that passes through x.

Theorem. *Let* $f, g : D \to R$ *be functions of class* C^1, *let* $X_x, Y_x \in T_x D$ *and* $a, b \in R$. *The following relations are satisfied*

$$D_{aX_x + bY_x} f = a D_{X_x} f + b D_{Y_x} f$$

$$D_{X_x}(af + bg) = a D_{X_x} f + b D_{X_x} g$$

$$D_{X_x}(fg) = g(x) D_{X_x} f + f(x) D_{X_Y} g.$$

The proof is based on the preceding lemma and on the properties of gradients.

Using the preceding notions, we can define the action of a vector field X on a scalar field f of class C^1 (both of them defined on D) as the scalar field denoted by $D_X f$ whose value at each point $x \in D$ is the number $D_{X(x)} f$. The scalar field $D_X f$ is called the *derivative of the scalar field* f *with respect to the vector field* X. In particular, for the case $n = 3$, we have

$$D_i f = \frac{\partial f}{\partial x}, \quad D_j f = \frac{\partial f}{\partial y}, \quad D_k f = \frac{\partial f}{\partial z}.$$

Basing on the preceding theorem, we deduce the following properties of the derivative $D_X f$:

$$D_X(af + bg) = a D_X f + b D_X g$$

$$D_X(fg) = f D_X g + g D_X f,$$

where f, g, h are real functions, X and Y are vector fields and a, b are real numbers.

Remark. The relation $D_X f = (\nabla f, X)$ implies that $D_X f = 0$ if and only if X is a vector field tangent to the sets of constant level of f.

The next notion generalizes the derivative $D_{X_Y} f$ and represents an operation on vector fields.

Let Y be a vector field defined on the open set D of R^n and X_x be a tangent vector to D at the point x. We assume that Y is of class C^1 and consider the composed function $t \to Y(x + tX)$, where I and $t \in I$ are determined by the condition $x + tX \in D$.

The vector

$$D_{X_x} Y = \frac{d}{dt} Y(x + tX)|_{t=0}$$

tangent to D at x is called the *covariant derivative of* Y *with respect to* X_x.

The covariant derivative $D_{X_x} Y$ measures the rate of modification of $Y(x)$ while the point x moves in the sense of X_x (Fig.21) and hence it represents an action of the vector X_x on the vector field Y.

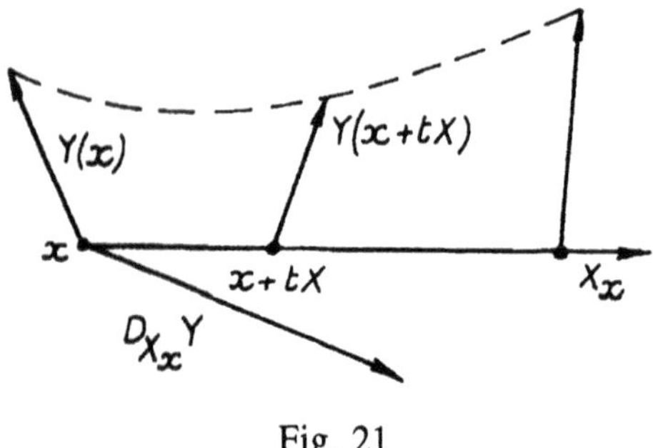

Fig. 21

Lemma. *If* $Y = Y_1 U_1 + \cdots + Y_n U_n$ *is a vector field of class* C^1 *and* X_x *is a tangent vector to* D *at* x, *then*

$$D_{X_x} Y = (D_{X_x} Y_1) U_1(x) + \cdots + (D_{X_x} Y_n) U_n(x).$$

Proof. We notice that

$$Y(x + tX) = Y_1(x + tX) U_1(x + tX) + \cdots + Y_n(x + tX) U_n(x + tX).$$

To differentiate such a vector field at $t = 0$ means to differentiate its components at $t = 0$. Taking account of the definition of the derivative with respect to a vector, the lemma becomes obvious.

The properties of the covariant derivative follow from this lemma and from the properties of the derivative $D_{X_x} f$.

Theorem. *Let* X *and* Y *be two vector fields of class* C^1 *on* D, *let* $V_x, W_x \in T_x D$ *and let* $a, b \in R$. *We have*

$$D_{aV_x + bW_x} Y = a D_{V_x} Y + b D_{W_x} Y$$

$$D_{V_x}(fY) = (D_{V_x} f) Y + f D_{V_x} Y$$

$$D_{V_x}(aX + bY) = a D_{V_x} X + b D_{V_x} Y$$

$$D_{V_x}(X, Y) = (D_{V_x} X, Y) + (X, D_{V_x} Y).$$

The above notion may be extended by considering the covariant derivative of a vector field Y of class C^1, with respect to the vector field X. The result is a vector field denoted by $D_X Y$ whose value at x is the vector $D_{X_x} Y$. If $Y = Y_1 U_1 + \cdots + Y_n U_n$, then

$D_X Y = (D_X Y_1) U_1 + \cdots + (D_X Y_n) U_n$. Based on the preceding facts, it follows that $D_X Y$ has the following properties:

$$D_{fV+gW} Y = f D_V Y + g D_W Y, \quad D_V (fY) = (D_V f) Y + f D_V Y,$$

$$D_V (aX + bY) = a D_V X + b D_V Y, \quad D_V (X, Y) = (D_V X, Y) + (X, D_V Y).$$

Remarks. 1) Consider the covariant derivative $D_X Y$. The role of X is an algebraic one, while Y is differentiated.

2) The covariant derivatives of the fundamental fields U_i, $i = 1, \dots, n$, are null since U_i are parallel vector fields.

3) Let X and Y be two vector fields of class C^1. The vector field defined by $[X, Y] = D_X Y - D_Y X$ is called the *bracket* of the fields X and Y.

Applications. 1) Let $x = (x_1, \dots, x_n)$, $f(x) = a_1 x_1^{\alpha_1} + \cdots + a_n x_n^{\alpha_n}$, where $\alpha_i > 0$, and $a_1, \dots, a_n$ is a geometric progression of ratio $r \neq 1$. Calculate $D_v f(x_0)$ for $v = \left(\frac{1}{\alpha_1}, \dots, \frac{1}{\alpha_n}\right)$ and $x_0 = (1, \dots, 1)$.

Solution. It is known that $D_v f(x_0) = (v, \nabla f(x_0))$. But

$$\nabla f(x) = (a_1 \alpha_1 x_1^{\alpha_1 - 1}, \dots, a_n \alpha_n x_n^{\alpha_n - 1}), \quad \nabla f(x_0) = (a_1 \alpha_1, \dots, a_n \alpha_n).$$

Therefore $D_v f(x_0) = a_1 + \cdots + a_n = \dfrac{a_1 (r^n - 1)}{r - 1}$. Let $r \in (0,1) \cup (1, \infty)$; if $a_1 > 0 (a_1 < 0)$, then f increases (decreases) in the direction and sense of v_{x_0}.

2) Verify that $X = U_1 + \cdots + U_n$ is a vector field tangent to the constant level sets of the function $f : R^n \to R$,

$$f(x_1, \dots, x_n) = \begin{vmatrix} 1 & 1 \dots 1 \\ x_1 & x_2 \dots x_n \\ \dots & \dots \\ x_1^{n-1} & x_2^{n-1} \dots x_n^{n-1} \end{vmatrix}.$$

Solution. We must verify the relation $D_X f = (\nabla f, X) = 0$, i.e., $\sum_{i=1}^{n} \frac{\partial f}{\partial x_i} = 0$. This fact can be established using the derivation rules of a determinant or writing $f(x)$ in the form

$f(x) = \prod\limits_{1 \le j < i \le n} (x_i - x_j)$, as being a Vandermonde determinant. However, the shortest way is to notice that

$$f(x_1, \dots, x_n) = \varphi(x_1 - x_n, x_2 - x_n, \dots, x_{n-1} - x_n);$$

then, denoting $u_1 = x_1 - x_n, \dots, u_{n-1} = x_{n-1} - x_n$, we find

$$\sum_{i=1}^{n} \frac{\partial f}{\partial x_i} = \sum_{j=1}^{n-1} \frac{\partial \varphi}{\partial u_j} - \sum_{j=1}^{n-1} \frac{\partial \varphi}{\partial u_j} = 0.$$

3) Consider the vector field $X = x_1 U_1 + \cdots + x_n U_n$ and $Y = \dfrac{X}{\|X\|}$. Determine $D_X Y$.

Solution. Based on the derivation rules, we may write

$$D_X Y = D_X\left(\frac{1}{\|X\|} X\right) = \left(D_X \frac{1}{\|X\|}\right) X + \frac{1}{\|X\|} D_X X$$

$$= \left(X, \nabla \frac{1}{\|X\|}\right) X + \frac{1}{\|X\|} X = \left(X, -\frac{1}{\|X\|^2} \frac{X}{\|X\|}\right) X + \frac{1}{\|X\|} X = 0.$$

Variant:

$$Y = \frac{x_1}{\sqrt{x_1^2 + \cdots + x_n^2}} U_1 + \cdots + \frac{x_n}{\sqrt{x_1^2 + \cdots + x_n^2}} U_n, \quad D_X Y = \sum_{i=1}^{n} D_X\left(\frac{x_i}{\sqrt{x_1^2 + \cdots + x_n^2}}\right) U_i$$

and

$$D_X \frac{x_i}{\sqrt{x_1^2 + \cdots + x_n^2}} = 0.$$

This result shows that X is a vector field tangent to the constant level sets attached to the functions

$$f_i : R^3 \setminus \{0\} \to R, \; f_i(x) = \frac{x_i}{\sqrt{x_1^2 + \cdots + x_n^2}},$$

i.e., to cones with the vertex O. The functions f_i are not functionally independent since $\sum\limits_{i=1}^{n} f_i^2 = 1$.

1.5. VECTOR FIELDS AS LINEAR OPERATORS AND DERIVATIONS

In this section, we shall use notations and conventions that are specific to Tensor Calculus. Thus, indices will occupy inferior or superior positions and consequently sums will be replaced by duplicating upper-lower indices (Einstein convention).

Let D be an open set of R^n. The set $C^\infty(D)$ of all real functions (scalar fields) of class C^∞ defined on D is a real vector space. Since multiplication of real functions is an R-bilinear operation that is commutative, the set $C^\infty(D)$ is a commutative algebra.

Let $x = (x^1, \dots, x^n) \in D$ and $f \in C^\infty(D)$. To a vector X_x, tangent to D at the point x, we associate the number $X_x(f) = D_{X_x} f$ named the *derivative of f with respect to* X_x (see 1.4). The derivative $X_x(f)$ has the following properties

$$X_x(af+bg) = aX_x(f) + bX_x(g)$$
$$X_x(fg) = (X_x(f))g(x) + f(x)X_x(g)$$
$$(aX_x+bY_x)(f) = aX_x(f) + bY_x(f),$$

where X_x, Y_x are tangent vectors to D at x, a and b are real numbers, $f, g \in C^\infty(D)$.

Let us now consider the facts from another point of view, namely the rule $f \to X_x(f)$ with convenient properties will determine X_x. We are this way led to the following alternative as a definition of the tangent vectors, unanimously accepted in the literature of Differential Geometry.

Let x be a fixed point of D. A function $X_x : C^\infty(D) \to R$ that satisfies the conditions:

1) is linear, i.e., $X_x(af+bg) = aX_x(f) + bX_x(g)$,

2) is a derivation, that is

$$X_x(fg) = (X_x(f))g(x) + f(x)X_x(g), \quad \text{where} \quad a, b \in R,\ f, g \in C^\infty(D),$$

is called *a tangent vector to D at the point x*.

We notice that the function defined by $0_x(f) = 0$, for any $f \in C^\infty(D)$, so the *null vector* and the partial differential operators $\frac{\partial}{\partial x^1}|_x, \dots, \frac{\partial}{\partial x^n}|_x$ are tangent vectors to D at the point x. Also, if $f = g = 1$, then $X_x(1) = 2X_x(1)$ and hence $X_x(1) = 0$. Furthermore, $X_x(c) = cX_x(1) = 0$, for any constant function c. Identifying the constant functions by their own values, we can assert that the values of any tangent vector for scalars are null.

Let $T_x D$ be the set of all the tangent vectors to D at x. The elements of $T_x D$ are real functions defined on $C^\infty(D)$, and then the sum of two tangent vectors and the multiplication of a tangent vector by a real number make sense. Furthermore, for any $x \in D$, the set $T_x D$ is a real vector space, called the *tangent space to* D *at the point* x.

Theorem. *The set* $\left\{\dfrac{\partial}{\partial x^i}\,,\ i = 1\,,\dots,n\right\}_{x_0}$ *is a basis of the vector space* $T_{x_0} D$ *(a frame at the point* x_0*).*

Proof. Obviously $\dfrac{\partial}{\partial x^i}|_{x_0}$, $i = 1\,,\dots,n$, belong to $T_{x_0} D$. Let us show that these vectors are linearly independent. To do this, we start from the relation $a^i \dfrac{\partial}{\partial x^i}|_{x_0} = 0$ and use the coordinate functions $x^j : D \to R$, $j = 1\,,\dots,n$. Based on the definition of the tangent vector as a linear derivation, and on the remark $\dfrac{\partial x^j}{\partial x^i} = \delta^j_i$, it follows that

$$0 = a^i \frac{\partial}{\partial x^i}|_{x_0}(x^j) = a^i \frac{\partial x^j}{\partial x^i}|_{x_0} = a^i \delta^j_i = a^j,\ j = 1\,,\dots,n.$$

Therefore, the tangent vectors $\dfrac{\partial}{\partial x^i}|_{x_0}$ are linearly independent.

It remains to show that $\left\{\dfrac{\partial}{\partial x^i}\,,\ i = 1\,,\dots,n\right\}_{x_0}$ generates $T_{x_0} D$. For this we notice that, on a convex neighborhood of x_0 and any $f \in C^\infty(D)$, we have

$$f(x) = f(x_0) + \frac{\partial f}{\partial x^i}(x_0)(x^i - x^i_0) + f_{ij}(x)(x^i - x^i_0)(x^j - x^j_0),\ f_{ij} = f_{ji}.$$

According to the definition of X_x and the remark that the values of X_x on constants are all null, we find

$$X_x f = X_x(x^i)\frac{\partial f}{\partial x^i}(x_0) + X_x(f_{ij}(x))(x^i - x^i_0)(x^j - x^j_0) + 2f_{ij}(x)X_x(x^i)(x^j - x^j_0).$$

Replacing $x = x_0$, we obtain

$$X_{x_0} f = X_{x_0}(x^i)\frac{\partial f}{\partial x^i}(x_0).$$

Considering that $f \in C^{\infty}(D)$ is arbitrary and denoting $X_{x_0}(x^i) = a^i$, we infer

$$X_{x_0} = a^i \frac{\partial}{\partial x^i}\Big|_{x_0}.$$

The numbers $X_{x_0}(x^i) = a^i$ are called the *components* of X_{x_0}, while the frame $\left\{\frac{\partial}{\partial x^i},\ i = 1, \ldots, n\right\}_{x_0}$ is called a *natural frame*.

If we relate $T_{x_0}D$ to the natural frame, then addition of two vectors reduces to addition of the corresponding components, while multiplication of a vector by a real number reduces to multiplication of the components of the vector by that number.

Example. For $X = \frac{\partial}{\partial x} - 2\frac{\partial}{\partial y}$, $Y = \frac{\partial}{\partial x} + 5\frac{\partial}{\partial y}$, $k \in R$, we find

$$X + Y = 2\frac{\partial}{\partial x} + 3\frac{\partial}{\partial y},\quad kX = k\frac{\partial}{\partial x} - 2k\frac{\partial}{\partial y}.$$

A function

$$X : D \to \bigcup_{x \in D} T_x D,\ X(x) \in T_x D$$

is called a *vector field* on D.

The addition of two vector fields and the product between a real function and a vector field are pointwise defined.

The vector fields defined by

$$x \to \frac{\partial}{\partial x^i}\Big|_x,\ i = 1, \ldots, n$$

and denoted by $\frac{\partial}{\partial x^i}$, $i = 1, \ldots, n$, are called *fundamental fields (partial differential operators)*. Their ensemble is called the *field of the natural frame*.

Theorem. *If X is a vector field on D, then there exist n real functions $X^i : D \to R$, $i = 1, \ldots, n$ such that*

$$X = X^i \frac{\partial}{\partial x^i}.$$

Proof. By definition, X associates with $x \in D$ a vector $X(x)$ tangent to D at the point

x. But $X(x) = X^i(x) \frac{\partial}{\partial x^i}|_x$ and the rules $x \to X^i(x)$, $x \in D$, define (uniquely) the functions $X^i : D \to R$.

The real functions X^i are called *components* of the field X. The vector field $X = X^i \frac{\partial}{\partial x^i}$ is called of *class* C^p if the functions X^i are of class C^p.

Example. $X(x,y) = x^2 \frac{\partial}{\partial x} + e^y \frac{\partial}{\partial y}$ is a vector field of class C^∞.

On the other hand, the vector field X may be considered as the application $X : C^\infty(D) \to C^\infty(D)$ satisfying the conditions:

1) is linear, that is

$$X(af+bg) = aX(f) + bX(g),$$

2) is a derivation, that is

$$X(fg) = (X(f))g + fX(g), \quad \text{where} \quad a,b \in R, \;\; f,g \in C^\infty(D).$$

Let X and Y be two vector fields of class C^∞ on D. The vector field $[X,Y]$ defined by

$$f \to [X,Y](f) = X(Y(f)) - Y(X(f))$$

is called the *bracket* of the fields X and Y.

Obviously $[X,Y] = -[Y,X]$. Also, for any three vector fields X, Y, Z of class C^∞ the Jacobi identity is satisfied, namely

$$[X,[Y,Z]] + [Y,[Z,X]] + [Z,[X,Y]] = 0.$$

The set $\mathcal{X}(D)$ of all the vector fields of class C^∞ on D is an infinite-dimensional real vector space. Since the bracket $[,]$: $\mathcal{X}(D) \times \mathcal{X}(D) \to \mathcal{X}(D)$ is bilinear over the real number field, is anticommutative and verifies the Jacobi identity, the set $\mathcal{X}(D)$ is called a *Lie algebra*.

Let $T_x D$ be the tangent space to D at x and ω_x a 1-form at x, that is a linear transformation $\omega_x : T_x D \to R$. The set of all 1-forms at x is a real vector space of dimension n, the *dual space* of $T_x D$. This vector space is called the *cotangent space to* D *at the point* x and is denoted by $T_x^* D$.

Let $f \in C^{\infty}(D)$. The function $df_x : T_x D \to R$ defined by $df_x(X_x) = X_x(f)$ is called *the differential* of f at the point x.

This definition with the definition of the tangent vectors shows that df_x is a 1-form at x.

Theorem. *Let* $x^j : D \to R$, $j = 1, \dots, n$, *be the coordinate functions on* D. *The set* $\{dx^j, j = 1, \dots, n\}_{x_0}$ *is a basis of* $T_{x_0} D$ *(a frame at the point* x_0*).*

Proof. Obviously $dx^j|_{x_0}$, $j = 1, \dots, n$ belong to $T_{x_0} D$. Let $\left\{\dfrac{\partial}{\partial x^i}, i = 1, \dots, n\right\}_{x_0}$ be the natural frame of $T_{x_0} D$. Taking account of the definition of the differential, we infer

$$dx^j|_{x_0}\left(\frac{\partial}{\partial x^i}\right)_{x_0} = \frac{\partial}{\partial x^i}|_{x_0}(x^j) = \frac{\partial x^j}{\partial x^i}|_{x_0} = \delta^j_i, \ i, j = 1, \dots, n,$$

and consequently $\{dx^j, j = 1, \dots, n\}_{x_0}$ is the dual basis.

The frame $\{dx^j, j = 1, \dots, n\}_{x_0}$ is called a *natural coframe* at x_0.

Let $X_x = a^i \dfrac{\partial}{\partial x^i}|_x$. Then $dx^j|_x(X_x) = a^i dx^j|_x\left(\dfrac{\partial}{\partial x^i}\right) = a^j$.

Also, any 1-form $\omega_x \in T_x D$ is written $\omega_x = \omega_j dx^j|_x$, ω_j being the components of ω_x with respect to the natural coframe. Then $\omega_x\left(\dfrac{\partial}{\partial x^i}\right)_x = \omega_i$, that is the components of the 1-form ω_x are the values of ω_x on the vectors of the natural frame at the point x.

Let $C^{\infty}(D)$ be the algebra of the real functions of class C^{∞} on D and $\mathcal{X}(D)$ the Lie algebra of the vector fields of class C^{∞} on D. A function $\omega : \mathcal{X}(D) \to C^{\infty}(D)$, with $\omega(X)$ of class C^{∞}, for any $X \subset \mathcal{X}(D)$ and $\omega(fX + gY) = f\omega(X) + g\omega(Y)$, $f, g \in C^{\infty}(D)$, for any $X, Y \in \mathcal{X}(D)$, is called a *differential 1-form* on D.

The addition of two differential 1-forms and the product of a real function and a differential 1-form are pointwise defined.

Let ω be a differential 1-form. The values ω_x are 1-forms at the points x. Therefore the local expression of a differential 1-form is $\omega_x = \omega_j(x) dx^j|_x$. For brevity, we may write $\omega = \omega_j dx^j$ since the differential 1-forms $dx^1, \dots, dx^n$ are dual to the fundamental fields $\dfrac{\partial}{\partial x^1}, \dots, \dfrac{\partial}{\partial x^n}$. The ensemble $\{dx^j,\ j = 1, \dots, n\}$ is called the *field of the natural coframe*. The set of all differential 1-forms on D will be denoted by $\mathcal{X}^*(D)$.

An ordered set $\{X_1, \dots, X_n\}$ of vector fields is called a *field of frames* on D if $\{X_1(x), \dots, X_n(x)\}$ is a basis in $T_x D$ for any point $x \in D$. Analogously, we define the field of coframes $\{\omega^1, \dots, \omega^n\}$. These frames are said to be *dual to each other* if $\omega^b(X_a) = \delta^b_a$. Although, in general, the field of frames (or coframes) exist only in a neighborhood of the point x of D, the fact that D is an open set of R^n ensures us of the existence of some global examples of such fields.

If $\{X_a,\ a = 1, \dots, n\}$ is a field of frames on D, then any other vector field V is of the form $V = V^a X_a$. Analogously, if $\{\omega^b,\ b = 1, \dots, n\}$ is a field of coframes, then any other differential 1 - form μ is expressed as $\mu = \mu_b \omega^b$.

Let x be a point in D characterized on the one hand by the coordinates $(x^1, \dots, x^n) = (x^i)$, and on the other hand by the coordinates $(x^{1'}, \dots, x^{n'}) = (x^{i'})$, the change of coordinates being $x^{i'} = x^{i'}(x^i)$ with inverse $x^i = x^i(x^{i'})$, on a neighborhood of the point $x \in D$. The basis $\left\{\dfrac{\partial}{\partial x^i}\right\}_x$ changes into $\left\{\dfrac{\partial}{\partial x^{i'}}\right\}_x$ with the link $\dfrac{\partial}{\partial x^i}\Big|_x = \dfrac{\partial x^{i'}}{\partial x^i}(x^i)\dfrac{\partial}{\partial x^{i'}}\Big|_x$; accordingly, the dual basis $\{dx^j\}_x$ changes into $\{dx^{j'}\}_x$ with the link $dx^j|_x = \dfrac{\partial x^j}{\partial x^{j'}}(x^{j'})\,dx^{j'}|_x$. Obviously

$$\frac{\partial x^{i'}}{\partial x^i}\frac{\partial x^i}{\partial x^{j'}} = \delta^{i'}_{j'}, \quad \frac{\partial x^i}{\partial x^{i'}}\frac{\partial x^{i'}}{\partial x^j} = \delta^i_j.$$

These relations imply

$$X^{i'} = \frac{\partial x^{i'}}{\partial x^i} X^i, \quad \omega_{j'} = \frac{\partial x^j}{\partial x^{j'}}\omega_j.$$

Remarks. 1) In this paragraph, the open set D can be replaced by any submanifold of dimension $m \geq 1$, with or without boundary, of R^n (see 1.3).

2) Let x be a fixed point of D and $C^\infty(D)_x$ the set of all the functions defined on a neighborhood of x which are of class C^∞ at the point x. The maximal domain of definition of a vector X_x is $C^\infty(D)_x$.

1.6. DIFFERENTIAL OPERATORS

Gradient. Let $C^{\infty}(D)$ be the algebra of the functions of class C^{∞}, while $\mathcal{X}(D)$ is the Lie algebra of the vector fields of class C^{∞} on the open set $D \subset R^n$.

The operator $C^{\infty}(D) \to \mathcal{X}(D)$, $f \to \operatorname{grad} f$, is called the *gradient*. The basic properties of the gradient have been presented in 1.4.

Let X be a vector field of class C^{∞} on D. If there exists a scalar field $f: D \to R$ of class C^{∞}, with $X = \operatorname{grad} f$, then X is called a *potential field*, the function f is called the *potential* of X and the constant level sets of f are called *equipotential sets*. The existence and uniqueness of the potential will be discussed in the following paragraph.

Hessian. Let $f \in C^{\infty}(D)$. The second-order differential

$$d^2 f(x) = \sum_{i,j=1}^{n} \frac{\partial^2 f}{\partial x_i \partial x_j}(x)\, dx_i\, dx_j$$

is called the *Hessian* of f and sometimes is denoted by $\operatorname{Hess} f$.

The Hessian is often used in extremum problems and convexity problems.

To a vector field $X = X_1 U_1 + \cdots + X_n U_n$, of class C^{∞} on $D \subset R^n$, we may attach the skew-symmetric matrix

$$\operatorname{rot} X = \left[\frac{\partial X_i}{\partial x_j} - \frac{\partial X_j}{\partial x_i} \right]$$

which is called the *rotor* (or *curl*) of X. Like every skew-symmetric matrix of order n, this matrix is determined by $\frac{n(n-1)}{2}$ possibly non-zero elements (those placed above the first diagonal).

Let $V = (V_1, \ldots, V_n)$ and $W = (W_1, \ldots, W_n)$ be two arbitrary vector fields on $D \subset R^n$. We denote by $V \wedge W$ the matrix with elements $V_j W_i - V_i W_j$, that is $V \wedge W = [V_j W_i - V_i W_j]$. By this convention and $\nabla = \left(\frac{\partial}{\partial x^1}, \ldots, \frac{\partial}{\partial x^n} \right)$ we can write symbolically $\operatorname{rot} X = \nabla \wedge X$. Using this symbol we may simply express certain properties of the curl. For example

$$\nabla \wedge (X + Y) = \nabla \wedge X + \nabla \wedge Y, \quad \nabla \wedge (fX) = \nabla f \wedge X + f \nabla \wedge X.$$

A vector field whose curl is everywhere null is called an *irrotational field*.

If $n = 3$ (thus in R^3), then $\frac{n(n-1)}{2} = 3$ and the matrix $\operatorname{rot} X$ is equivalent to the vector field

$$\mathrm{rot}\boldsymbol{X} = \left(\frac{\partial X_3}{\partial x_2} - \frac{\partial X_2}{\partial x_3}\right)\boldsymbol{i} + \left(\frac{\partial X_1}{\partial x_3} - \frac{\partial X_3}{\partial x_1}\right)\boldsymbol{j} + \left(\frac{\partial X_2}{\partial x_1} - \frac{\partial X_1}{\partial x_2}\right)\boldsymbol{k}.$$

Thus, on R^3 (and only on it), to each vector field $\boldsymbol{X} = (X_1, X_2, X_3)$ we may attach another vector field $\mathrm{rot}\boldsymbol{X}$ called the *rotor* or *curl*. We may write symbolically

$$\mathrm{rot}\boldsymbol{X} = \begin{vmatrix} \boldsymbol{i} & \boldsymbol{j} & \boldsymbol{k} \\ \dfrac{\partial}{\partial x_1} & \dfrac{\partial}{\partial x_2} & \dfrac{\partial}{\partial x_3} \\ X_1 & X_2 & X_3 \end{vmatrix} = \nabla \times \boldsymbol{X},$$

where $\times$ is the sign of the *vector product*.

Remark. Any vector field on R^2 can be viewed as a vector field on R^3 with the third component equal to zero, and in this sense its rotor is a vector field on R^3.

Divergence. Let $\boldsymbol{X} = X_1 \boldsymbol{U}_1 + \cdots + X_n \boldsymbol{U}_n$ be a vector field of class C^∞ on $D \subset R^n$. This vector field determines the scalar field

$$\mathrm{div}\, \boldsymbol{X} = \sum_{i=1}^{n} \frac{\partial X_i}{\partial x_i} = (\nabla, \boldsymbol{X}),$$

called the *divergence* of $\boldsymbol{X}$. The operator $\mathrm{div} : \mathcal{X}(D) \to C^\infty(D)$ defined by

$$\boldsymbol{X} = (X_1, \ldots, X_n) \to \sum_{i=1}^{n} \frac{\partial X_i}{\partial x_i}$$

is called the *divergence*.

Let $F : D \to R^n$, $F(x) = (X_1(x), \ldots, X_n(x))$ be a function of class C^∞. We notice that $\mathrm{div}\, \boldsymbol{X}$ coincides with the trace of the Jacobi matrix attached to the function F.

The simplest properties of divergence are

$$\mathrm{div}\,(\boldsymbol{X} + \boldsymbol{Y}) = \mathrm{div}\boldsymbol{X} + \mathrm{div}\boldsymbol{Y}, \ \mathrm{div}(f\boldsymbol{X}) = (\nabla f, \boldsymbol{X}) + f\mathrm{div}\boldsymbol{X}.$$

If $\mathrm{div}\boldsymbol{X} = 0$, then the vector field $\boldsymbol{X}$ is called *solenoidal*.

The divergence of a vector field defines the *speed of contraction-dilation* of the volumes by the flow generated by the vector field (see 3.7).

Laplace Operator (Laplacian). The operator Δ defined by $\Delta f = \mathrm{div}(\mathrm{grad} f)$ is called the *Laplace Operator* or *Laplacian*. Obviously Δf coincides with the trace of the Hessian of f, that is

$$\Delta f = \frac{\partial^2 f}{\partial x_1^2} + \cdots + \frac{\partial^2 f}{\partial x_n^2}.$$

A function $f: D \to R$ of class C^2 with $\Delta f = 0$ is called a *harmonic function*.

Remark. The hypothesis of "class C^∞" is imposed by reasons of mathematical formalism (being nonaltered by derivation). In concrete situations, the scalar and vector fields will be of class C^p, where the least value of p is imposed by the context.

Application. The intensity of the electric field generated by an electric dipole is defined by the formula

$$\boldsymbol{E} = \frac{1}{4\pi\epsilon_0}\left[\frac{3(\boldsymbol{p},\boldsymbol{r})\boldsymbol{r}}{r^5} - \frac{\boldsymbol{p}}{r^3}\right],$$

where $\boldsymbol{p}$ is the dipole moment (parallel vector field), $\boldsymbol{r} = x\boldsymbol{i} + y\boldsymbol{j} + z\boldsymbol{k}$, $r = (x^2+y^2+z^2)^{\frac{1}{2}}$ and $\epsilon_0 \approx 8{,}86 \cdot 10^{-12} F/m$ is the dielectric constant of vacuum. The vector field $\boldsymbol{E}$ is defined on $R^3 \setminus \{0\}$, symmetric with respect to an axis of direction $\boldsymbol{p}$. Fixing $\boldsymbol{p} = c\boldsymbol{k}$ at the origin and the plane $y = 0$, we get the representation in Fig.22.

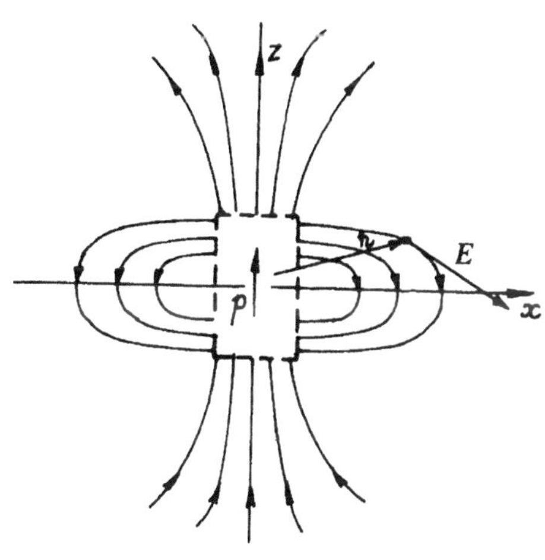

Fig. 22

1) Check that $f: R^3 \setminus \{0\} \to R$, $f(x,y,z) = -\dfrac{(\boldsymbol{p},\boldsymbol{r})}{r^3}$ is the potential of $4\pi\epsilon_0\boldsymbol{E}$.

2) Calculate $\text{rot}\boldsymbol{E}$ and $\Delta f = \text{div}\boldsymbol{E}$.

Solution. 1)

$$\text{grad} f = -\nabla\frac{(\boldsymbol{p},\boldsymbol{r})}{r^3} = -\frac{(\boldsymbol{p},\boldsymbol{r})\nabla r^3 - r^3\nabla(\boldsymbol{p},\boldsymbol{r})}{r^6} = \frac{(\boldsymbol{p},\boldsymbol{r})3r^2\dfrac{\boldsymbol{r}}{r} - r^3\boldsymbol{p}}{r^6} = 4\pi\varepsilon_0\boldsymbol{E}.$$

2) $4\pi\varepsilon_0 \mathrm{rot}\boldsymbol{E} = \mathrm{rotgrad} f = \nabla \times (\nabla f) = 0$;

$$4\pi\varepsilon_0 \mathrm{div}\,\boldsymbol{E} = \nabla \frac{3(p,r)r}{r^5} - \nabla \frac{p}{r^3} = 3\left[\left(\frac{r}{r^5}, \nabla(p,r)\right) + (p,r)\left(\nabla\frac{1}{r^5}, r\right) + \frac{3(p,r)}{r^5}\right] - \left(\nabla\frac{1}{r^3}, p\right)$$

$$= 3\,\frac{(p,r)}{r^5} - 15\,\frac{(p,r)}{r^5} + \frac{9(p,r)}{r^5} + \frac{3(p,r)}{r^5} = 0.$$

Thus, $\boldsymbol{E}$ is an irrotational and solenoidal vector field; the function f is harmonic.

1.7. PROPOSED PROBLEMS

1. Let S be a convex set of R^n and $f: S \to R$ be a real valued function. If $f((1-t)x+ty) \leq (1-t)f(x) + tf(y)$, for any $x, y \in S$, any $t \in [0,1]$, then the function f is said to be *convex*.

1) We assume that f is of class C^2 on S. Show that f is convex if and only if the Hessian of f is positive semidefinite at every point of S.

2) Let $\mathcal{F}(D)_x \subset C^\infty(D)_x$ the set of all functions $f \in C^\infty(D)_x$ that, in a neighborhood of $x \in D \subset R^n$, can be expressed by $f = c + \sum_{\alpha=1}^{n} f_\alpha g_\alpha$, c = constant, while $f_\alpha, g_\alpha \in C^\infty(D)_x$ satisfy $f_\alpha(x) = g_\alpha(x) = 0$. Prove that a linear operator $v: C^\infty(D)_x \to R$ is a derivation if and only if it vanishes on $\mathcal{F}(D)_x$.

The preceding problem gives an alternative of the definition of the tangent vectors that can be easily extended for n-th order tangent vectors [7].

3. Let $p \in D \subset R^n$ and the pair (x,a), where x is a chart of D whose domain contains p, while $a \in R^n$. We say that (x,a) is equivalent with (y,b), if $a = (J(\phi)(z))b$, where $z = y(p)$, $\phi = x \circ y^{-1}$ and $J(\phi)$ is the Jacobi matrix. Prove that this definition determines an equivalence relation and the quotient set V is a vector space.

Let $\{x,a\}$ be the equivalence class that contains (x,a). Show that the function $\{x,a\} \to a^i \frac{\partial}{\partial x^i}\Big|_p$ is an isomorphism between V and T_pD, independent of the fixed particular pair.

The preceding problem gives an alternative for the definition of the tangent vectors. The main part is also good for the infinite-dimensional manifolds [7, 24].

4. Prove that if the vector fields X and Y are tangent to a hypersurface, then also $[X,Y]$ is a tangent vector field to the respective hypersurface.

5. Determine the functions $F: R^n \to R^n$ of class C^∞ for which the Jacobi matrix

is the n-th order unit matrix. Solve the same problem for the case in which the Jacobi matrix is a diagonal matrix of the form $\operatorname{diag}(\varphi_1(x_1), \varphi_2(x_2), \ldots, \varphi_n(x_n))$.

6. Determine the harmonic polynomials of two variables.

Hint. The polynomial solutions of the Laplace equation are called *harmonic polynomials*. A basis $\{P_n(x,y), Q_n(x,y), n \in N\}$ of the vector space of all the harmonic polynomials of two variables may be defined by $(x+iy)^n = P_n(x,y) + iQ_n(x,y)$. We find

$$\left.\begin{matrix} P_0 = 1 \\ Q_0 = 0 \end{matrix}\right\}, \quad \left.\begin{matrix} P_1 = x \\ Q_1 = y \end{matrix}\right\}, \quad \left.\begin{matrix} P_2 = x^2 - y^2 \\ Q_2 = 2xy \end{matrix}\right\}, \quad \left.\begin{matrix} P_3 = x^2 - 3xy^2 \\ Q_3 = 3x^2y - y^3 \end{matrix}\right\}, \quad \left.\begin{matrix} P_4 = x^4 - 6x^2y^2 + y^4 \\ Q_4 = 4x^3y - xy^3 \end{matrix}\right\},$$

$$\left.\begin{matrix} P_5 = x^5 - 10x^3y^2 + 5xy^4 \\ Q_5 = y^5 - 10x^2y^3 + 5x^4y \end{matrix}\right\}, \quad \left.\begin{matrix} P_6 = x^6 - 15x^4y^2 + 15x^2y^4 - y^6 \\ Q_6 = 6x^5y - 20x^3y^3 + 6xy^5 \end{matrix}\right\},$$

$$\left.\begin{matrix} P_7 = x^7 - 21x^5y^2 + 35x^3y^4 - 7xy^6 \\ Q_7 = 7x^6 - 35x^4y^3 + 21x^2y^5 - y^7 \end{matrix}\right\}, \quad \left.\begin{matrix} P_8 = x^8 + y^8 - 28x^2y^2(x^4+y^4) + 70x^4y^4 \\ Q_8 = 8x^7y - 56x^5y^3 + 56x^3y^5 - 8xy^7 \end{matrix}\right\}.$$

The recurrence formulas are

$$\left.\begin{matrix} P_0 = 1 \\ Q_0 = 1 \end{matrix}\right\}, \quad \left.\begin{matrix} P_{n+1} = xP_n - yQ_n \\ Q_{n+1} = yP_n + xQ_n \end{matrix}\right\} \quad \text{or} \quad \left.\begin{matrix} P_{n+2} = 2xP_{n+1} - (x^2+y^2)P_n \\ Q_{n+2} = 2xQ_{n+1} - (x^2+y^2)Q_n \end{matrix}\right\}.$$

7. Show that any harmonic function f (i.e., solution of the Laplace equation) of two variables can be expanded about a regular point into a series of harmonic polynomials having the form

$$f(x,y) = \sum_{n=0}^{\infty} [a_n P_n(x,y) + b_n Q_n(x,y)].$$

8. Check that the mean curvature of the surface $z = f(x,y)$ may be written in the form

$$H = \frac{1}{2} \operatorname{div} \frac{\operatorname{grad} f}{\sqrt{1 + \|\operatorname{grad} f\|^2}}.$$

9. Show that the function defined by the formulas $x = \cos t$, $y = \sin t$, $t \in R$, is a non-injective immersion from R to R^2 whose image is a circle.

10. Show that the function defined by the formulas

$$x = \cos\varphi \cos\theta, \; y = \cos\varphi \sin\theta, \; z = \sin\varphi, \; (\theta, \varphi) \in R^2$$

is not an immersion, but its image is a sphere.

11. Show that the function $f: R^3 \to R$, $f(x,y,z) = x^2 + y^2 + z^2$ is not a submersion, but $f^{-1}(1)$ is a sphere.

2. PARTICULAR VECTOR FIELDS

In this chapter we develope the theory of local representation of vector fields and establish some links between vector fields with certain physical significance and vector fields with geometric significance.

The irrotational vector fields of class C^1 *are locally potentials and the potentials are found using a curvilinear integral of the second type. In the case in which we work on some n-dimensional intervals or on convex sets, it is sufficient to use the simple integral, and the results are global. The exterior magnetic field generated by an electric current in a cylindrical conductor is irrotational (see 2.1).*

Vector fields with spherical symmetry are global potential fields, the most frequently met being Newtonian and electrostatic fields (see 2.2).

Each solenoidal vector field of class C^1 *on open sets of* R^3 *admits a local vector potential.*

The solenoidal vector fields of class C^∞ *on open sets of* R^n, $n \geq 3$, *admit the local representation*

$$X = \mathrm{grad} f_1 \times \cdots \times \mathrm{grad} f_{n-1}.$$

The field of velocities of an incompressible fluid and the Biot-Savart-Laplace field are solenoidal (see 2.3).

Any vector field of class C^∞ *on an open and connected set of* R^3 *admits the Monge local representation,* $X = \mathrm{grad} h + f \mathrm{grad} g$ *and the Stokes local representation* $X = \mathrm{grad} h + \mathrm{rot} Y$ *(see 2.4).*

The vector fields which are irrotational and solenoidal are called harmonic fields, the most suggestive example being the field of velocities of an incrompressible fluid (see 2.5).

For Killing vector fields (see 2.6), conformal vector fields (see 2.7), and affine or projective vector fields (see 2.8) on R^n, *we have some explicit expressions. Finally, the torse forming vector fields (see 2.9) are interesting at least in particular cases: concircular fields, concurrent fields, recurrent fields and parallel fields. Newtonian fields and electrostatic fields, with spherical symmerty, are torse forming.*

In 2.10 we give some problems referring to special vector fields, Monge and Stokes potentials, harmonic functions, circulation, flux etc.

2.1. IRROTATIONAL VECTOR FIELDS

Let X be a continuous vector field on an open set $D \subset R^n$. If there exists a scalar field $f: D \to R$ of class C^1 with the property $X = \mathrm{grad} f$, then X is called a *potential field*, f is called the *potential* of X and the sets of constant level of f are called *equipotential sets* (see Fig.23).

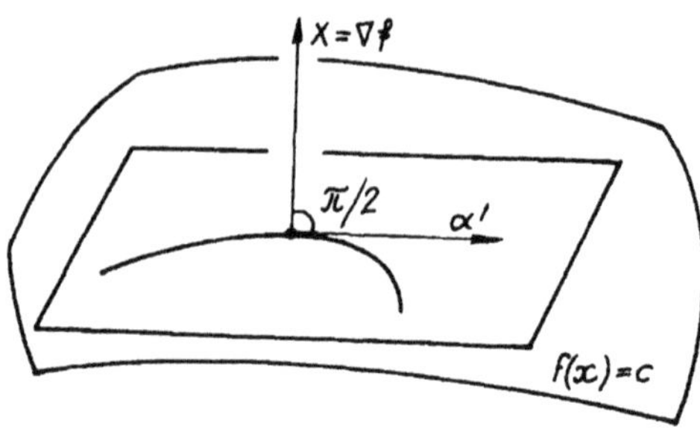

Fig. 23

Let us show that on an open connected set, one potential is unique modulo an arbitrary additive constant.

Theorem. *Let X be a vector field on an open and connected set $D \subset R^n$. If X admits on D one potential f, then this potential is uniquely determined, modulo an arbitrary additive constant.*

Proof. We assume that X admits on D two potential functions f and g, i.e., $X = \operatorname{grad} f = \operatorname{grad} g$. It follows $\operatorname{grad}(f - g) = 0$.

Let us show that $f - g = c$. To do this we denote $\psi = f - g$ and assume that any two points x, y from D can be joined by a curve $\alpha : [a,b] \to D$ of class C^1. We have $\alpha(a) = x$, $\alpha(b) = y$ and $(\psi \circ \alpha)'(t) = (\operatorname{grad}\psi(\alpha(t)), \alpha'(t)) = 0$, for any $t \in [a,b]$. It follows that $\psi \circ \alpha(t) = c$, for any $t \in [a,b]$, thus $\psi(\alpha(a)) = \psi(\alpha(b))$, that is $\psi(x) = \psi(y)$. Fixing y, we deduce $\psi(x) = c$, for any $x \in D$.

The manner of transferring the preceding reasoning to the case of piecewise C^1 curves (D being a connected set) is obvious.

Let $X = (X_1, \ldots, X_n)$ be a vector field and $\operatorname{rot} X = \left[\dfrac{\partial X_i}{\partial x_j} - \dfrac{\partial X_j}{\partial x_i}\right]$ its curl. If $\operatorname{rot} X$ doesn't vanish identically, then X is called a *rotational field* and if $\operatorname{rot} X$ is identically null, i.e. $\dfrac{\partial X_i}{\partial x_j}(x) = \dfrac{\partial X_j}{\partial x_i}(x)$, for any $x \in D$, $i, j = 1, \ldots, n$, then X is called an *irrotational field*. The following theorem shows that any irrotational field X of class C^1 admits the local representation $X = \operatorname{grad} f$, that is for any $x_0 \in D$ there exists an open set $U \subset D$ that contains x_0 and $f : U \to R$ of class C^2 such that $X = \operatorname{grad} f$ on U.

Theorem. *Let $X = (X_1, \ldots, X_n)$ be a vector field of class C^1 on D.*

1) If X is a potential field, then X is an irrotational field.

2) If D is an open n-dimensional interval and X is an irrotational field, then X is a potential field with the potential

$$f: D \to R,\ f(x) = \int_{x_{10}}^{x_1} X_1(x_1, \dots, x_n)\,dx_1 + \int_{x_{20}}^{x_2} X_2(x_{10}, x_2, \dots, x_n)\,dx_2$$

$$+ \dots + \int_{x_{n0}}^{x_n} X_n(x_{10}, \dots, x_{n-10}, x_n)\,dx_n\,,\ x_0 = (x_{10}, \dots, x_{n0}) \in D.$$

3) If D is a convex set and X is an irrotational field, then X is a potential field with the potential $f: D \to R$,

$$f(x) = \int_0^1 (X(x_0 + t(x - x_0)),\ x - x_0)\,dt, \quad x_0 = (x_{10}, \dots, x_{n0}) \in D.$$

Proof. 1) Let $X = \operatorname{grad} f$, i.e., $X_i = \dfrac{\partial f}{\partial x_i}$. It follows that

$$\frac{\partial X_i}{\partial x_j} = \frac{\partial^2 f}{\partial x_j \partial x_i} = \frac{\partial^2 f}{\partial x_i \partial x_j} = \frac{\partial X_j}{\partial x_i}$$

and then X is irrotational.

2) One can notice that

$$\frac{\partial f}{\partial x_1}(x) = X_1(x),\ \frac{\partial f}{\partial x_2}(x) = \frac{\partial}{\partial x_2}\int_{x_{10}}^{x_1} X_1(x_1, \dots, x_n)\,dx_1 + X_2(x_{10}, x_2, \dots, x_n)$$

$$= \int_{x_{10}}^{x_1} \frac{\partial X_1}{\partial x_2}(x_1, \dots, x_n)\,dx_1 + X_2(x_{10}, x_2, \dots, x_n) = \int_{x_{10}}^{x_1} \frac{\partial X_2}{\partial x_1}(x_1, \dots, x_n)\,dx_1 +$$

$$+ X_2(x_{10}, x_2, \dots, x_n) = X_2(x)$$

etc.

3) We specify that the set D is said to be *convex* if together with any two of its points it also contains the line segment determined by them.

We denote

$$u_i(t) = x_{i0} + t(x_i - x_{i0}),\ i = 1, \dots, n,\ u(t) = (u_1(t), \dots, u_n(t)).$$

It follows that

$$\frac{\partial f}{\partial x_k} = \int_0^1 \left(\left(\frac{\partial}{\partial x_k} X(u(t)), x - x_0 \right) + X_k(u(t)) \right) dt = \int_0^1 \left(\left(\sum_{j=1}^n \frac{\partial X}{\partial u_j}(u(t)) \frac{\partial u_j}{\partial x_k}(t), x - x_0 \right) + X_k(u(t)) \right) dt$$

$$= \int_0^1 t \left(\frac{\partial X}{\partial u_k}(u(t)), x - x_0 \right) dt + \int_0^1 X_k(u(t))dt - \int_0^1 t \sum_{i=1}^n \frac{\partial X_i}{\partial u_k}(u(t))(x_i - x_{i0})dt + \int_0^1 X_k(u(t))\,dt$$

$$= \int_0^1 t \sum_{i=1}^n \frac{\partial X_k}{\partial x_i}(u(t))(x_i - x_{i0})\,dt + \int_0^1 X_k(u(t))\,dt = \int_0^1 \left(t \frac{d}{dt} X_k(u(t)) + X_k(u(t)) \right) dt$$

$$= X_k(u(1)) - X_k(x).$$

Remarks. 1) The foregoing theorem can be formulated another way: a vector field X of class C^1 is locally potential if and only if it is irrotational.

2) The potentials are analogous to the antiderivatives from functions of a single variable.

Example. The vector field

$$X = (2xyz + z^2 - 2y^2 + 1)i + (x^2z - 4xy)j + (x^2y + 2xz - 2)k$$

is an irrotational field on R^n. Indeed,

$$\operatorname{rot} X = \begin{vmatrix} i & j & k \\ \dfrac{\partial}{\partial x} & \dfrac{\partial}{\partial y} & \dfrac{\partial}{\partial z} \\ 2xyz + z^2 - 2y^2 + 1 & x^2z - 4xy & x^2y + 2xz - 2 \end{vmatrix} = 0.$$

The above theorem gives some methods to determine the potential of X. However we prefer to find this potential f by the method of antiderivatives. Integrating the first equation of the system

$$\frac{\partial f}{\partial x} = 2xyz + z^2 - 2y^2 + 1, \ \frac{\partial f}{\partial y} = x^2z - 4xy, \ \frac{\partial f}{\partial z} = x^2y + 2xz - 2$$

with respect to x, we get $f(x,y,z) = x^2yz + z^2x - 2y^2x + x + \varphi(y,z)$. Replacing f in the second equation, we deduce $\dfrac{\partial \varphi}{\partial y} = 0$, that is $\varphi(y,z) = \psi(z)$; replacing f in the third equation of the initial system, we find $\dfrac{d\psi}{d}z = -2$, whence $\psi(z) = -2z + C$. Thus

$$f(x,y,z) = x^2yz + z^2x - 2y^2x + x - 2z + C.$$

Obviously, this is a global potential for X.

On n-dimensional intervals or convex sets, the potentials can be found by the usual integral. On an open and connected set that does not belong to the above mentioned classes, there does not always exist a potential function defined on the whole set. If there are any such, then founding of these potentials requires the curvilinear integral of the second type.

Let D be an open set of R^n and $\alpha : [a,b] \to D$ be an oriented curve of class C^1. Let X be a continuous vector field defined on D. The restriction of X to the image of α, i.e., $X \circ \alpha$, is a continuous function. The number

$$\int_\alpha (X, d\alpha) = \int_a^b (X(\alpha(t)), \ \alpha'(t))\, dt$$

is called *the integral of* X *along the curve* α *or a curvilinear integral of the second type or the circulation of* X *along the curve* α (Fig.24). This definition naturally extends to piecewise C^1 curves.

If $X = (X_1, \dots, X_n)$ and $\alpha = (x_1, \dots, x_n)$, then for circulation we use the notation

$$\int_\alpha X_1\, dx_1 + \dots + X_n\, dx_n .$$

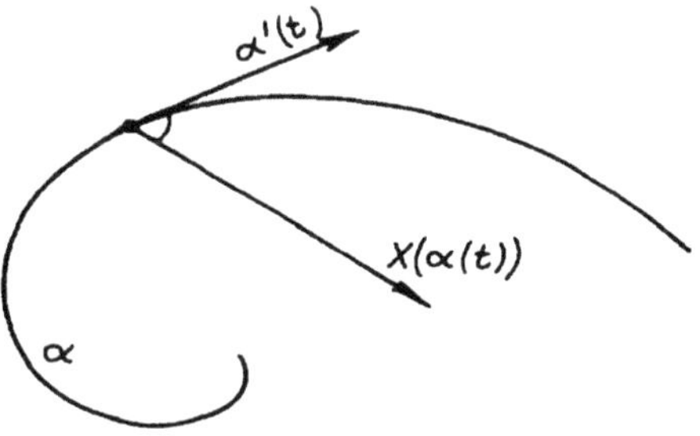

Fig. 24

Theorem. *Let $D \subset R^n$ be a connected open set, and X a continuous vector field on D. The following assertions are equivalent:*

1) X possesses a potential function on D;

2) for any $x, y \in D$, the circulation of X along the curve $\alpha : [a,b] \to D$, $\alpha(a) = x$, $\alpha(b) = y$ does not depend on the curve α;

3) the circulation of X along any closed curve in D is equal to zero.

Proof. Since D is a connected set, any two points of D can be joined by a piecewise C^1 curve in D. 1) → 2). We assume that 1) is true and that f is the potential of X, i.e., $X = \text{grad} f$. For any piecewise C^1 curve $\alpha : [a,b] \to D$, $\alpha(a) = x$, $\alpha(b) = y$, we find

$$\int_\alpha (X, dx) = \int_a^b (\text{grad} f, \alpha'(t))dt = f(\alpha(t))\Big|_a^b = f(y) - f(x).$$

In other words, the integral depends only on the points x and y, and not on the curve that joins them. Therefore 2) is true.

2) ⇒ 3), obvious.

3) ⇒ 2). Let $\alpha : [a,b] \to D$, $\beta : [a,b] \to D$ be two curves of class C^1 which join the points $\alpha(a) = \beta(a) = x$, $\alpha(b) = \beta(b) = y$. The curve $\{\alpha, \beta^-\}$ is closed (piecewise of C^1 class) and by hypothesis $\int_\alpha + \int_{\beta^-} = 0$. It follows that $\int_\alpha = \int_\beta$.

2) ⇒ 1). Consider the points $x_0 = (x_{10}, \ldots, x_{n0})$ and $x = (x_1, \ldots, x_n)$ of D. Since $\int_\alpha (X, d\alpha)$ does not depend on the curve α that joins the points x_0 and x, we can use the notation $\int_{x_0}^x (X, d\alpha)$.

We fix x_0 and define $f(x) = \int_{x_0}^x (X, d\alpha)$. Let us show that f is a potential of

$X = (X_1, \dots, X_n)$ that is $\dfrac{\partial f}{\partial x_i} = X_i$, $i = 1, \dots, n$. Denoting $e_i = (0, \dots, 0, 1, 0, \dots, 0)$, we notice that

$$f(x + he_i) - f(x) = \int_{x_0}^{x+he_i} (X, d\alpha) - \int_{x_0}^{x} (X, d\alpha) = \int_{x}^{x+he_i} (X, d\alpha).$$

The independence of the integral on the curve joining two points, and the fact that we can consider the points x and $x + he_i$ sufficiently close (to each other) enables us to make the particular choice $\alpha(t) = x + th_i$, $t \in [0, 1]$, that is the segment of a line joining the points x and $x + he_i$ (Fig.25). It follows that

$$\frac{f(x + he_i) - f(x)}{h} = \frac{1}{h} \int_0^1 (X + the_i), he_i) dt = \frac{1}{h} \int_0^h X_i(x + ue_i) du$$

(we used $u = ht$). We pass to the limit for $h \to 0$ and find $\dfrac{\partial f}{\partial x_i} = X_i$.

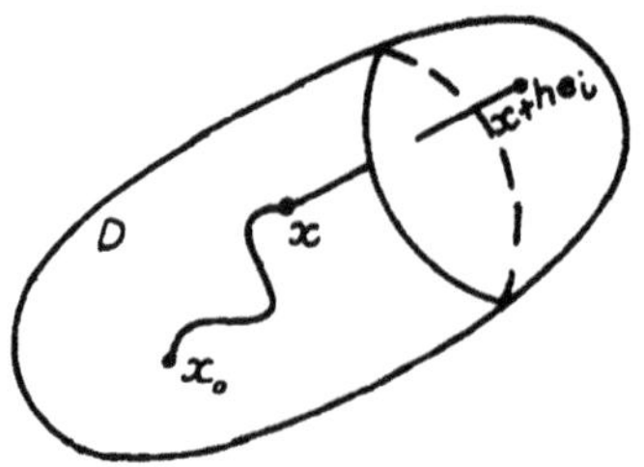

Fig. 25

Remarks. 1) For vector fields $X = (X_1, \dots, X_n)$ of class C^1, existence of the potential is equivalent to the fact that $X_1\, dx_1 + \cdots + X_n\, dx_n$ is everywhere the differential of a scalar field.

2) There are irrotational vector fields that are not globally potential. For example, the vector field

$$X = (X_1, X_2),\ X_1(x, y) = \frac{y}{x^2 + y^2},\ X_2(x, y) = -\frac{x}{x^2 + y^2},\ (x, y) \neq (0, 0),$$

is irrotational on $R^2 \setminus \{(0,0)\}$ (a domain that is not simply connected, Fig.26). On the other hand

(1) there exists the scalar field $f: R^2 \setminus \{(x, 0), x \in R\} \to R$, $f(x, y) = \arctan\dfrac{x}{y}$ such that $X_1 = \dfrac{\partial f}{\partial x}$, $X_2 = \dfrac{\partial f}{\partial y}$ on $R^2 \setminus \{(x, 0),\ x \in R\}$;

(2) there exists the scalar field $g: R^2 \setminus (\{0, y),\ y \in R\} \to R$, $g(x, y) = -\arctan\dfrac{y}{x}$ such

that $X_1 = \frac{\partial g}{\partial x}$, $X_2 = \frac{\partial g}{\partial y}$ on $R^2 \setminus \{(0,y),\ y \in R\}$, that is X is a potential vector field on any domain that does not contain the origin.

But there exists no scalar field $\varphi : R^2 \setminus \{(0,0)\} \to R$ such that $X_1 = \frac{\partial \varphi}{\partial x}$, $X_2 = \frac{\partial \varphi}{\partial y}$ on $R^2 \setminus \{(0,0)\}$. Indeed, if there exists such a field, then using the circle $\alpha : x = \cos t,\ y = \sin t,\ t \in [0, 2\pi]$ (a closed curve around the origin) we find the contradiction

$$0 = \varphi(\alpha(t))\Big|_0^{2\pi} = \int_0^{2\pi} d\varphi(\alpha(t)) = \int_\alpha (\operatorname{grad}\varphi, d\alpha)$$

$$= \int_\alpha (X, d\alpha) = \int_\alpha \frac{y\,dx - x\,dy}{x^2 + y^2}$$

$$= \int_0^{2\pi} (-\sin^2 t - \cos^2 t)\,dt = -2\pi.$$

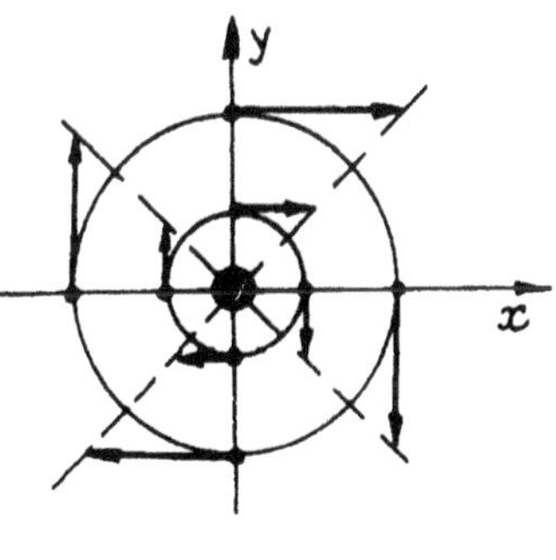

Fig. 26

Application. Let C be a rectilinear conductor with circular section of radius a and a current of intensity I (Fig.27). We fix the origin O as in the figure and denote $\boldsymbol{r} = x\boldsymbol{i} + y\boldsymbol{j} + z\boldsymbol{k}$, $r = (x^2 + y^2 + z^2)^{\frac{1}{2}}$. The current generates the magnetic field

$$\boldsymbol{H} = \begin{cases} (\boldsymbol{I} \times \boldsymbol{r}) / (2\pi a^2) & \text{for } (x,y,z) \in \operatorname{Int} C \cup \partial C \\ (\boldsymbol{I} \times \boldsymbol{r}) / (2\pi r^2) & \text{for } (x,y,z) \in \operatorname{Ext} C, \end{cases}$$

whose field lines are circles with their centres on the axis of the cylinder and contained in planes perpendicular to this straight line. By calculus we find

$$\operatorname{rot} \boldsymbol{H} = \begin{cases} \boldsymbol{I} / (\pi a^2) & \text{for } (x,y,z) \in \operatorname{Int} C \cup \partial C \\ 0 & \text{for } (x,y,z) \in \operatorname{Ext} C. \end{cases}$$

In other words, the restriction of $\boldsymbol{H}$ to $\operatorname{ext} C$ is an irrotational vector field.

Fixing a Cartesian frame such that the axis Oz coincides with the axis of the cylinder, oriented in the opposite sense of I, it follows

$$\boldsymbol{H} = \begin{cases} \dfrac{y\boldsymbol{i} - x\boldsymbol{j}}{2\pi a^2} & \text{for } (x,y,z) \in \operatorname{Int} C \cup \partial C \\ \dfrac{y\boldsymbol{i} - x\boldsymbol{j}}{2\pi(x^2 + y^2)} & \text{for } (x,y,z) \in \operatorname{Ext} C. \end{cases}$$

This expression shows that the restriction of $\boldsymbol{H}$ to $\operatorname{Ext} C$ cannot be a globally potential vector field.

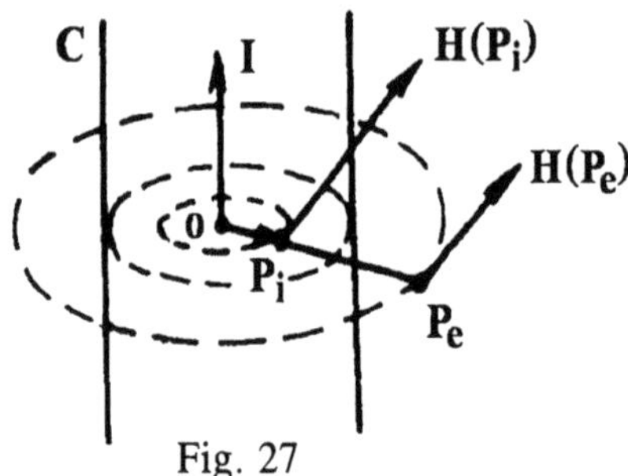

Fig. 27

Complements. 1) Let X be a vector field on an open and connected set of R^n. We assume that there exist two scalar fields h and f such that $X = h\,\mathrm{grad} f$. If h and f are functionally independent, then the vector field X is said to be *biscalar*. If h and f are functionally dependent, then it can be proved that X is a potential field; indeed $h(f)\,\mathrm{grad} f = \mathrm{grad}\,\varphi$ is equivalent with $h(f)\,df = d\varphi$ and then

$$\varphi(x) = \int_{x_0}^{x} h(f)\,df.$$

2) The potential theory [57] allows us to determine the conditions under which a given family of constant level hypersurfaces is attached to a harmonic function.

Theorem. *Let D be an open and connected set of R^n and $h : D \to R$ be a scalar field of class C^2 without critical points. The constant level hypersurfaces $h(x) = c$ attached to a harmonic scalar field $f : D \to R$ if and only if there exists a real function φ of class C^2 and a continuous real function ψ such that*

$$\frac{\Delta h}{\|\nabla h\|^2} = -\frac{\varphi''(h)}{\varphi'(h)} = \psi(h).$$

Proof. The implication $h(x) = c \Rightarrow f(x) = a$ is equivalent to the existence of a real function φ of class C^2 such that $f = \varphi(h)$. Then $df = \varphi'(h)$, $d^2 f = \varphi''(h)\,dh^2 + \varphi'(h)\,d^2 h$. Retaining only the trace of the Hessian, we find $\Delta f = \varphi''(h)\|\nabla h\|^2 + \varphi(h)\Delta h$ and $\Delta f = 0$ shows that the relation from the theorem is necessary.

Conversely, from $\dfrac{\varphi''(h)}{\varphi'(h)} + \psi(h) = 0$ we deduce $\varphi'(h) = A\exp(-\int \psi(h)\,dh)$ and then $f = \varphi(h) = A\int \exp(-\int \psi(h)\,dh)\,dh + B$, where A and B are constants.

Application. We refer to R^3 and ask if a family of right circular semicones, with the same axis and vertex, is a family of constant level hypersurfaces of a harmonic scalar field.

Without sacrificing generality, we may assume that the family of semicones is described by $x^2 + y^2 = cz^2$, $z < 0$. It follows $h(x, y, z) = \dfrac{x^2 + y^2}{z^2}$, $z > 0$ and the condition from the theorem becomes

$$\frac{\varphi''(h)}{\varphi'(h)} = -\frac{\frac{2}{z^2}+\frac{2}{z^2}+\frac{6(x^2+y^2)}{z^4}}{\frac{4x^2}{z^4}+\frac{4y^2}{z^4}+\frac{4(x^2+y^2)}{z^6}} = -\frac{2+3h}{2h(h+1)} = -\frac{1}{h}-\frac{1}{2(h+1)}.$$

Therefore $\ln|\varphi'(h)| + \ln|h| + \frac{1}{2}\ln|h+1| = \ln A$ or $d\varphi = \frac{A\,dh}{h\sqrt{h+1}}$. Putting $h = \tan^2\theta$ we find $d\varphi = \frac{2A\,d\theta}{\sin\theta}$ and $f = \varphi(h) = 2A\ln\left|\tan\frac{\theta}{2}\right| + B$, where A and B are arbitrary constants. Obviously, θ is the semiangle of a cone.

2.2. VECTOR FIELDS WITH SPHERICAL SYMMETRY

Let $y = (y_1, \dots, y_n)$ be a fixed point and $x = (x_1, \dots, x_n)$ a variable point of R^n. We denote $\boldsymbol{r} = \boldsymbol{yx}$ and $r = \|\boldsymbol{yx}\| = \|\boldsymbol{x}-\boldsymbol{y}\| = \sqrt{(x_1-y_1)^2 + \cdots + (x_n-y_n)^2}$.

Let $f: (0,\infty) \to R$ be a function of class C^∞. The scalar field defined on $R^n \setminus \{y\}$ by $f(r)$ is called a *scalar field with spherical symmetry of centre of symmetry* y (since it depends only on the distance between y and x. The constant level hypersurfaces of a spherically symmetrical scalar field are spheres.

The gradient of a spherically symmetrical scalar field $f(r)$ is $\operatorname{grad} f(r) = f'(r)\,\frac{\boldsymbol{r}}{r}$.

Let $\varphi(r)$ be a spherically symmetrical scalar field with symmetry centre y. The vector field X defined on $R^n \setminus \{y\}$ by

$$X(x) = \varphi(r)\,\frac{\boldsymbol{r}}{r}$$

is called a *vector field with spherical symmetry of centre of symmetry* y.

Any spherically symmetrical vector field with symmetry centre y is a potential field on $R^n \setminus \{y\}$ having as equipotential hypersurfaces the spheres centred at y. Indeed, for any function $\varphi : (0,\infty) \to R$ of class C^∞ there exists a C^∞ function $f: (0,\infty) \to R$ such that $f' = \varphi$, and the set of equations $f(r) = \text{const}$ is equivalent with the set of equations $r = \text{const}$.

Let X be a spherically symmetrical vector field. One observes that $\operatorname{div}\boldsymbol{X}(x) = \frac{r\varphi'(r) - (n-1)\varphi(r)}{r}$ and then X is solenoidal if and only if $\varphi(r) = \frac{c}{r^{n-1}}$, where c is a constant.

Newtonian fields. a) According to Newton's law, in R^3, the universal attraction law by which a mass m placed at the fixed point $y(y_1, y_2, y_3)$ acts on the unit mass placed at the variable point $x(x_1, x_2, x_3)$ is

$$X(x) = -\frac{m}{r^2}\frac{\boldsymbol{r}}{r},$$

where $\boldsymbol{r} = \boldsymbol{yx}$, $r = \sqrt{(x_1 - y_1)^2 + (x_2 - y_2)^2 + (x_3 - y_3)^2}$.

The field X is a vector field on $R^3 \setminus \{y\}$ called a *Newtonian field* or a *gravitational field* (Fig.28). Having spherical symmetry, it obviously is a potential field with the potential

$$f(\mathrm{r}) = \frac{m}{r}.$$

Variant. The Newtonian field

$$X(x_1, x_2, x_3) = -\frac{(x_1 - y_1)\boldsymbol{i} + (x_2 - y_2)\boldsymbol{j} + (x_3 - y_3)\boldsymbol{k}}{((x_1 - y_1)^2 + (x_2 - y_2)^2 + (x_3 - y_3)^2)^{\frac{3}{2}}},$$

$(x_1, x_2, x_3) \in R^3 \setminus \{(y_1, y_2, y_3)\}$, is an irrotational field whose domain of definition is connected and simply connected but not convex. Using the formulas from 2.1, second theorem, on an open parallelepiped or on an open convex set $D \subset R^3 \setminus \{(y_1, y_2, y_3)\}$, we find the potential $f(x_1, x_2, x_3) = [(x_1 - y_1)^2 + (x_2 - y_2)^2 + (x_3 - y_3)]^{-1/2}$, $(x_1, x_2, x_3) \in D$. One finds that f can be differentiable extended to $R^3 \setminus \{(y_1, y_2, y_3)\}$ and therefore the Newtonian field X is a potential field on $R^3 \setminus \{(y_1, y_2, y_3)\}$.

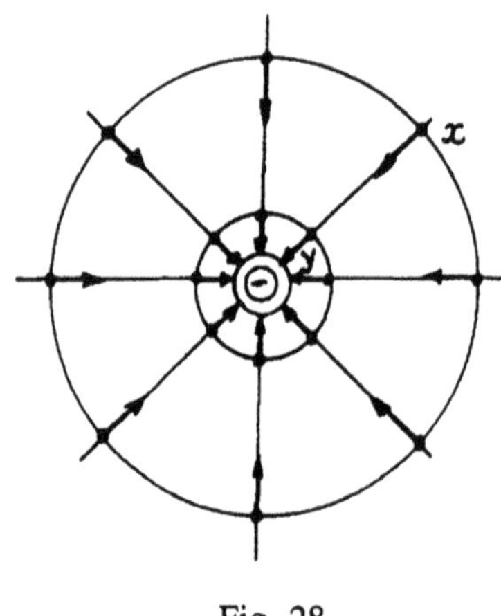

Fig. 28

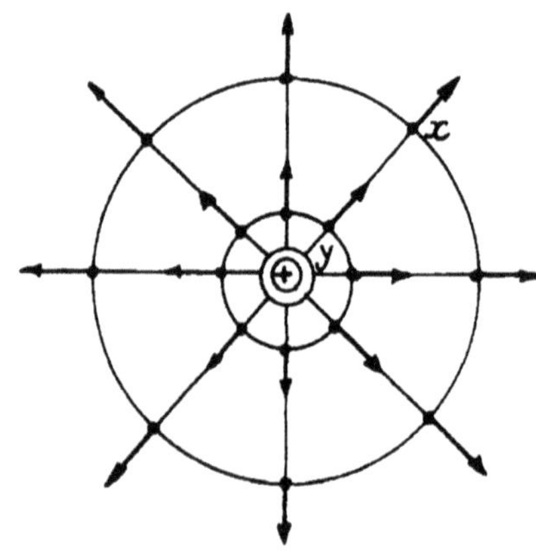

Fig. 29

b) In R^3 we consider the *gravitational field* generated by the masses $m_1, \ldots, m_k$ placed at the points $y^1, \ldots, y^k$ and acting on the unit mass placed at the point x. This field is given by

$$X(x) = -\sum_{i=1}^{k} \frac{m_i}{r_i^2} \frac{r_i}{r_i}, \quad x \in R^3 \setminus \{y^1, \dots, y^k\},$$

and possesses the potential

$$f(x) = \sum_{i=1}^{k} \frac{m_i}{r_i},$$

where $r_i = y^i x$, $r_i = \|r_i\|$.

c) Let D be an open, connected and bounded set in R^3, with a piecewise smooth boundary ∂D. We consider a distribution of masses on $D = D \cup \partial D$, with continuous density $\mu(y)$. The total gravitational force

$$X(x) = -\int_D \frac{\mu(y)}{r^2} \frac{r}{r}\, dy, \quad r = (y,x)$$

defines a *Newtonian field* X on R^3 (in the case in which $x \in D$, the foregoing integral is improper, but absolutely convergent). The potential of the vector field X is

$$f(x) = \int_D \frac{\mu(y)}{r}\, dy.$$

d) The notion of Newtonian field extends to R^n. For example, if D is an open, connected and bounded set of R^n, with piecewise smooth boundary ∂D and $\mu : D \to R$ is a continuous function, then the vector field defined on R^n by

$$X(x) = -\int_D \frac{\mu(y)}{r^{n-1}} \frac{r}{r}\, dy, \quad r = (y,x),$$

is called a *Newtonian field*. One can see that it possesses the potential

$$f(x) = \begin{cases} \dfrac{1}{n-2} \displaystyle\int_D \frac{\mu(y)}{r^{n-1}}\, dy & \text{for } n > 2, \\ \displaystyle\int_D \mu(y) \ln \frac{1}{r}\, dy & \text{for } n = 2. \end{cases}$$

Electrostatic fields

a) Coulomb concluded that the interaction force between two point charges is proportional to the product of the charges and inversely proportional to the square of the distance between the points. According to this law, the (repulsive or attractive) force by which the charge q from the fixed point $y = (y_1, y_2, y_3)$ acts on the unit charge $+1$ placed at the arbitrary point $x = (x_1, x_2, x_3)$ is

$$E(x) = \frac{1}{4\pi\varepsilon_0} \frac{q}{r^2} \frac{r}{r}, \quad x \in R^3 \setminus \{y\},$$

where $\varepsilon_0 \simeq 8{,}86 \cdot 10^{-12}\, F/m$ is the dielectric constant of vacuum, while $r = yx$.

The force E determines a vector field on $R^3 \setminus \{y\}$ called an *electric field*. This is a spherically symmetrical field (for $q < 0$ see Fig.28, for $q > 0$ see Fig.29). The corresponding potential is $f(r) = -\frac{1}{4\pi\varepsilon_0}\frac{q}{r}$.

b) The *electrostatic field* generated by the charges $q_1, \dots, q_k$ located at the points $y^1, \dots, y^k$ and acting on the unit charge placed at x is

$$E(x) = \frac{1}{4\pi\varepsilon_0}\sum_{i=1}^{k}\frac{q_i}{r_i^2}\frac{r_i}{r_i}, \quad x \in R^3 \setminus \{y^1, \dots, y^k\},$$

where $r_i = y^i x$. This field possesses the potential

$$f(x) = -\frac{1}{4\pi\varepsilon_0}\sum_{i=1}^{k}\frac{q_i}{r_i}.$$

2.3. SOLENOIDAL VECTOR FIELDS

A C^1 vector field X on R^n is said to be *solenoidal* if $\operatorname{div} X = 0$.

Examples. 1) The Newtonian field

$$X = -\frac{xi + yj + zk}{(x^2 + y^2 + z^2)^{\frac{3}{2}}}, \quad (x,y,z) \in R^3 \setminus \{0\},$$

is irrotational and solenoidal.

2) The vector field $X = \operatorname{grad} f$ is solenoidal if and only if f is a harmonic function, i.e., $\Delta f = 0$.

3) The vector field

$$X = \frac{y}{x^2 + y^2}i - \frac{x}{x^2 + y^2}j, \quad (x,y) \in R^2 \setminus \{(0,0)\},$$

is irrotational and solenoidal, but not globally potential.

4) If $f, g : R^3 \to R$ are of class C^2, then the vector field

$$X = \operatorname{grad} f \times \operatorname{grad} g$$

is solenoidal on R^3.

5) If Y is a vector field of class C^2 on R^3, then the vector field

$$X = \operatorname{rot} Y,$$

is solenoidal.

6) Let $R^6 = \{(x_1, x_2, x_3, v_1, v_2, v_3)\}$ considered as the phase space associated to the Lorentz equation describing the motion of a particle with charge q and mass m, in some stationary electromagnetic field generated by the electric field

$$E(x) = (E_1(x), E_2(x), E_3(x))$$

and the magnetic field

$$B(x) = (B_1(x), B_2(x), B_3(x)), \ x = (x_1, x_2, x_3) \in R^3.$$

The vector field

$$X = \left(v_1, v_2, v_3, \frac{q}{m}(E_1 + v_2 B_3 - v_3 B_2), \frac{q}{m}(E_2 + v_3 B_1 - v_1 B_3), \frac{q}{m}(E_3 + v_1 B_2 - v_2 B_1) \right),$$

which locally represents the evolution velocity of the phenomenon in R^6, is solenoidal. Indeed,

$$\operatorname{div} X = \frac{\partial X_1}{\partial x_1} + \frac{\partial X_2}{\partial x_2} + \frac{\partial X_3}{\partial x_3} + \frac{\partial X_4}{\partial v_1} + \frac{\partial X_5}{\partial v_2} + \frac{\partial X_6}{\partial v_3} = 0.$$

In the sequel we shall prove that any solenoidal field of class C^1 on an open set of R^3 reduces locally to a curl field, that is (locally) $X = \operatorname{rot} Y$. The vector field Y is uniquely determined modulo an arbitrary additive gradient, and Y is called the *vector potential* of X.

Theorem. *Let X be a vector field on an open convex set $D \subset R^3$. If X possesses on D a vector potential Y of class C^1, then this potential is uniquely determined up to an additive gradient.*

Proof. Let $X = \operatorname{rot} Y_1$ and $X = \operatorname{rot} Y_2$. It follows $\operatorname{rot} Y_1 = \operatorname{rot} Y_2$ and then $\operatorname{rot}(Y_1 - Y_2) = 0$. Since $Y_1 - Y_2$ is an irrotational vector field of class C^1, according to the second theorem from section 2.1, there exists a scalar field f on D such that $Y_1 - Y_2 = \operatorname{grad} f$.

Theorem. *Let $D \subset R^3$ be an open set and X a vector field of class C^1 on D. The following assertions are equivalent:*

1) X is solenoidal;

2) for any point $p \in D$ there exists an open neighborhood $U \subset D$ of p and a vector field Y on U such that $X = \operatorname{rot} Y$ on U;

3) the flux of X through the boundary of any spherical body included in D is null.

Proof. 1) ⇒ 2). Let $X = (P, Q, R)$. The hypothesis $\operatorname{div} X = 0$ on D is transcribed as

$$\frac{\partial P}{\partial x} + \frac{\partial Q}{\partial y} + \frac{\partial R}{\partial z} = 0, \quad \text{for any} \quad (x,y,z) \in D.$$

Let $(x_0, y_0, z_0) \in D$ and U be an open ball centred at (x_0, y_0, z_0) placed in D (or an open tridimensional interval). The functions

$$f, g : U \to R,\ f(x,y,z) = \int_{x_0}^{x} Q(x,y,t)\,dt,\ g(x,y,z) = -\int_{x_0}^{x} P(x,y,t)\,dt + \int_{x_0}^{x} R(t,y,z_0)\,dt$$

determine on U the vector field $Y = (f, g, 0)$ with the property $\operatorname{rot} Y = X$.

Remark. The vector potential $Y = (f, g, 0)$ with f, g defined as above, is of class C^1 and with $\frac{\partial f}{\partial z}, \frac{\partial g}{\partial z}, \frac{\partial g}{\partial x} - \frac{\partial f}{\partial y}$ of class C^1. If X is a solenoidal vector field on R^3, then the representation $X = \operatorname{rot} Y$, $Y = (f, g, 0)$ is global.

2) ⇒ 1). Obviously, $\operatorname{div} \operatorname{rot} Y = 0$.

1) ⇒ 3). We apply the Gauss-Ostrogradski formula

$$\iint_{\Sigma} (X, N)\, d\sigma = \iiint_{\Omega} (\operatorname{div} X)\, dx\, dy\, dz.$$

3) $\Rightarrow$ 1). Let $p \in D$ and Ω a spherical body of centre p and of radius ε, included in D. The Gauss-Ostrogradski formula implies

$$\iiint_\Omega (\mathrm{div}\, X)\, dx\, dy\, dz = 0.$$

We use the Mean Value formula and we pass to the limit for $\varepsilon \to 0$. It follows that $(\mathrm{div} X)(p) = 0$, for any $p \in D$.

Euler's Theorem. *Let X be a vector field of class C^∞ on an open and connected set $D \subset R^3$. If X is solenoidal, then for any point $(x_0, y_0, z_0) \in D$ with $X(x_0, y_0, z_0) \neq 0$, there exists an open set $U \subset D$ that contains (x_0, y_0, z_0) and two scalar fields f, g of class C^∞ on U such that (Fig.30)*

$$X|_U = \mathrm{grad} f \times \mathrm{grad} g,$$

where $X|_U$ is the restriction of X to U.

The scalar fields f, g are called *Euler potentials* of X. They are not unique.

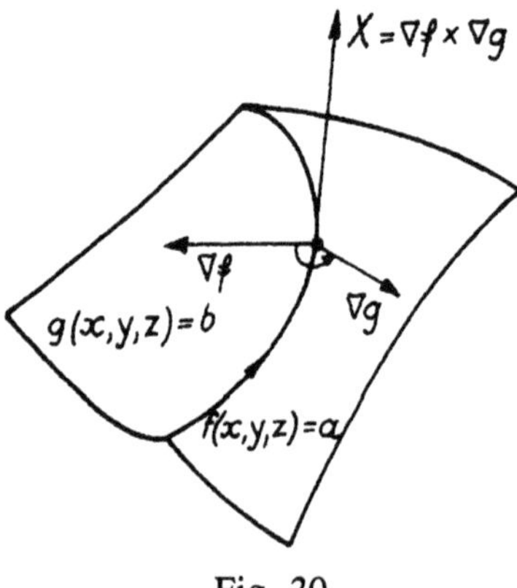

Fig. 30

The classical proof of Euler's Theorem is specific for the tridimensional space using the notion of vector potential. Therefore we prefer the generalization and proof that are good for any dimension $n \geq 3$. These will be given in 3.2.

Applications. 1) Determine the field of velocities of an incompressible fluid due to a source q placed at the point M_0.

Solution. The fluid particles which spring from M_0 describe some rays of origin M_0; this is equivalent to the fact that the velocity V is a spherically symmetrical vector field on $R^3 \setminus \{M_0\}$, i.e., $V(M) = \varphi(r)\dfrac{\boldsymbol{r}}{r}$, where $\boldsymbol{r} = \overline{M_0 M}$. The debit q of the source placed at M_0 is $q = \iint_S (N, V)\, d\sigma$, where S is a sphere of centre M_0 and radius r. It follows that

$q = \varphi(r) 4\pi r^2$ and then $V(M) = \dfrac{1}{4\pi}\dfrac{q}{r^2}\dfrac{r}{r}$. This is a solenoidal vector field.

2) **The Biot-Savart-Laplace vector field**

Let D be an open connected set of R^3 and ∂D its boundary, which is assumed to be piecewise smooth. We denote by X a vector field of class C^1 on $\bar{D} = D \cup \partial D$. The vector field defined on R^3 by

$$Y(x) = \iiint_D \frac{1}{r^3} X(y) \times r dy, \ r = (y,x),$$

is called the *Biot-Savart-Laplace vector field*. The name comes from the fact that for the case in which D is filled out with electric charges in a certain motion, $X(y)$ being the current density, then the magnetic field Y generated by this current is given by the Biot-Savart-Laplace law (the foregoing equality).

Generally the field Y is not irrotational but solenoidal. Its vector potential is

$$Z(x) = \iiint_D \frac{X(y)}{r} dy.$$

2.4. MONGE AND STOKES REPRESENTATIONS

Monge's Theorem. *If X is a vector field of class C^∞ on some open and connected set $D \subset R^3$, then for any $x_0 \in D$ with $\mathrm{rot}X(x_0) \neq 0$, there exists an open set $U \subset D$ containing x_0 and three scalar fields h, f, g of class C^∞ on U such that*

$$X|_U = \mathrm{grad}h + f\mathrm{grad}g.$$

The scalar fields h, f, g are called *Monge potentials* of X. They are not unique.

Proof. The field $\mathrm{rot}X$ is solenoidal on D since always $\mathrm{div}(\mathrm{rot}X) = 0$. Taking account of Euler's theorem for solenoidal fields, it follows that for every $x_0 \in D$ with $\mathrm{rot}X(x_0) \neq 0$, there exists an open set $U_1 \subset D$ containing x_0 and two scalar fields f, g of class C^∞ on U_1 such that

$$\mathrm{rot}\,X = \mathrm{grad}f \times \mathrm{grad}g \text{ on } U_1.$$

This equality is transcribed as $\mathrm{rot}(X - f\mathrm{grad}g) = 0$ and then the vector field $X - f\mathrm{grad}g$ is irrotational on U_1. Therefore there exists a neighborhood $U \subset U_1$ of x_0 and a scalar field h of class C^∞ on U such that

$$X - f\mathrm{grad}g = \mathrm{grad}h \text{ on } U.$$

Stokes' Theorem. *If X is a vector field of class C^1 with $\mathrm{div}X$ of class C^1 on an open and connected set $D \subset R^3$, then for every $x_0 \in D$ there exists an open set $U \subset D$ which* *contains* x_0, *a scalar field* h *of class* C^2 *on* U *and a vector field* Y *of class* C^2 *and with* $\mathrm{rot}\,Y$ *of class* C^1 *on* U *such that* $X|_U = \mathrm{grad}h + \mathrm{rot}Y$.

The scalar field h and the vector field Y are called *Stokes potentials* of X. They are not unique.

Proof. It will be sufficient to show that there exists a local scalar field of class C^2 such that $X - \mathrm{grad}h =$ a solenoidal field. But $\mathrm{div}(X - \mathrm{grad}h) = 0$ shows that h must be a solution of the Poisson equation $\Delta h = \mathrm{div}X$.

Such an equation admits infinitely many local solutions. For example, if U is an open, connected and bounded set with a piecewise smooth boundary ∂U, and a is a vector parameter, then

$$h_a(x) = (a, X) - \frac{1}{4\pi}\iiint_U \frac{\mathrm{div}X(x)}{\|x - y\|}\,dy,\ x \in U,$$

are solutions of the Poisson equation $\Delta h = \mathrm{div}X$.

Notice. If X is of class C^∞, then the Stokes representation is equivalent to the representation $X|_U = \mathrm{grad}h + \mathrm{grad}f \times \mathrm{grad}g$. For $n > 3$, this variant generalizes to

$$X|_U = \mathrm{grad}f_n + \mathrm{grad}f_1 \times \cdots \times \mathrm{grad}\,f_{n-1},$$

where $U \subset R^n$.

2.5. HARMONIC VECTOR FIELDS

A C^2 vector field $X = (X_1, \dots, X_n)$ is said to be *harmonic* if it is irrotational and solenoidal or, equivalently, if $\Delta X = 0 = (\Delta X_1, \dots, \Delta X_n)$.

Example. The Newtonian field $X = -m\dfrac{xi + yj + zk}{(x^2 + y^2 + z^2)^{\frac{3}{2}}}$, $m > 0$, is harmonic on $R^3 \setminus \{0\}$.

Theorem. *If* $D \subset R^n$ *is an open and convex set and* X *is a field of class* C^2 *on* D, *then the following assertions are equivalent:*

1) X *is harmonic on* D;

2) there exists a C^3 *harmonic scalar field* $f: D \to R$ *such that* $X = \mathrm{grad}f$.

Proof. 1) $\Rightarrow$ 2). From $\mathrm{rot}X = 0$, we get the conclusion that there exists $f: D \to R$ such that $X = \mathrm{grad}f$. But $\mathrm{div}X = 0$ imposes $\mathrm{div}(\mathrm{grad}f) = 0$, i.e., $\Delta f = 0$. In other words, f is harmonic.

2) $\Rightarrow$ 1). The hypotheses $X = \mathrm{grad}f$, $\Delta f = 0$ imply $\mathrm{rot}X = 0$ and $\mathrm{div}X = 0$. Therefore, X is harmonic on D.

Application. A part of a fluid can be identified with an open set $D \subset R^3$. The density of the fluid $\mu(x,y,z,t)$ and the velocity of the fluid $v(x,y,z,t)$ are assumed to be functions of class C^2 on $D \times R$.

The part of the fluid corresponding to the spherical body $\Omega \subset D$, with $\partial\Omega = \Sigma$, has the mass

$$m(t) = \iiint_{\Omega} \mu(x,y,z,t)\,dx\,dy\,dz,$$

a function of class C^1 of t. It follows that

$$m'(t) = \iiint_{\Omega} \frac{\partial\mu}{\partial t}\,dx\,dy\,dz.$$

Physical reasons show that $m'(t)$ must be the flux of μv through Σ, that is

$$m'(t) = \iint_{\Sigma} (\mu v, n)d\sigma = \iiint_{\Omega} \operatorname{div}(\mu v)\,dx\,dy\,dz.$$

From $\iiint_{\Omega}\left(\frac{\partial\mu}{\partial t} - \operatorname{div}(\mu v)\right)dx\,dy\,dz = 0$, for any $\Omega \subset D$, we obtain the continuity equation $\operatorname{div}(\mu v) = \frac{\partial\mu}{\partial t}$.

If μ = constant and $v = \operatorname{grad} f$, then we say that the fluid is incompressible, while f is called the *velocity potential*. Then, the continuity equation reduces to $\operatorname{div}\mu v = 0$, i.e., $\Delta f = 0$ and therefore μv is a harmonic field on D.

2.6. KILLING VECTOR FIELDS

A vector field $X = (X_1, \dots, X_n)$ of class C^∞ on R^n is called a *Killing field* if it satisfies Killing equations (partial differential equations, see also Chapter 3)

$$\frac{\partial X_i}{\partial x_j} + \frac{\partial X_j}{\partial x_i} = 0,\ i,j = 1, \dots, n. \tag{1}$$

Obviously, the PDEs system (1) implies $\frac{\partial X_i}{\partial x_i} = 0$, $i = 1, \dots, n$, that is $X_i = X_i(x_1, \dots, x_{i-1}, x_{i+1}, \dots, x_n)$. This means that for $n = 1$, the Killing vector fields reduce to parallel fields. Generally, $\operatorname{div} X = 0$ and hence any Killing field is a solenoidal field.

Let $n \geq 2$. Partially differentiating (1) and permuting indices, we find

$$\frac{\partial^2 X_i}{\partial x_k \partial x_j} + \frac{\partial^2 X_j}{\partial x_k \partial x_i} = 0,\quad \frac{\partial^2 X_j}{\partial x_i \partial x_k} + \frac{\partial^2 X_k}{\partial x_i \partial x_j} = 0,\quad \frac{\partial^2 X_k}{\partial x_j \partial x_i} + \frac{\partial^2 X_i}{\partial x_j \partial x_k} = 0.$$

We add the first two equalities and subtract the third from the sum; based on the complete integrability conditions, $\frac{\partial^2 X_i}{\partial x_j \partial x_k} = \frac{\partial^2 X_i}{\partial x_k \partial x_j}$ we find $\frac{\partial^2 X_j}{\partial x_k \partial x_i} = 0$. It follows that

$\frac{\partial X_j}{\partial x_i} = a_{ji}$ (constants) and (1) imposes the skew-symmetry condition for the matrix $[a_{ij}]$. Thus a Killing field on R^n has components of the form

$$X_j = \sum_{i=1}^{n} a_{ji} x_i + c_j , \quad j = 1 , \ldots , n,$$

where $a_{ij} = -a_{ji}$ and c_j are arbitrary constants. Since the dimension of the vector space of all skew-symmetric matrices $[a_{ji}]$ of order n is $\frac{n(n-1)}{2}$, and the dimension of the vector space of all column matrices $[c_j]$ is n, it follows that on R^n there exist $\frac{n(n-1)}{2} + n = \frac{n(n+1)}{2}$ linearly independent Killing fields in $\mathcal{X}(R^n)$ (this is not the same with pointwise linear independence in R^n).

The bracket of two Killing vector fields is a Killing vector field, too. This can be proved either by showing that if $X = (X_1, \ldots, X_n)$, $Y = (Y_1, \ldots, Y_n)$ are solutions of the system (1), then $[X, Y] = (X(Y_i) - Y(X_i))$ is a solution, too, or by putting

$$X = \left(\sum_k a_{jk} x_k + c_j \right) , \quad Y = \left(\sum_k b_{jk} x_k + d_j \right)$$

and calculating

$$[X, Y] = \left(\sum_k \sum_j (a_{jk} b_{ij} - b_{jk} a_{ij}) x_k \right) = \left(\sum_k d_{ik} x_k \right) ,$$

where $[d_{ik}]$ is obviously a skew-symmetric matrix. It follows that the set of all Killing vector fields on R^n is a Lie algebra of dimension $\frac{n(n+1)}{2}$.

Remark. If $A = ai + bj + ck$ is a parallel field and $X = xi + yj + zk$, then $A \times X = (bz - cy)i + (cx - az)j + (ay - bx)k$ is a Killing field on R^3. Conversely, any Killing field Y on R^3 which is not a parallel field can be written as $A \times X$. This result arises from Euler's representation theorem for a solenoidal vector field (see 2.3).

Application (Fig.31). We consider the rotation motion of a solid S with angular velocity ω around an axis Δ passing through the origin. A point (x, y, z) of the solid S describes a circle C whose centre is on the axis and radius is d, laying on a plane perpendicular to the axis. The tangential velocity is a vector $V(x, y, z)$ tangent to the circle, directed towards the sense of the motion and having modulus $V = \omega d$.

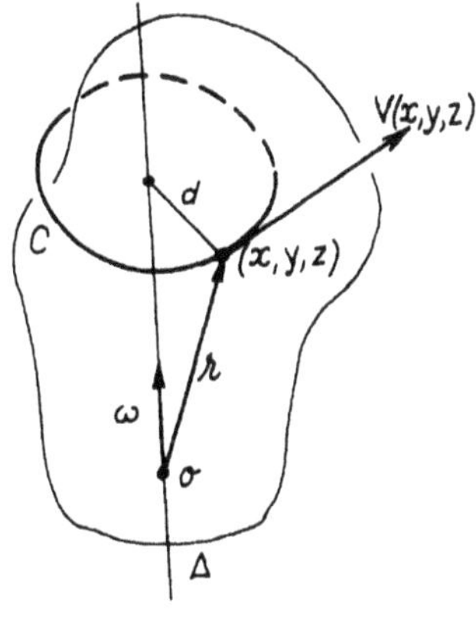

Fig. 31

We denote by ω the vector of modulus ω, having the direction of the axis and oriented by the right-hand rule, the sense being induced on the axis by the rotation of the solid. Then $V(x,y,z) = \omega \times r$, where $r = xi + yj + zk$. The vector field V is a Killing field.

2.7. CONFORMAL VECTOR FIELDS

A vector field $X = (X_1, \dots, X_n)$ of class C^∞ on R^n is called a *conformal field* if it satisfies the partial differential equations (see also Chapter 3)

$$\frac{\partial X_i}{\partial x_j} + \frac{\partial X_j}{\partial x_i} = \psi\, \delta_{ij}, \quad i,j = 1, \dots, n, \tag{2}$$

where δ_{ij} is Kronecker's symbol, and $\psi : R^n \to R$. If ψ is a constant, then the conformal field is called a *homothetic field*. If $\psi = 0$, then the conformal field is a Killing field.

The PDEs system (2) implies $\dfrac{\partial X_1}{\partial x_1} = \dots = \dfrac{\partial X_n}{\partial x_n} = \dfrac{\psi}{2}$, and then $\psi = \dfrac{2 \operatorname{div} X}{n}$. In particular, we notice that if $n = 1$, then the conformal fields identify with the functions of class C^∞.

We assume that ψ does not reduce to a constant and $n \geq 2$. Computing partial derivatives of (2) and permuting indices, we obtain

$$\frac{\partial^2 X_i}{\partial x_k \partial x_j} + \frac{\partial^2 X_j}{\partial x_k \partial x_i} = \frac{\partial \psi}{\partial x_k}\delta_{ij}, \quad \frac{\partial^2 X_j}{\partial x_i \partial x_k} + \frac{\partial^2 X_k}{\partial x_i \partial x_j} = \frac{\partial \psi}{\partial x_i}\delta_{jk},$$

$$\frac{\partial^2 X_k}{\partial x_j \partial x_i} + \frac{\partial^2 X_i}{\partial x_j \partial x_k} = \frac{\partial \psi}{\partial x_j}\delta_{ki}.$$

We add the first two equalities and subtract the third; based on the complete integrability conditions

$$\frac{\partial^2 X_i}{\partial x_j \partial x_k} = \frac{\partial^2 X_i}{\partial x_k \partial x_j},$$

we obtain

$$2\frac{\partial^2 X_j}{\partial x_k \partial x_i} = \frac{\partial \psi}{\partial x_k}\delta_{ij} + \frac{\partial \psi}{\partial x_i}\delta_{jk} - \frac{\partial \psi}{\partial x_j}\delta_{ki}. \tag{3}$$

We impose again the complete integrability conditions,

$$\frac{\partial^3 X_j}{\partial x_k \partial x_i \partial x_l} = \frac{\partial^3 X_j}{\partial x_k \partial x_l \partial x_i}.$$

We find

$$\frac{\partial^2 \psi}{\partial x_k \partial x_l}\delta_{ij} - \frac{\partial^2 \psi}{\partial x_j \partial x_l}\delta_{ki} = \frac{\partial^2 \psi}{\partial x_k \partial x_i}\delta_{lj} - \frac{\partial^2 \psi}{\partial x_j \partial x_i}\delta_{kl}.$$

Summing upon i and j, we get

$$(2-n)\frac{\partial^2 \psi}{\partial x_k \partial x_l} = (\Delta \psi)\delta_{kl}.$$

A new summation with respect to k and l gives $(1-n)\Delta\psi = 0$.

Let $n > 2$. It follows that $\dfrac{\partial^2 \psi}{\partial x_k \partial x_l} = 0$ and then $\psi(x) = \sum_{l=1}^{n} c_l x_l + c$. By this relation, the system (3) is written as

$$2\frac{\partial^2 X_j}{\partial x_k \partial x_i} = c_k\delta_{ij} + c_i\delta_{jk} - c_j\delta_{ki}.$$

Integrating, we obtain

$$\frac{\partial X_j}{\partial x_i} = \frac{1}{2}\left(\delta_{ij}\sum_{k=1}^{n} c_k x_k + c_i x_j - c_j x_i\right) + c_{ji}.$$

The equations (2) impose on the matrix $[c_{ji}]$ the conditions $c_{ij} + c_{ij} = c\delta_{ij}$. A new integration gives

$$X_j = \frac{1}{2}\int_{x_0}^{x}\sum_i\left(\delta_{ij}\sum_k c_k x_k + c_i x_j + c_j x_i\right)dx_i + \sum_i c_{ji}x_i$$

$$= \frac{1}{2}\int_{x_0}^{x} d\left[\left(\sum_k c_k x_k\right)x_j - \frac{1}{2}c_j\sum_i x_i^2\right] + \sum_i c_{ji}x_i$$

$$= \frac{1}{2} x_j \sum_k c_k x_k - \frac{1}{4} c_j \sum_k x_k^2 + \sum_k c_{jk} x_k + d_j ,$$

where d_j are arbitrary constants. Since the dimension of the vector space of the matrices $[c_{ij}]$ of order n is $\frac{n^2 - n}{2} + 1$ and we have two arbitrary matrix vectors $[c_k]$, $[d_j]$, it follows that on R^n, $n > 2$, there exist

$$\frac{n^2 - n}{2} + 1 + n + n = \frac{(n+1)(n+2)}{2}$$

linearly independent conformal fields in $\mathcal{X}(R^n)$.

An analogous reasoning shows that the bracket of two conformal fields is a conformal field too. Therefore, the set of all conformal vector fields on R^n, $n > 2$, is a Lie algebra of dimension $\frac{(n+1)(n+2)}{2}$.

Let $n = 2$. The equations (2) become

$$2 \frac{\partial X_1}{\partial x_1} - \psi, \; 2 \frac{\partial X_2}{\partial x_2} = \psi, \; \frac{\partial X_1}{\partial x_2} + \frac{\partial X_2}{\partial x_1} - 0.$$

It follows that $X = (X_1, X_2)$ satisfies on R^2 the Cauchy-Riemann conditions

$$\frac{\partial X_1}{\partial x_1} = \frac{\partial X_2}{\partial x_2}, \; \frac{\partial X_1}{\partial x_2} = - \frac{\partial X_2}{\partial x_1},$$

and then X_1, X_2 respectively are the real and the imaginary part of a holomorphic function $f: C \rightarrow C$. In other words, the set of conformal fields on R^2 is equivalent with the set of the holomorphic functions on C.

We assume that $X = (X_1, \ldots, X_n)$ is a homothetic vector field, i.e., $\psi(x) = c$, for any $x \subset R^n$. In this case we find $X_j = \sum_{i=1}^{n} c_{ji} x_i + d_j$, $j = 1, \ldots, n$, where c_{ij} are constants that satisfy the relations $c_{ij} + c_{ji} = \delta_{ij}$, while d_j are arbitrary constants. Let $c \neq 0$; then on R^n there are $\frac{n^2 - n}{2} + 1 + n = \frac{n(n+1)}{2} + 1$ homothetic vector fields, which are linearly independent in $\mathcal{X}(R^n)$.

Notice. The equations (2) are a natural generalization of the Cauchy-Riemann conditions.

2.8. AFFINE AND PROJECTIVE VECTOR FIELDS

A vector field $X = (X_1, \dots, X_2)$ of class C^∞ on R^n which satisfies the partial differential equations

$$\frac{\partial^2 X_i}{\partial x_j \partial x_k} = 0, \ i, j, k = 1, \dots, n, \tag{4}$$

is called an *affine vector field.*

The PDEs system (4) implies $\frac{\partial}{\partial x_j} \operatorname{div} X = 0$ and therefore any affine vector field has constant divergence. From (4) we also notice that $\frac{\partial X_i}{\partial x_j} = a_{ij}$ (constant). Therefore, an affine vector field on R^n has components of the form

$$X_i = \sum_{j=1}^{n} a_{ij} x_j + c_i, \ i = 1, \dots, n,$$

where c_i are constants.

The dimension of the vector space of quadratic matrices $[a_{ij}]$ of order n is n^2, while the dimension of the vector space of column matrices $[c_i]$ is n. It follows therefore that on R^n there exist $n^2 + n$ affine vector fields that are linearly independent in $\mathcal{X}(R^n)$.

If X and Y are affine vector fields, then the bracket $[X, Y] = D_X Y - D_Y X$ is an affine vector field. Therefore the set of affine vector fields on R^n is a Lie algebra of dimension $n^2 + n$. Let us notice that any Killing vector field is an affine vector field.

A vector field $X = (X_1, \dots, X_n)$ of class C^∞ on R^n for which there exists a vector field $Y = (Y_1, \dots, Y_n)$ of class C^∞ on R^n such that

$$\frac{\partial^2 X_i}{\partial x_j \partial x_k} = Y_j \delta_{ik} + Y_k \delta_{ij}, \ i, j, k = 1, \dots, n, \tag{5}$$

where δ_{ij} is Kronecker's symbol, is called a *projective vector field.*

Any affine vector field is a *projective vector field.* Therefore from (5) it follows $\frac{\partial}{\partial x_j} \operatorname{div} X = (n+1) Y_j$, that is Y is necessarily a potential field.

For $n = 1$, the projective vector fields identify with the functions of class C^∞. For $n \geq 2$, we impose complete integrability conditions for the system of partial differential equations (5), that is

$$\frac{\partial^3 X_i}{\partial x_l \partial x_j \partial x_k} = \frac{\partial^3 X_i}{\partial x_j \partial x_l \partial x_k}.$$

Since

$$\frac{\partial^3 X_i}{\partial x_l \partial x_j \partial x_k} = \frac{\partial Y_j}{\partial x_l}\delta_{ik} + \frac{\partial Y_k}{\partial x_l}\delta_{ij},$$

we get

$$\frac{\partial Y_j}{\partial x_l}\delta_{ik} + \frac{\partial Y_k}{\partial x_l}\delta_{ij} = \frac{\partial Y_l}{\partial x_j}\delta_{ik} + \frac{\partial Y_k}{\partial x_j}\delta_{il}.$$

Summing with respect to i and j, we find $n\dfrac{\partial Y_k}{\partial x_l} = \dfrac{\partial Y_l}{\partial x_k}$. But $\dfrac{\partial Y_k}{\partial x_l} = \dfrac{\partial Y_l}{\partial x_k}$, so that $(n-1)\dfrac{\partial Y_k}{\partial x_l} = 0$ or $\dfrac{\partial Y_k}{\partial x_l} = 0$. The last partial differential equations claim that $\boldsymbol{Y}$ is a parallel vector field, that is $Y_k = c_k$, $k = 1, \dots, n$. By this remark, the PDEs system (5) becomes

$$\frac{\partial^2 X_i}{\partial x_j \partial x_k} = c_j\,\delta_{ik} + c_k\,\delta_{ij}.$$

It follows that

$$\frac{\partial X_i}{\partial x_k} = \delta_{ik}\sum_{j=1}^{n} c_j x_j + c_k x_i + a_{ik},$$

and finally

$$X_i = \int_{x_0}^{x}\sum_{k=1}^{n}\left(\delta_{ik}\sum_{j=1}^{n} c_j x_j + c_k x_i\right) dx_k + \sum_{k=1}^{n} a_{ik} x_k$$

$$= \int_{x_0}^{x} d\left[x_i \sum_{j=1}^{n} c_j x_j\right] + \sum_{j=1}^{n} a_{ij} x_j = x_i \sum_{j=1}^{n} c_j x_j + \sum_{j=1}^{n} a_{ij} x_j + d_i.$$

The dimension of the vector space of matrices $[a_{ij}]$ of order n is n^2 and the column vectors $[c_j]$, $[d_i]$ are arbitrary. This means that on R^n, $n \geq 2$, there exist $n^2 + 2n$ projective vector fields that are linearly independent in $\mathcal{X}(R^n)$.

It can be proved that the bracket of two projective vector fields is a projective vector field. This means that the set of projective vector fields on R^n, $n \geq 2$, is a Lie algebra of dimension $n^2 + 2n$.

2.9. TORSE FORMING VECTOR FIELDS

A vector field $X = (X_1, \dots, X_n)$ of class C^∞ on an open and connected set $D \subset R^n$ is said to be *torse forming* if there exists a scalar field $a : D \to R$ of class C^∞ and a vector field $Y = (Y_1, \dots, Y_n)$ of class C^∞ on D such that

$$\frac{\partial X_i}{\partial x_j} = a\delta_{ij} + X_i Y_j, \quad i, j = 1, \dots, n, \tag{6}$$

where δ_{ij} is Kronecker's symbol. Obviously, the relations (6) are equivalent to $D_Z X = aZ + (Y, Z)X$, for any $Z \in \mathcal{X}(D)$.

From the definition one can notice that a torse forming vector field X can be identically null only in the case in which a is the identically null function. By definition, it also follows that

$$\text{rot}X = X \wedge Y, \ \text{div}X = \text{an} + (X, Y).$$

Therefore, a torse forming vector field is: (1) *irrotational* if and only if Y and X are collinear, (2) *solenoidal* if and only if $an + (X, Y) = 0$, (3) *potential* or *biscalar*.

For $n = 1$, the torse forming vector fields reduce to solutions of first-order linear differential equations. For $n \geq 2$, the complete integrability conditions of the PDEs system (6),

$$\frac{\partial^2 X_i}{\partial x_j \partial x_k} = \frac{\partial^2 X_i}{\partial x_k \partial x_j},$$

are written as

$$\frac{\partial a}{\partial x_k}\delta_{ij} + a\delta_{ik}Y_j + X_i\frac{\partial Y_j}{\partial x_k} = \frac{\partial a}{\partial x_j}\delta_{ik} + a\delta_{ij}Y_k + X_i\frac{\partial Y_k}{\partial x_j}. \tag{7}$$

Summing with respect to i and j, we deduce the consequence

$$\sum_{i=1}^{n} X_i\left(\frac{\partial Y_i}{\partial x_k} - \frac{\partial Y_k}{\partial x_i}\right) = (1-n)\left(\frac{\partial a}{\partial x_k} - aY_k\right). \tag{8}$$

The summations with respect to i and k, or j and k do not give any supplementary conditions.

For $n \geq 2$, the most interesting particular cases of torse forming vector fields are:

1) *Concircular field*, if Y is a potential field. The relations (8) show that if $a \neq 0$,

then necessarily $Y = \operatorname{grad}\ln|a|$. From (6) it follows that $d\dfrac{X_i}{a} = dx_i$ and then $X_i(x) = a(x)(x_i + c_i)$ are the components of a concircular field.

2) *Concurrent field* (Fig.32), if $a \neq 0,\ Y = 0$. In this case, the relations (8) imply that a is constant and $X_i(x) = a(x_i + c_i)$. The change of variables $y_i = ax_i,\ i = 1, \dots, n,$ shows that we do not lose generality if we assume $a = 1$.

3) *Recurrent field*, if $a = 0$. In this hypothesis, the equations (6) become $\dfrac{\partial \ln|X_i|}{\partial x_j} = Y_j$ and then Y is necessarily an irrotational vector field (a fact resulting from (7)). Further, $\ln|X_i| = \displaystyle\int_{x_0}^{x} \sum_{j=1}^{n} Y_j\, dx_j$.

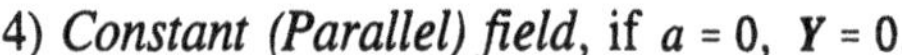

4) *Constant (Parallel) field*, if $a = 0,\ Y = 0$.

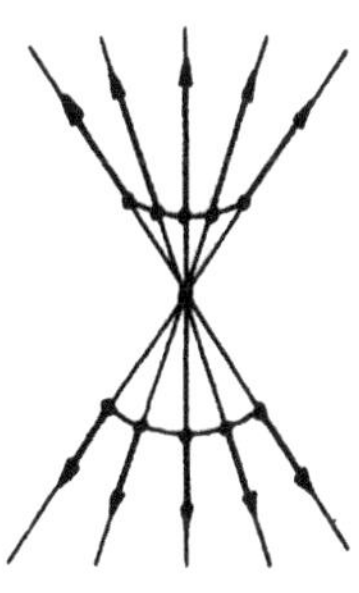

Fig. 32

The reader should check that, except for some particular cases, a torse forming field on R^n can be neither a Killing field nor a conformal field. What about being an affine or projective field?

The bracket of two torse forming vector fields X and Y is a vector field coplanar to X and Y.

Indeed, the relations

$$D_Z X = aZ + (U, Z)X,\ D_Z Y = bZ + (V, Z)Y,$$

for any $Z \in \mathcal{X}(D)$, imply

$$[X, Y] = D_X Y - D_Y X = (b - (U, Y))X + ((V, X) - a)Y.$$

Examples. 1) Let us determine the concircular vector field for which $Y_j = x_j,\ j = 1, \dots, n$. According to the preceding explanations, we find

$$a(x) = b\exp\left(\frac{1}{2}\sum_{k=1}^{n} x_k^2\right),\ b = \text{constant}$$

and

$$X_i(x) = b\exp\left(\frac{1}{2}\sum x_k^2\right)(x_i + c_i),\ c_i = \text{constant}.$$

2) Any vector field with spherical symmetry is torse forming. Indeed, if

$$X = (X_1, \dots, X_n),\ X_i(x) = f(r)(x_i - y_i),\ f(r) = \frac{\varphi(r)}{r},$$

$$r = \sqrt{(x_i - y_i)^2 + \cdots + (x_n - y_n)^2},\ x \in R^n \setminus \{y\},$$

then

$$\frac{\partial X_i}{\partial x_j} = f(r)\delta_{ij} + \frac{f'(r)}{r}(x_i - y_i)(x_j - y_j) = f(r)\delta_{ij} + \frac{f'(r)}{rf^2(r)}X_i X_j.$$

Obviously, X may be considered as a concircular vector field with $Y = \mathrm{grad}\ln|f(r)|$.

In particular, the Newtonian vector fields and the electrostatic vector fields, which are also fields with spherical symmetry , are torse forming fields (concircular; collinear to concurrent fields). These torse forming fields are irrotational and solenoidal.

Counterexample. The Newtonian vector field $X = (X_1, \dots, X_n)$,

$$X_i(x) = -\int_D \frac{\mu(y)}{r^{n-1}} \frac{x_i - y_i}{r} dy; \; r = \sqrt{(x_1 - y_1)^2 + \cdots + (x_n - y_n)^2}, \; D \subset R^n$$

is not a torse forming field on R^n since

$$\frac{\partial X_i}{\partial x_j}(x) = \int_D \mu(y) \left(-\frac{1}{r^n}\delta_{ij} + n r^{n-2} \frac{x_i - y_i}{r^n} \frac{x_j - y_j}{r^n} \right) dy = a(x)\delta_{ij} + \psi_{ij}(x),$$

and $\psi_{ij}(x)$ can't be written as conveniently as for torse forming vector fields.

2.10. PROPOSED PROBLEMS

1. Study which of the following vector fields are potential fields and, if so, find the potential.

1) $X = (\sin xy + xy\cos xy)i + (x^2\cos xy)j$;

2) $X = 3y^4z^2 i + 4x^3z^2 j - 3x^2y^2 k$;

3) $X = (y^2\cos x + z^2)i - (4 - 2y\sin x)j + (2xz + 1)k$.

2. Show that the family of ellipsoids $u(x,y,z) = \text{const} \geq 0$ defined by the equation

$$\frac{x^2}{a^2 + u} + \frac{y^2}{b^2 + u} + \frac{z^2}{c^2 + u} = 1$$

represent the equipotential surfaces of the field produced by an ellipsoid conductor of semiaxes $a > b > c$.

3. Determine some Monge potentials and Stokes potentials for the vector field

$$X = x^2 y i + y^2 z j + z^2 x k.$$

4. Let $\varphi(x) = f(r)$, $r = \sqrt{x_1^2 + \ldots + x_n^2}$ be a scalar field with spherical symmetry on $R^n \setminus \{0\}$, $n \geq 2$, of class C^2.

1) Show that $\Delta\varphi = f''(r) + \frac{n-1}{r} f'(r)$.

2) Find the solutions with spherical symmetry of the Laplace equation $\Delta\varphi = 0$.

Answer.

$$\varphi(x) = f(r) = \begin{cases} A\ln r + B & \text{for } n = 2 \\ A r^{2-n} + B & \text{for } n > 2, \end{cases}$$

A, B = constants.

5. Let $V = f((a, r))(a \times r)$, where f is a function of convenient class.
1) Find f such that $\mathrm{rot} V$ is collinear to r.
2) Calculate the flux of V through a closed surface.

6. Let $V = f(\|a \times r\|)(a \times r)$, where f is a function of convenient class.
1) Calculate $\mathrm{grad}\|a \times r\|$, $\mathrm{rot} V$ and $\mathrm{div}\, V$.
2) Determine f such that V is irrotational and find a local potential.

7. On R^3 we give the vector field $V = \varphi(r)(a \times r) + \psi(r)r$, where a is a constant vector collinear to j, r is the position vector, and φ, ψ are functions of class C^1.

1) Compute the circulation of V on a circle Γ of centre O placed in the plane xOy and the flux of V through the disk bounded by Γ.

2) Find the function φ and ψ such that the flux of the field V through any closed surface is null, and $\mathrm{rot} V$ is collinear to r.

8. Determine the harmonic vector fields on R^2, the potentials of which are harmonic polynomials on R^2.

9. Check the assertions: 1) the bracket of two conformal vector fields is a conformal vector field, 2) the bracket of two affine vector fields is an affine vector field, 3) the bracket of two projective vector fields is a projective vector field.

Hint. $[X,Y] = D_X Y - D_Y X$.

10. We consider a torse forming vector field defined in a neighborhood of the origin of R^n. Using Taylor's formula, find the linear and quadratic approximations of this field around the origin.

11. Are there any harmonic torse forming vector fields ?

12. Study which of the torse forming vector fields are (respectively): Killing vector fields, conformal vector fields, affine vector fields, projective vector fields.

13. Show that the set of all solenoidal vector fields of class C^∞ on $D \subset R^n$ is a Lie algebra.

3. FIELD LINES

The field lines of a vector field of class C^1 are oriented curves of class C^2 having the property that the values of the vector field on these curves are self-distributed as tangent vectors to curves. The parallel, torse forming, Newtonian, electrostatic, etc vector fields serve as examples for finding analytic expressions of the field lines (see 3.1, 3.2).

The rectification theorem of a vector field is equivalent to the theorem of existence of local first integrals, while the orbits may be locally represented as intersections of families of constant level hypersurfaces attached to functionally independent (local) first integrals. Global first integrals occur only for some exceptional cases e.g., Hamiltonian vector fields, Killing fields (see 3.2), etc.

For some vector fields, field lines can be easily described by formulas (see 3.1, 3.2), the simplest example being linear vector fields (see 3.3). When it is not possible to find them using formulas, then we use certain numerical calculus techniques, as for example the Runge-Kutta method (see 3.4).

The completeness of the vector fields problem generates special interest both theoretically and practically. The explanations from 3.5 are exemplified by Newtonian vector fields and by electrical vector fields with spherical symmetry, by conformal vector fields, by torsional vector fields and by Lorenz equations for the motion of a fluid. In particular, the completeness problem is posed for the Hamiltonian vector fields that play an important role in describing some phenomena of nature (see 3.6).

The flows generated by vector fields have some interesting physical-and-geometric properties among which we mention Liouville's theorem (see 3.7) and the characterization of the Killing, affine (see 3.8), conformal (see 3.9), projective (see 3.10) irrotational, solenoidal or torse forming (see 3.11) vector fields. The volume conservation theorem is exemplified by the stationary electromagnetic fields, the stationary magnetic fields, the Biot-Savart-Laplace fields, the Hamiltonian fields and the Newtonian fields (see 3.7). We also find the flows generated by the Killing, affine (see 3.8), conformal (see 3.9) projective (see 3.10) and irrotational, solenoidal or torse forming (see 3.11) vector fields and we exemplify the procedure of obtaining the vector fields from the local groups of diffeormorphisms (see 3.12).

The problems of 3.13 refer to the rectification theorem of vector fields, first integrals, analytic expressions of the solutions of certain differential systems, the Runge-Kutta methods, completeness and flows.

3.1. FIELD LINES

Let $D \subset R^n$ be an open connected set and X be a vector field of class C^1 on D. A curve $\alpha : I \to D$ of class C^1 whose tangent vector field α' coincides with $X \circ \alpha$ is called a *field line* of X. The image $\alpha(I) \subset D$ of a field line is called an *orbit* of X (Fig.33).

The field lines of the vector field X are characterized by the differential equation $\alpha'(t) = X(\alpha(t))$ or by the integral equation $\alpha(t) = \alpha(t_0) + \int_{t_0}^{t} X(\alpha(s))\,ds$. Since X and α are functions of class C^1, the field lines of X are necessarily of class C^2.

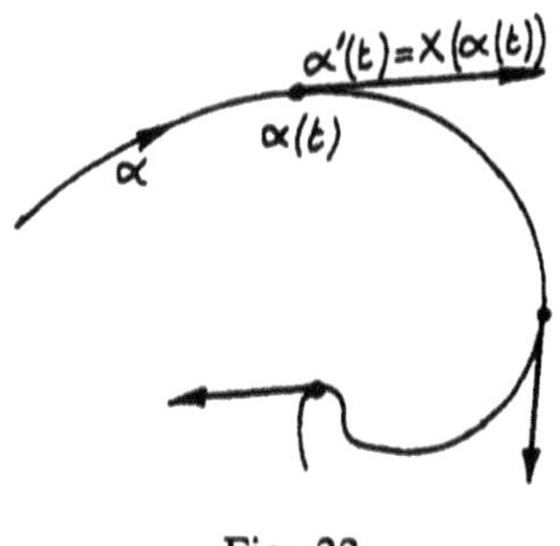

Fig. 33

Theorem. *If X is a vector field of class C^1 on a connected and open set $D \subset R^n$, then for any $x_0 \in D$, $t_0 \in R$, there exists an open interval I and a field line $\alpha : I \to D$ of X such that:*

1) $\alpha(t_0) = x_0$,

2) any other field line $\beta : J \to D$ of X with $\beta(t_0) = x_0$ has the property $J \subseteq I$ and $\beta(t) = \alpha(t)$, for any $t \in J$.

In this case α is called a *maximal field line* of X through x_0.

Proof. Here we have a reformulation of the Existence and Uniqueness Theorem for solutions of a first-order differential system [1]. Indeed, using the notations

$$X(x) = (X_1(x), \dots, X_n(x)),\ X_i : D \to R,$$

$$\alpha(t) = (x_1(t), \dots, x_n(t)),\ x_i : I \to R,$$

$$\alpha'(t) = \left(\frac{dx_1}{dt}(t), \dots, \frac{dx_n}{dt}(t)\right),$$

the vector differential equation $\alpha'(t) = X(\alpha(t))$, for any $t \in I$, is also written as an autonomous differential system

$$\frac{dx_1}{dt} = X_1(x_1, \ldots, x_n), \ldots, \frac{dx_n}{dt} = X_n(x_1, \ldots, x_n). \tag{1}$$

The existence theorem shows that there exists a neighborhood I_1 of t_0 and n functions $x_i : I_1 \to R$ of class C^1 that satisfy the system (1) and the initial conditions $x_i(t_0) = x_{i0}$, $i = 1, \ldots, n$, $x_0 = (x_{10}, \ldots, x_{n0})$. The ensemble $\beta_1(t) = (x_1(t), \ldots, x_n(t))$ defines a field line $\beta_1 : I_1 \to D$ of X with $\beta_1(t_0) = x_0$.

The uniqueness theorem shows that if $\tilde{x}_i : I_2 \to R$, $i = 1, \ldots, n$, is another solution of the system (1) that satisfies the initial conditions $\tilde{x}_i(t_0) = x_{i0}$, then $\tilde{x}_i(t) = x_i(t)$, for any $t \in I_1 \cap I_2$. Equivalently, if $\beta_2 = (x_1, \ldots, x_n) : I_2 \to D$ is another field line of X with $\beta_2(t_0) = x_0$, then $\beta_1(t) = \beta_2(t)$, for $t \in I_1 \cap I_2$.

From these it follows: (1) there is a unique maximal field line α of X, with $\alpha(t_0) = x_0$, defined on the union of the domains of definition of the field lines of X, which maps t_0 into x_0 (the domain of definition of a maximal field line is an open interval of R); (2) any other field line $\beta : J \to D$ of X, with $\beta(t_0) = x_0$, is a restriction of α.

The solutions of the algebraic system

$$X_1(x_1, \ldots, x_n) = 0, \ldots, X_n(x_1, \ldots, x_n) = 0, \tag{2}$$

that is the *zeros* of the vector field $X = (X_1, \ldots, X_n)$, generate solutions of the differential system (1). Indeed, if $a = (a_1, \ldots, a_n)$ is a solution of (2), then $x(t) = a$, for any $t \in R$, is a solution (constant with respect to the time t) of (1). Such a solution is called an *equilibrium point*.

The length $\|X(x)\|$ is, in fact, the speed of passing of a solution of the system (1) through the point x.

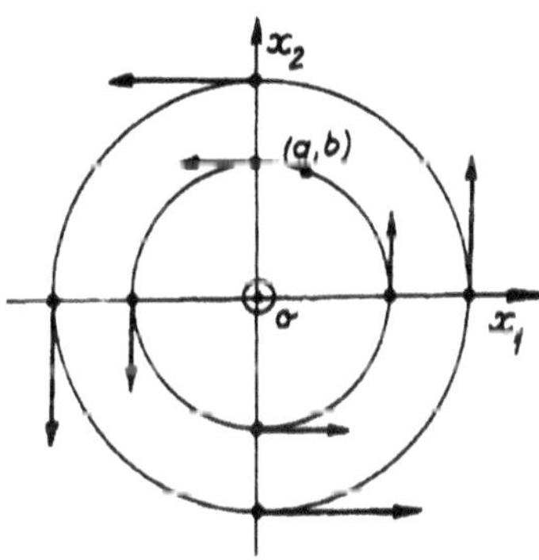

Fig. 34

Applications. 1) Let $X(x_1, x_2) = (-x_2, x_1)$. The field lines are solutions of the system

$$\frac{dx_1}{dt} = -x_2, \quad \frac{dx_2}{dt} = x_1,$$

that is $x_1(t) = 0,\ x_2(t) = 0,\ t \in R$ (equilibrium point), and

$$x_1(t) = c_1 \cos t + c_2 \sin t,\ x_2(t) = c_1 \sin t - c_2 \cos t,\ t \in R$$

(the general solution). The maximal field line passing through the point $x_1(0) = a,\ x_2(0) = b$ is

$$\alpha(t) = (a\cos t - b\sin t, a\sin t + b\cos t), \quad t \in R.$$

Obviously, $\| \alpha(t) \|^2 = a^2 + b^2$, for any $t \in R$ and then the orbit is a circle of radius $\sqrt{a^2 + b^2}$ (Fig. 34). Also $\lim\limits_{\substack{a \to 0 \\ b \to 0}} x_1(t) = \lim\limits_{\substack{a \to 0 \\ b \to 0}} x_2(t) = 0$ for any $t \in R$ (the equilibrium point), while $\lim\limits_{t \to \pm\infty} \alpha(t)$ does not exist.

2) Let $X = (a_1, \dots, a_n)$ be a parallel vector field on R^n. The system that gives the field lines, $\frac{dx_i}{dt} = a_i,\ i = 1, \dots, n$ admits the general solution $x_i = a_i t + c_i,\ t \in R$. Consequently, the field lines of a parallel vector field are parallel straight lines.

3) Let us find the field lines of a torse forming vector field $X = (X_1, \dots, X_n)$ on an open, connected set D of R^n. By definition, we have

$$\frac{\partial X_i}{\partial x_j} = a\,\delta_{ij} + X_i Y_j,\ i, j = 1, \dots, n.$$

Starting from

$$\frac{dx_i}{dt} = X_i(x),\ i = 1, \dots, n$$

and differentiating, we find

$$\frac{d^2 x_i}{dt^2} = \sum_{j=1}^{n} \frac{\partial X_i}{\partial x_j} \frac{dx_j}{dt} = (a + \langle X, Y \rangle)(x) \frac{dx_i}{dt}.$$

Substituting

$$s = c_1 + c_2 \int_{t_0}^{t} \exp\left(\int_{t_0}^{r} (a + \langle X, Y \rangle) \circ \alpha(u)\, du \right) dr,\ c_1, c_2 = \text{const},$$

we get $\frac{d^2 x_i}{ds^2} = 0$ and then $x_i = a_i + b_i s,\ s \in I \subset R,\ a_i, b_i = \text{const},\ i = 1, \dots, n$. Thus the field lines of a torse forming field (which are not equilibrium points) are included in the family of portions of straight lines reparametrized by the parameter s.

Particular cases. 1) The field lines of a concurrent vector field on R^n (different from the equilibrium point) are open semi-straight lines, all of them having the equilibrium position as origin. Indeed, in this case $(X, Y) = 0$, $a = 1$ and $x_i = a_i + d_i e^t$, $t \in R$, d_i being arbitrary constants.

The equilibrium point $x_i = a_i$ is an asymptotic point of all the other field lines since $\lim_{t \to -\infty} x_i = a_i$ (Fig.32).

2) The orbits of a vector field with spherical symmetry,

$$X = (X_1, \dots, X_n),\ X_i(x) = \varphi(r)(x_i - y_i)/r,$$

$$r = \sqrt{(x_1 - y_1)^2 + \cdots + (x_n - y_n)^2},\quad x \in R^n \setminus \{y\},$$

are open semi-straight lines, while the point y occurs as an asymptotic point for them. The sense on the orbits is imposed by the sign of φ. In this context we have the Newtonian vector fields with spherical symmetry (attraction fields) and the electrical vector fields with spherical symmetry (attraction or repulsion fields).

Lemma. *Let X be a vector field of class C^1 on an open and connected set $D \subset R^n$, and $\alpha : I \to D$ be a field line of X. If s is a fixed point of I and $\tau_s : J \to I$, $\tau_s(t) = t + s$ (translation in R by s), then the curve $\beta = \alpha \circ \tau_s$ is a field line of X defined on the interval $J = \tau_{-s}(I)$.*

Proof (Fig.35). If $\alpha(t)$ is a field line, then also $\alpha(t+s)$ is another field line. Indeed,

$$\frac{d\alpha}{dt}(t+s)\Big|_{t=t_0} = \frac{d\alpha}{dt}(t)\Big|_{t=t_0+s} = X(\alpha(t_0+s)) = X(\alpha(t+s))\Big|_{t=t_0}.$$

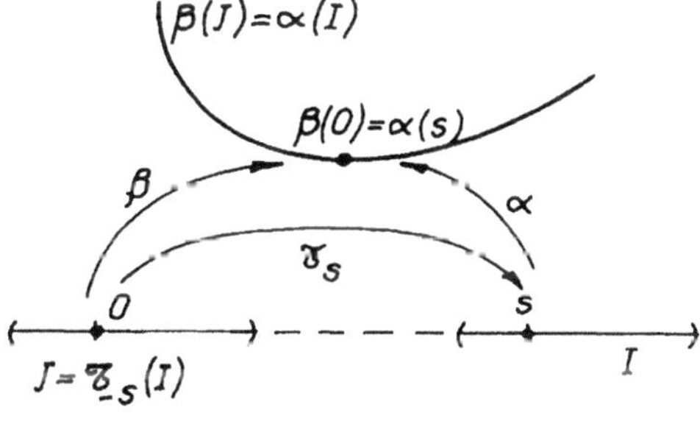

Fig. 35

Theorem. *Let X be a vector field of class C^1 on a connected, open set $D \subset R^n$, let $x_0 \in D$ and $\alpha_{x_0} : I(x_0) \to D$ the maximal field line of X through x_0. If s is a fixed point of*

$I(x_0)$, *then* $\alpha_{x_0} \circ \tau_s : \tau_{-s} I(x_0) \to D$ *is the maximal field line of* X *through* $\alpha_{x_0}(t_0 + s)$.

Proof. According to the lemma, $\alpha_{x_0} \circ \tau_s$ is a field line through $x_1 = \alpha_{x_0}(t_0 + s)$ defined on $\tau_{-s} I(x_0)$.

Since it must coincide in this domain with the maximal field line α_{x_1}, it is necessary that $\tau_{-s} I(x_0) \subset I(x_1)$. It follows that $t_0 - s \in I(x_1)$.

We apply again the lemma showing that $\alpha_{x_1} \circ \tau_{-s}$ is the field line through $\alpha_{x_1}(t_0 - s) = x_0$ defined on $\tau_s I(x_1)$. Therefore $\tau_s I(x_1) \subset I(x_0)$. It follows that the domain of definition of $\alpha_{x_0} \circ \tau_s$ is equal to $I(x_1)$ and consequently $\alpha_{x_0} \circ \tau_s = \alpha_{x_1}$.

Let X be a vector field of class C^1 on $D \subset R^n$. The preceding theorems show that two different maximal field lines of X do not intersect (if they had a common point, they would have an entire common part). Consequently, no equilibrium point can be an initial value of a solution that is different from it, but the equilibrium point can be an asymptotic point of this one (the limit with respect to t) or the limit of the solution with respect to the initial point.

There exist self-intersecting field lines only if they are closed curves. In particular, the equilibrium points of the system belong to this type of curve. A closed field line has the shape from Fig.36 (a smooth curve) and not the one from Fig.37, since the tangent vector to the curve at every point is unique (a value of the field X). The preceding theorem shows that any maximal field line is either injective, or simple and closed, or even constant.

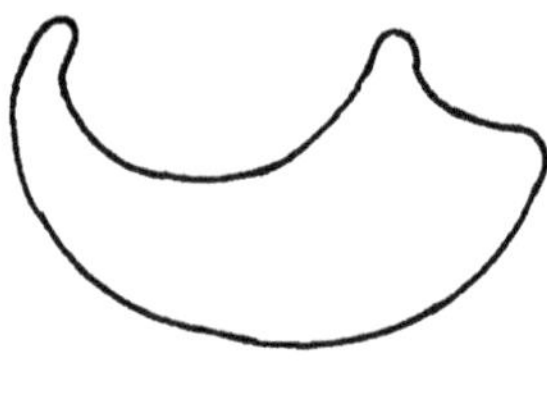

Fig. 36

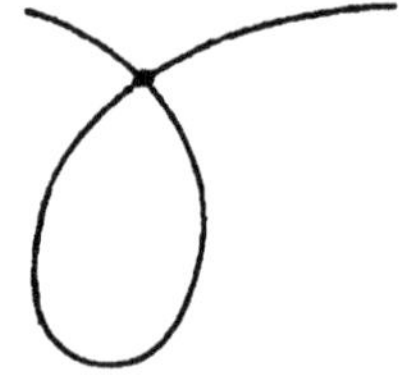

Fig. 37

Theorem. *Let* X *be a vector field of class* C^1 *on* $D \subset R^n$. *If* $\alpha : I \to D$ *is a field line of* X *with* $\alpha(t_1) = \alpha(t_2)$, $t_1, t_2 \in I$, $t_1 < t_2$ *(i.e.,* α *is closed), then* α *can be extended to the whole axis* R, *the prolongation* $\tilde{\alpha} : R \to D$ *being periodic of period* $T \in (0, t_2 - t_1]$.

Proof. Any $s \in R$ can be uniquely represented in the form $s = t + n(t_2 - t_1)$, $t \in [t_1, t_2]$, $n \in Z$. The function $\tilde{\alpha} : R \to D$, $\tilde{\alpha}(s) = \alpha(t)$ is periodic of period

$$\min\{T |\, \tilde{\alpha}(s + T) = \tilde{\alpha}(s)\} \in (0, t_2 - t_1].$$

On the other side, based on the preceding theorem, $\tilde{\alpha} : R \to D$ is a field line. Moreover,

$\tilde{\alpha}(t_1) = \alpha(t_1)$.

It is well known that for a periodic continuous function the set of all periods coincides either with the real straight line (case in which the function is constant) or with the set of all integer multipliers of the least period [1].

Theorem. *Let X be a vector field of class C^1 on an open and connected set D of R^n, and $M \subset D$ a closed submanifold with the property that for every point $x \in M$, the vector $X(x)$ is tangent to M at x. If I is an interval of R and $\alpha : I \to D$ is a field line of X such that $\alpha(t_0) \in M$, then $\alpha(t)$ belongs to M for every $t \in I$.*

Proof. From the Existence and Uniqueness Theorem it follows that there exists a single field line α defined on a neighborhood of t_0, with values in M. Let $J = \{t \in I \mid \alpha(t) \in M\}$. The set J is open, since it cannot contain a point without containing a whole neighborhood of it; the continuity of α shows that the set J is also closed, $J = \alpha^{-1}(M)$. Therefore $J = I$, since I is connected.

Remarks. 1) The field lines are in fact oriented curves. Indeed, if $\alpha(t)$, $t \in [a,b]$, is a field line of the vector field X that joins the point $\alpha(a)$ with the point $\alpha(b)$, then $\alpha(a+b-u)$, $u \in [a,b]$, is a field line of $-X$ that joins the point $\alpha(b)$ with $\alpha(a)$.

2) The field lines of the vector field $X = (X_1, \dots, X_n)$ of class C^2 are (naturally parametrized) straight lines if and only if $D_X X = 0$. Indeed, from $\frac{dx_i}{dt} = X_i(x)$ we get

$$\frac{d^2 x_i}{dt^2} = \sum_{j=1}^{n} \frac{\partial X_i}{\partial x_j} X_j = D_X X_i, \text{ while } \frac{d^2 x_i}{dt^2} = 0 \text{ is equivalent to } x_i = a_i + b_i t,\ t \in R,\ i = 1, \dots, n.$$

Extension Theorem. *Let X be a vector field of class C^1 on an open and connected set $D \subset R^n$. Let $K \subset D$ be a compact set and $x_0 \in K$. The field line α_{x_0} of X fixed by the initial condition $\alpha_{x_0}(t_0) = x_0$ can be extended into the future (or into the past) either boundless, or up to the boundary ∂K. The extension is unique in the sense that any two field lines with the same initial condition coincide on the intersection of the intervals of definition.*

Proof. Let α be the maximal field line of X fixed by the initial condition $\alpha(t_0) = x_0$, and denote

$$A = \{\tau \in R \mid \alpha(t) \in K, \forall t \in [t_0, \tau]\},\ T = \sup A.$$

If $T = \infty$, then the field line α can be extended without bound into future. However, $T < \infty$. According to the Existence and Uniqueness Theorem for any $x \subset D$, there exists a neighborhood V_x and $\varepsilon(x) > 0$, such that for every $y \in V_x$ there exists a field line β, defined for $|t-t_0| < \varepsilon(x)$, with $\beta(t_0) = y$. Since K is compact we can extract a finite covering of K by sets like V_x, and we can replace $\varepsilon(x)$ by $\varepsilon = \min_{x\in K} \varepsilon(x)$. By the definition of T there exists $\tau \in A$ with $T-\varepsilon < \tau < T$. As the point $\alpha(\tau)$ of K is in one of the neighborhoods V_x, there exists a field line $\beta(\tau-\varepsilon,\tau+\varepsilon) \to D$ for which $\beta(\tau) = \alpha(\tau)$. By the Uniqueness Theorem it follows that α is defined at least on the interval $[t_0, \tau+\varepsilon)$, i.e. , there exists $\alpha(T)$ which is, by continuity, a point of K. On the other hand for any $\delta > 0$, there exist $t \in (T, T+\delta)$ with $\alpha(t) \notin K$ and therefore $\alpha(T) \in \partial K$.

Differentiability Theorem. *Let X be a vector field of class C^∞ on an open and connected set $D \subset R^n$, let $x_0 \in D$ and $\alpha_x : I \to D$ be the field line of X fixed by the initial condition $\alpha_x(t_0) = x$. The function $(t,x) \to \alpha_x(t)$ is of class C^∞ on a neighborhood of the point (t_0, x_0) in $I \times D$.*

Proof. We consider the extended differential system

$$\frac{dx}{dt} = X(x)\,,\ x \in D\,;\ \frac{dz}{dt} = X_*(x)z\,,\ z \in End(R^n)$$

with the initial conditions

$$\alpha(t_0) = x\ ,\ \zeta(t_0) = E,$$

where $X_*(x)$ is the Jacobian matrix of X at x. By the method of successive approximations, we obtain

$$\alpha_{n+1}(t,x) = x + \int_{t_0}^{t} X(\alpha_n(\tau,x))d\tau$$

$$\zeta_{n+1}(t,x) = E + \int_{t_0}^{t} X_*(\alpha_n(\tau,x))\zeta_n(\tau,x)d\tau\ .$$

Since $\alpha_*(t_0,x) = \zeta(t_0) = E$, by induction, we obtain $(\alpha_{n+1})_*(t_0,x) = \zeta_{n+1}$. On the other hand, the sequence $\{\zeta_n\}$ converges uniformly, as well as $\{\alpha_n\}$ to α_x, and therefore $\alpha_x(t) = \alpha(t,x)$ is of class C^∞ on D.

Finally, the formula

$$\alpha(x,t) = x + \int_{t_0}^{t} X(\alpha(\tau,x))d\tau$$

shows that the function $(t,x) \to \alpha_x(t) = \alpha(t,x)$ is of class C^∞ in a neighborhood of the point $(t_0, x_0) \in I \times D$.

3.2. FIRST INTEGRALS

Let us assume that $\varphi : D \to D_*$, $y = \varphi(x)$ is a diffeomorphism of class C^1, where D and D_* are open sets in R^n. Then the autonomous differential system

$$\frac{dx_i}{dt} = X_i(x),\ i = 1, \dots, n, \tag{1'}$$

on D is equivalent to the autonomous differential system

$$\sum_{j=1}^{n} \frac{\partial x_i}{\partial y_j}(y)\,\frac{dy_j}{dt} = X_i(\varphi^{-1}(y)),\ i = 1, \dots, n,$$

or

$$\frac{dy_j}{dt} = \sum_{i=1}^{n}\left(\frac{\partial y_j}{\partial x_i}X_i\right)(\varphi^{-1}(y)),\ j = 1, \dots, n,$$

or

$$\frac{dy_j}{dt} = (D_X\, y_j)(\varphi^{-1}(y)),\ j = 1, \dots, n, \quad \text{on} \quad D_* = \varphi(D).$$

The following theorem gives some conditions that ensure the existence of a local diffeomorphism $y = \varphi(x)$ with the property

$$D_X\, y_i = \begin{cases} 0 & \text{for} \quad j = 1, \dots, n-1 \\ 1 & \text{for} \quad j = n. \end{cases} \tag{1''}$$

Rectification theorem. *If $X = (X_1, \dots, X_n)$ is a C^1 vector field on D and $x_0 \in D$ is a point at which $X(x_0) \neq 0$, then there exists a neighborhood U of x_0 and a C^1 diffeomorphism $\varphi : U \to U_*$, $y = \varphi(x)$ such that the autonomous differential system*

$$\frac{dx_i}{dt} = X_i(x),\ i = 1, \dots, n \text{ on } U$$

reduces to the autonomous differential system

$$\frac{dy_1}{dt} = 0, \dots, \frac{dy_{n-1}}{dt} = 0,\ \frac{dy_n}{dt} = 1 \text{ on } U_* = \varphi(U).$$

Proof. It will be sufficient to find a local diffeormorphism that changes the parallel vector field $e_n = (0, \dots, 0, 1)$ into the vector field X. In this context, we consider the tangent space $T_{x_0} R^n \approx R^n$ to be the direct sum between the horizontal part

$$H = \{h \in R^n \mid (h, X(x_0)) = 0\} \approx R^{n-1}$$

and the vertical part

$$V = \{tX(x_0) \mid t \in R\} \approx R,$$

where $\approx$ means identification through the canonical isomorphism. We consider in H the ball $H_\rho : \|h\| < \rho$, while in V we consider the segment $V_\rho : |t| < \rho$.

The continuity of X and the hypothesis $X(x_0) \neq 0$ ensure the existence of a neighborhood of x_0 in which there are no equilibrium points. We attach to each pair $(h,t) \in H_\rho \times V_\rho$ the point $\phi(h,t) = \alpha_h(t) \in R^n$, where $\alpha_h(t)$ is the solution of the system $(1')$ fixed by the initial condition $\phi(h,0) = \alpha_h(0) = h$. We'll show that the C^1 function $(h,t) \to \phi(h,t)$ [1], [39] is the local diffeomorphism we are searching for.

The relation $H \perp V$ imposes the orthogonal decomposition

$$\phi(h,t) = u(h,t) + v(h,t)X(x_0),$$

where $u(h,t)$ is the horizontal part and $v(h,t)X(x_0)$ is the vertical part. Since $v(h,t) = (\phi(h,t), X(x_0)) / \|X(x_0)\|^2$, we obtain $\dfrac{\partial v}{\partial t}(0,0) = 1, \dfrac{\partial u}{\partial t}(0,0) = 0$. Identifying $\phi(h,t)$ with the pair $(u(h,t), v(h,t))$, we find the Jacobi matrix

$$\begin{bmatrix} E & 0 \\ \dfrac{\partial v}{\partial h}(0,0) & 1 \end{bmatrix}$$

which is nonsingular. According to the Inverse Function Theorem, the function $(h,t) \to \phi(h,t)$ is a diffeomorphism on a neighborhood $U_* \subset H_\rho \times V_\rho$ of the point $(0,0)$. Denoting $y = (h,t)$, $x = \phi(y)$, we find $\varphi = \phi^{-1}$ and $U = \phi(U_*)$. Moreover

$$0\,\frac{\partial x_i}{\partial y_1}(\phi(y)) + \cdots + 0\,\frac{\partial x_i}{\partial y_{n-1}}(\phi(y)) + 1\,\frac{\partial x_i}{\partial y_n}(\phi(y))$$

$$= \frac{\partial x_i}{\partial y_n}(\phi(h)) = \frac{\partial \phi_i}{\partial t}(\phi(h,t)) = X_i(\phi(h,t)) = X_i(x),\ i = 1, \ldots, n.$$

A function $f: D \to R$ of class C^1 is called a *first integral* of the differential system $(1')$ if $D_X f = 0$, where D_X is the derivation with respect to the vector field $X = (X_1, \ldots, X_n)$. The defining relation $D_X f = 0$ is equivalent to each of the following two properties:

- the function f is constant along each solution $\alpha : I \to D$ of the system $(1')$, that is $f \circ \alpha$ = constant, since

$$D_X f \circ \alpha = \frac{d}{dt}(f \circ \alpha);$$

- each orbit of X is included in only one level set of the function f (see Fig. 38).

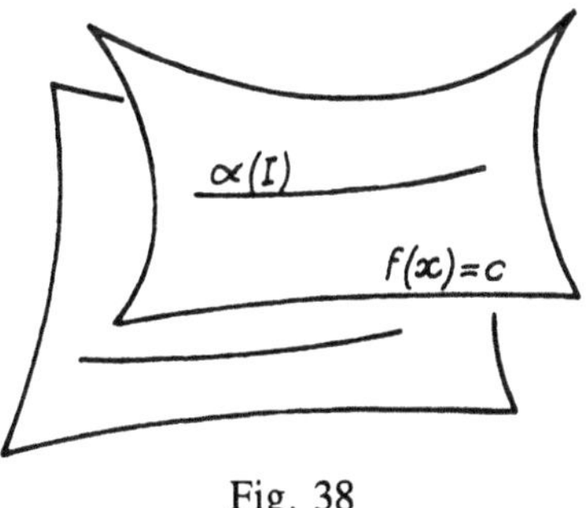

Fig. 38

A first integral represents a *law of conservation*.

Applications. 1) Hamilton has shown that some problems of mechanics, optics, variational calculus etc., can be modeled by the following system of differential equations

$$\frac{dx_i}{dt} = -\frac{\partial H}{\partial y_i}, \quad \frac{dy_i}{dt} = \frac{\partial H}{\partial x_i}, \quad i = 1, \ldots, n,$$

where $H: R^{2n} \to R$ is a C^2 function of $2n$ variables $x_1, \ldots, x_n;\ y_1, \ldots, y_n$. The law of conservation of energy is equivalent to the fact that H is a first integral of the preceding differential system. Indeed, if we denote

$$X_i = -\frac{\partial H}{\partial y_i}, \quad X_{n+i} = \frac{\partial H}{\partial x_i}, \quad X = (X_i, X_{n+i}),$$

then

$$D_X H = \sum_{i=1}^{n} X_i \frac{\partial H}{\partial x_i} + \sum_{i=1}^{n} X_{n+i} \frac{\partial H}{\partial y_i} = -\sum_{i=1}^{n} \frac{\partial H}{\partial y_i}\frac{\partial H}{\partial x_i} + \sum_{i=1}^{n} \frac{\partial H}{\partial x_i}\frac{\partial H}{\partial y_i} = 0.$$

The function H is an example of a global first integral, a quite rare case.

2) Let $A = [a_{ij}]$ be a skew-symmetric matrix of order n and $X = (X_1, \ldots, X_n)$, $X_i = \sum_j a_{ij} x_j$, a Killing vector field. The system that gives the field lines

$$\frac{dx_i}{dt} = \sum_i a_{ij} x_j, \quad i = 1, \ldots, n$$

(a homogeneous linear differential system with constant coefficients) admits the global first integrals $f_m(x) = \|A^m x\|^2$, $m = 0, 1, \ldots, n-2$. Indeed,

$$D_{Ax} f_0(x) = D_{Ax}(x,x) = 2(x, D_{Ax} x) = 2(x, Ax) = 0,$$

$$D_{Ax} f_1(x) = D_{Ax}(Ax, Ax) = 2(Ax, D_{Ax} Ax) = 2(Ax, A^2 x) = 2(Ax, A(Ax)) = 0,$$

and generally

$$D_{Ax} f_m(x) = D_{Ax}(A^m x, A^m x) = 2(A^m x, A^m D_{Ax} x) = 2(A^m x, A(A^m x)) = 0,$$

based on the skew symmetry of the matrix A. The following theorem shows that we cannot have more than $n-1$ functionally independent first integrals.

The level hypersurfaces of the function $f_0(x) = \|x\|^2$ are hyperspheres. Therefore, the orbits of the Killing vector field $X_i = \sum_i a_{ij} x_j$ belong to some hyperspheres.

The level hypersurfaces of the functions $f_m(x) = \|A^m x\|^2$, $m = 1, \dots, n-2$, can be diffeomorphic with some hyperspheres (if A is nonsingular and so n is even) or are cylindrical submanifolds of revolution (if A is singular). Indeed, they are characterized by equations of the form $y_1^2 + \dots + y_n^2 = c$, where

$$y_i = \sum_{j=1}^{n} \alpha_{ij} x_j, \; i = 1, \dots, n,$$

are linear forms, either linearly independent, or linearly dependent.

Generally there exist no global first integrals but there exist local first integrals, in the sense of the following theorem.

Theorem. *If X is a C^1 field on D and $x_0 \in D$ is a point at which $X(x_0) \neq 0$, then there exists a neighborhood D of x_0 such that the system $(1')$ admits $n-1$ functionally independent first integrals $f_1, \dots, f_{n-1}$ on U, and any other first integral is a C^1 function of them. Within these conditions, the orbits on U of the vector field X are described by*

$$f_1(x_1, \dots, x_n) = c_1, \dots, f_{n-1}(x_1, \dots, x_n) = c_{n-1}.$$

Proof. Within the hypotheses, there exists a rectifying diffeomorphism

$$y_1 = f_1(x), \dots, y_{n-1} = f_{n-1}(x), \; y_n = f_n(x), \; x \in U,$$

that is a diffeomorphism satisfying the relations $(1')$. Obviously, the functions $f_1, \dots, f_{n-1}$ are the $n-1$ functionally independent first integrals of the system $(1')$ on U.

Let $f_1, \dots, f_{n-1}$ be functionally independent first integrals of the system $(1')$ on an open set U. If f is another first integral on U, then $X = (X_1, \dots, X_n)$ satisfies

$$X_1 \frac{\partial f}{\partial x_1} + \dots + X_n \frac{\partial f}{\partial x_n} = 0$$

$$X_1 \frac{\partial f_1}{\partial x_1} + \dots + X_n \frac{\partial f_1}{\partial x_n} = 0$$

$$\dots \dots \dots \dots \dots \dots \dots \dots \dots \dots$$

$$X_1 \frac{\partial f_{n-1}}{\partial x_1} + \dots + X_n \frac{\partial f_{n-1}}{\partial x_n} = 0.$$

But this is a homogeneous linear system of n equations that admits by assumption the nontrivial solution $(X_1, \dots, X_n)$. It follows that the determinant of the system must be null on U, $\dfrac{D(f, f_1, \dots, f_{n-1})}{D(x_1, x_2, \dots, x_n)} = 0$, and then $f, f_1, \dots, f_{n-1}$ are functionally dependent, that is, there exists ψ such that $f = \psi(f_1, \dots, f_{n-1})$. Conversely, any function of class C^1 of type $f = \psi(f_1, \dots, f_{n-1})$ is a first integral of the differential system $(1')$. Indeed,

$$D_X f = \sum_{j=1}^{n-1} \frac{\partial \psi}{\partial f_j} D_X f_j = 0.$$

The arbitrary orbits around x_0 of the vector field X are described by the system of implicit Cartesian equations (Fig.39)

$$f_1(x) = c_1, \dots, f_{n-1}(x) = c_{n-1},$$

since the orbit passing through x_0 is the one for which $c_i = f_i(x_0)$, $i = 1, \dots, n-1$.

Variant. The notions of first integral and functional independence are invariant with respect to diffeomorphisms (i.e., they do not depend on the chosen system of coordinates). Therefore it will be sufficient to prove the assertions of the theorem on the system in $y = (y_1, \dots, y_n)$ given by the Rectification Theorem. In this case, it is obvious that the coordinate functions $g_i(y) = y_i$, $i = 1, \dots, n-1$, are $n-1$ functionally independent first integrals and that any first integral is a C^1 function of $n-1$ first integrals $y_1, \dots, y_{n-1}$.

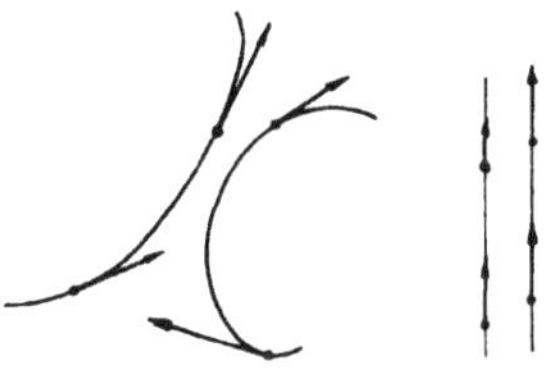

Fig. 39

The orbits on U are line segments of implicit Cartesian equations $y_1 = c_1, \dots, y_{n-1} = c_{n-1}$ (Fig.39).

Sometimes the autonomous differential system $(1')$ is replaced by the symmetric differential system

$$\frac{dx_1}{X_1(x_1, \dots, x_n)} = \dots = \frac{dx_n}{X_n(x_1, \dots, x_n)} = dt. \tag{3}$$

For convenience, if a denominator is a zero function, then the corresponding numerator must be equal to zero. Those points at which all the denominators vanish generate the equilibrium points.

The symmetric form (3) enables us to determine a first integral by the method of *integrable combinations* (see also Chapter 8). If there exist functions $\lambda_j : D \to R$, $j = 1, \dots, n$, of class C^0, such that

$$\sum_{j=1}^{n} \lambda_j dx_j = df \quad \text{and} \quad \sum_{j=1}^{n} \lambda_j X_j = 0,$$

then from

$$\frac{dx_1}{X_1} = \dots = \frac{dx_n}{X_n} = \frac{\sum_{j=1}^{n} \lambda_j dx_j}{\sum_{j=1}^{n} \lambda_j X_j} = \frac{df}{0}$$

will follow the exact Pfaff equation $df = 0$ with the general solution $f(x) = c$. In other words, the function $f: D \to R$, $x \to f(x)$ is a first integral. The differential $\sum_j \lambda_j dx_j = df$ with the condition $\sum_j \lambda_j X_j = 0$, establishing orthogonality of the vector fields $\Lambda = (\lambda_1, \dots, \lambda_n)$ and $X = (X_1, \dots, X_n)$, is called an *integrable combination*.

Example (Fig.40; see also 2.6). Let

$$\frac{dx}{bz - cy} = \frac{dy}{cx - az} = \frac{dz}{ay - bx} = \frac{adx + bdy + cdz}{0} = \frac{xdx + ydy + zdz}{0}.$$

It follows that

$$adx + bdy + cdz = 0,\ xdx + ydy + zdz = 0$$

and thus

$$ax + by + cz = c_1,\ x^2 + y^2 + z^2 = c_2.$$

To the first integrals defined by $f_1(x,y,z) = ax + by + cz$, respectively $f_2(x,y,z) = x^2 + y^2 + z^2$, we attach the Jacobi matrix

$$J = \begin{bmatrix} a & b & c \\ 2x & 2y & 2z \end{bmatrix}$$

with

$$\operatorname{rank} J = \begin{cases} 1 & \text{on} \quad A = \left\{(x,y,z) \mid \dfrac{x}{a} = \dfrac{y}{b} = \dfrac{z}{c}\right\} \\ 2 & \text{on} \quad R^3 \setminus A. \end{cases}$$

It follows that the general solution of the system on $R^3 \setminus A$ is the family of circles $ax + by + cz = c_1$, $x^2 + y^2 + z^2 = c_2$. Obviously, A coincides with the set of equilibrium points and is the normal passing through the origin of the family of parallel planes $ax + by + cz = c_1$. Both the general solution and the equilibrium points belong to the family of sets depicted by the equations $ax + by + cz = c_1$, $x^2 + y^2 + z^2 = c_2$.

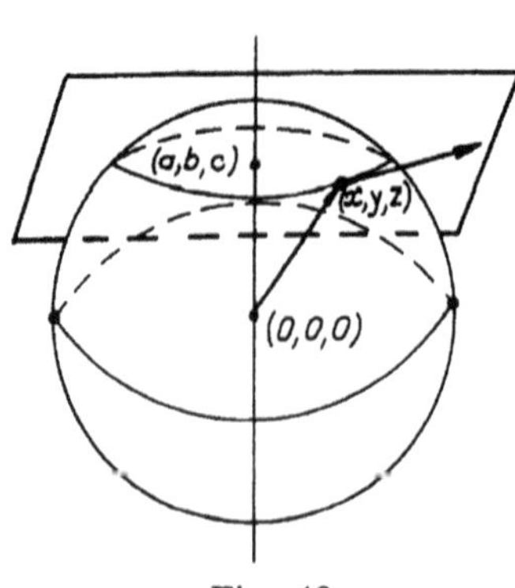

Fig. 40

Remarks. 1) Let X be a C^∞ vector field on $D \subset R^n$, $n \geq 3$ with no zeros. If $f_1(x) = c_1, \dots, f_{n-1}(x) = c_{n-1}$ are the orbits of X on $U \subset D$, then there exists $f_n : U \to R$ such that $X|_U = f_n \operatorname{grad} f_1 \times \cdots \times \operatorname{grad} f_{n-1}$.

2) $k(\leq n-1)$ independent first integrals determine a submanifold of R^n with dimension $n - k$, while the field lines (orbits) are completely included in this submanifold.

3) If we find $n-2$ functionally independent first integrals $f_1, \dots, f_{n-2}$ of the differential system (3), then finding the general solution reduces to finding the general solution of a first-order differential equation.

To prove the preceding claim, let us consider the bidimensional submanifold described by

$$f_1(x_1, \dots, x_n) = c_1, \dots, f_{n-2}(x_1, \dots, x_n) = c_{n-2}.$$

We have a system of $n - 2$ equations that define $x_1, \dots, x_{n-2}$ depending upon x_{n-1}, x_n:

$$x_k = \varphi_k(x_{n-1}, x_n; c_1, \dots, c_{n-2}),\ k = 1, \dots, n-2.$$

But $\dfrac{dx_{n-1}}{X_{n-1}} = \dfrac{dx_n}{X_n}$. Replacing x_k, we obtain a first-order differential equation with the solution

$$\phi(x_{n-1}, x_n; c_1, \dots, c_{n-2}) = c_{n-1}.$$

Putting $c_k = f_k$, it follows that $f_{n-1}(x) = c_{n-1}$ and thus we find a new first integral, which is functionally independent of the others.

Example. Let there be given the differential system

$$\frac{dx}{x^2} = \frac{dy}{-xy} = \frac{dz}{y^2}.$$

From $\dfrac{dx}{x} = \dfrac{dy}{-y}$ it follows that $xy = c_1$. From $\dfrac{dy}{-xy} = \dfrac{dz}{y^2}$, we find $\dfrac{dx}{c_1} + \dfrac{dz}{y^2} = 0$ or $\dfrac{y^3}{3} + c_1 z = \dfrac{1}{3} c_2$, that is $y^3 + 3xyz = c_2$. The general solution and the equilibrium points (the axis $Oz: x = 0, y = 0$) of the given system belong to the family of sets described by the equations $xy = c_1$, $y^3 + 3xyz = c_2$. Indeed, to the first integrals defined by $f_1(x,y,z) = xy$, $f_2(x,y,z) = y^3 + 3xyz$ will correspond the Jacobi matrix

$$J = \begin{bmatrix} y & x & 0 \\ 3yz & 3y^2 + 3xz & 3xy \end{bmatrix}, \quad \text{with} \quad \operatorname{rank} J = \begin{cases} 1 & \text{on } A - \{(x,y,z) | y = 0\} \\ 2 & \text{on } R^3 \setminus A. \end{cases}$$

4) We consider two collinear vector fields. The symmetric differential system (3) shows that, if we omit the equilibrium points that can be introduced by the factor of collinearity, then the two collinear vector fields have the same orbits.

5) For the case of three-dimensional space one can also use the notations

$$V(x,y,z) = v_1(x,y,z)\boldsymbol{i} + v_2(x,y,z)\boldsymbol{j} + v_3(x,y,z)\boldsymbol{k},$$

$$\boldsymbol{r} = x\boldsymbol{i} + y\boldsymbol{j} + z\boldsymbol{k},\ d\boldsymbol{r} = dx\boldsymbol{i} + dy\boldsymbol{j} + dz\boldsymbol{k},\ r = \sqrt{x^2 + y^2 + z^2},$$

and the differential symmetric system

$$\frac{dx}{v_1(x,y,z)} = \frac{dy}{v_2(x,y,z)} = \frac{dz}{v_3(x,y,z)} \tag{4}$$

is equivalent with the vector equation $\boldsymbol{V} \times d\boldsymbol{r} = 0$.

Application. Let

$$\boldsymbol{E} = \frac{q_0}{4\pi\varepsilon} \cdot \frac{\boldsymbol{r}}{r^3},\ (x,y,z) \in \boldsymbol{R}^3 \setminus \{0\}$$

be the electrostatic field produced by the charge q_0. The field lines are the solutions of the differential system

$$\frac{dx}{x} = \frac{dy}{y} = \frac{dz}{z},\ (x,y,z) \in \boldsymbol{R}^3 \setminus \{0\},$$

that is the family of semi-straight lines (rays)

$$x = c_1 y,\ x = c_2 z;\ y = 0,\ z = 0;\ (x,y,z) \in \boldsymbol{R}^3 \setminus \{0\}.$$

Moreover $\lim_{r \to \infty} E = 0$ and thus the point from ∞ in $\boldsymbol{R}^3$ may be considered an equilibrium point (Fig.41).

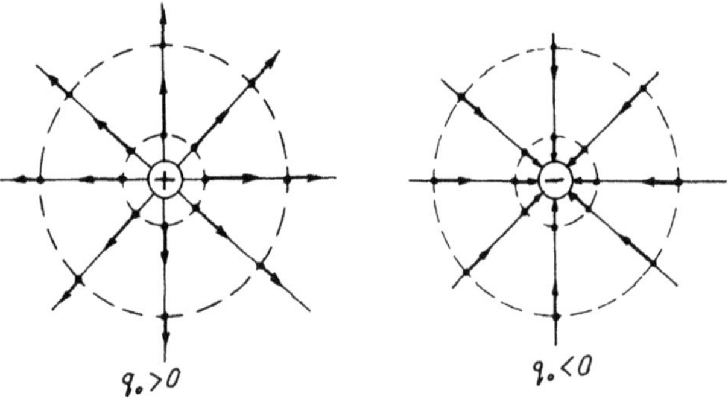

Fig. 41

Comment. The existence of first integrals of the vector field $X = (X_1, \dots, X_n)$ is equivalent to the existence of a rectifying diffeomorphism. If we assume the existence of the first integrals $f_1, \dots, f_{n-1}$, then the rectifying diffeomorphism φ may be obtained in the following way: the implicit Cartesian system $f_1(x) = c_1, \dots, f_{n-1}(x) = c_{n-1}$ determines the function of components

$$x_1 = \chi_1(x_n, c_1, \dots, c_{n-1}), \dots, x_{n-1} = \chi_{n-1}(x_n, c_1, \dots, c_{n-1});$$

we denote

$$h_n = \chi_n \circ (\chi_1, \dots, \chi_{n-1})$$

and define

$$\varphi : y_1 = f_1(x), \dots, y_{n-1} = f_{n-1}(x),\ y_n = \left(\int \frac{dx_n}{h_n(x_n, c_1, \dots, c_{n-1})} \right)_{c_i = f_i(x)} .$$

Application. Determine a local diffeomorphism that rectifies the vector field

$$X = (X_1, X_2, X_3),\ X_1 = x^3 + 3xy^2,\ X_2 = 2y^3,\ X_3 = 2y^2 z$$

and check the result by direct calculation.

Solution. The symmetric system $\dfrac{dx}{x^3 + 3xy^2} = \dfrac{dy}{2y^3} = \dfrac{dz}{2y^2 z}$ and the hypothesis $X_3 = 2y^2 z \neq 0$ yield $\dfrac{z}{y} = c_1$ and the Bernoulli equation $\dfrac{dx}{dy} - \dfrac{x^3}{2y^3} - \dfrac{3x}{2y} = 0$. The Bernoulli equation becomes a linear equation by the substitution $u = \dfrac{1}{x^2}$, $x \neq 0$. The general solution follows,

$$\frac{5y^2 + x^2}{5x^2 y^5} = c_3 .$$

From $X_3 = 2y^2 z$, $\dfrac{z}{y} = c_1$, $\dfrac{5y^2 + x^2}{5x^2 y^5} = c_2$ we get $h_3 = \dfrac{2z^3}{c_1^2}$ and

$$\int_{z_0}^{z} \frac{dz}{h_3} = -\frac{c_1}{4z^2} = -\frac{1}{4y^2} .$$

The diffeomorphism we seek is defined by $x' = \dfrac{z}{y}$, $y' = \dfrac{5y^2 + x^2}{5x^2 y^5}$, $z' = -\dfrac{1}{4y^2}$ (to prove that this really is indeed a diffeomorphism, one can use the inverse function theorem).

In order to verify our solution, we denote by $X_{1'}, X_{2'}, X_{3'}$ the components of X with respect to the new coordinates x', y', z', and taking account of the rule of change of components of a vector field at a change of coordinates (see 1.5), we obtain

$$X_{1'} = X_1 \frac{\partial x'}{\partial x} + X_2 \frac{\partial x'}{\partial y} + X_3 \frac{\partial x'}{\partial z} = 0,$$

$$X_{2'} = X_1 \frac{\partial y'}{\partial x} + X_2 \frac{\partial y'}{\partial y} + X_3 \frac{\partial y'}{\partial z} = 0,$$

$$X_{3'} = X_1 \frac{\partial z'}{\partial x} + X_2 \frac{\partial z'}{\partial y} + X_3 \frac{\partial z'}{\partial z} = 1.$$

Extension of Euler's Theorem. *Let X be a C^∞ vector field on a connected open set $D \subset R^n$, $n \geq 3$. If X is solenoidal, then for any point $x_0 \in D$ with $X(x_0) \neq 0$, there exist an open set $U \subset D$ that contains x_0 and $n-1$ C^∞ scalar fields $f_1, \ldots, f_{n-1}$ such that*

$$X|_U = \operatorname{grad} f_1 \times \cdots \times \operatorname{grad} f_{n-1}.$$

Proof. There exists a neighborhood $U_1 \subset D$ of x_0 and $n-1$ C^∞ functionally independent first integrals $g_1, \ldots, g_{n-1} : U_1 \to R$; any other first integral is a C^∞ function of these integrales. Since the orbits of X on U_1 have the implicit Cartesian equations $g_1(x) = c_1, \ldots, g_{n-1}(x) = c_{n-1}$, there exists a C^∞ function, $g_n : U_1 \to R$, such that $X = g_n \operatorname{grad} g_1 \times \cdots \times \operatorname{grad} g_{n-1}$ on U_1. The relation

$$\operatorname{div}(\operatorname{grad} g_1 \times \cdots \times \operatorname{grad} g_{n-1}) = 0$$

implies

$$\operatorname{div} X = (\operatorname{grad} g_n, \operatorname{grad} g_1 \times \cdots \times \operatorname{grad} g_{n-1})$$

and thus the condition that X be solenoidal is equivalent to the functional dependence of the scalar fields $g_1, \ldots, g_{n-1}, g_n$. Therefore, there exists a neighborhood $U \subset U_1$ of x_0 such that $g_n|_U$ is a C^∞ function of $g_1, \ldots, g_{n-1}$, that is, $g_n|_U$ is a first integral.

We consider a C^∞ local diffeomorphism that accomplishes the passage from the first integrals $g_1, \ldots, g_{n-1}$ to the first integrals

$$f_1 = f_1(g_1, \ldots, g_{n-1}), \ldots, f_{n-1} = f_{n-1}(g_1, \ldots, g_{n-1})$$

on a neighborhood of the point $(g_1(x_0), \dots, g_{n-1}(x_0))$. We denote the local inverse by $g_1 = g_1(f_1, \dots, f_{n-1}), \dots, g_{n-1} = g_{n-1}(f_1, \dots, f_{n-1})$. Then

$$X = g_n(g_1(f_1, \dots, f_{n-1}), \dots, g_{n-1}(f_1, \dots, f_{n-1})) \cdot$$

$$\cdot \frac{D(g_1, \dots, g_{n-1})}{D(f_1, \dots, f_{n-1})} \operatorname{grad} f_1 \times \cdots \times \operatorname{grad} f_{n-1} .$$

Fixing $f_1, \dots, f_{n-1}$ by the condition

$$\frac{D(f_1, \dots, f_{n-1})}{D(g_1, \dots, g_{n-1})} = g_n(g_1, \dots, g_{n-1}),$$

we get

$$X|_U = \operatorname{grad} f_1 \times \cdots \times \operatorname{grad} f_{n-1}.$$

Example. Let us consider the solenoidal vector field $X = (x^2 - y^2)(yz, zx, xy)$. The orbits of X are described by the implicit Cartesian equations $x^2 - y^2 = c_1$, $x^2 - z^2 = c_2$. Hence, $g_1 = x^2 - y^2$, $g_2 = x^2 - z^2$ and from $X = g_3 \operatorname{grad} g_1 \times \operatorname{grad} g_2$ it follows that $g_3 = \frac{g_1}{4}$. Putting $f_1 = \frac{g_1^2}{8}$, $f_2 = g_2$ we find $X = \operatorname{grad} f_1 \times \operatorname{grad} f_2$. Obviously, we can take $f_{1'} = \frac{g_1^2}{8}$, $f_{2'} = g_1 + g_2$ and then $X = \operatorname{grad} f_{1'} \times \operatorname{grad} f_{2'}$.

3.3. FIELD LINES OF LINEAR VECTOR FIELDS

A vector field $X = (X_1, \dots, X_n)$ on R^n is called *linear* if all the components X_i are linear functions on R^n, that is $X_i = \sum_{j=1}^{n} a_{ij} x_j$, $i = 1, \dots, n$, where a_{ij} are n^2 given real numbers. A vector field that is not linear is called *a nonlinear vector field*. A linear vector field is called:

1) *potential*, if $a_{ij} = a_{ji}$ (one potential is a quadratic form with coefficients $\frac{1}{2} a_{ij}$);

2) *solenoidal*, if $a_{11} + \cdots + a_{nn} = 0$;

3) *harmonic*, if $a_{ij} = a_{ji}$, $a_{11} + \cdots + a_{nn} = 0$,

4) *Killing*, if $a_{ij} = - a_{ji}$;

5) *homothetic*, if $a_{ij} + a_{ji} = \psi \, \delta_{ij}$, $\psi =$ constant $\neq 0$.

The bracket of two linear vector fields Ax and Bx is the linear vector field $[Ax,Bx] = D_{Ax}Bx - D_{Bx}Ax = (BA-AB)x$. Therefore, the set of linear vector fields on R^n is a Lie algebra of dimension n^2 (the dimension of the real vector space of the real quadratic matrices of order n).

The field lines of a linear vector field are the solutions of the homogeneous linear differential system with constant coefficients

$$\frac{dx_i}{dt} = \sum_{j=1}^{n} a_{ij}x_j,\ i = 1, \dots, n.$$

Using matrix notations $A = [a_{ij}]$, $x = {}^t[x_1, \dots, x_n]$, we write

$$\frac{dx}{dt} = Ax. \tag{5}$$

The equilibrium points of the differential system (5) are generated by solutions of the homogeneous linear algebraic system $Ax = 0$.

The field lines of the linear vector field Ax can be found in an explicit form using the exponential matrix

$$e^{tA} = \sum_{n=0}^{\infty} \frac{(tA)^n}{n!},\ t \in R,$$

which is an analytic function.

Theorem. *The field line of* Ax *passing through* x_0 *at the moment* t_0 *is defined by*

$$x(t) = e^{(t-t_0)A}x_0,\ t \in R.$$

Proof. Since

$$\frac{dx}{dt} = Ae^{(t-t_0)A}x_0 = Ax,\ \ x(t_0) = e^{(t_0-t_0)A}x_0 = x_0,$$

the given function is a solution of the Cauchy problem $\frac{dx}{dt} = Ax$, $x(t_0) = x_0$. This solution is unique, according to the Uniqueness Theorem [1, 28, 39].

Taking account of the fact that the exponential matrix is nonsingular, the set $\{x(t) = e^{(t-t_0)A}x_0 \mid x_0 \in R^n\}$ is a vector space isomorphic to R^n.

Application. Find the field line of Ax,

$$A = \begin{bmatrix} -1 & 2 & 2 \\ 2 & 2 & 2 \\ -3 & -6 & -6 \end{bmatrix},$$

passing through the point $(-1,2,0)$ at the moment $t = 0$.

Solution. The characteristic equation $\det(A - \lambda I) = 0$ has the solutions $\lambda_1 = -3$, $\lambda_2 = -2$, $\lambda_3 = 0$. The corresponding proper vectors are

$$e_1 = {}^t[1,0,-1],\ e_2 = {}^t[2,-1,0],\ e_3 = {}^t[0,1,-1].$$

The matrix of proper vectors

$$S = \begin{bmatrix} 1 & 2 & 0 \\ 0 & -1 & 1 \\ -1 & 0 & -1 \end{bmatrix}$$

is the diagonalizing matrix of A, that is

$$D = S^{-1}AS = \begin{bmatrix} -3 & 0 & 0 \\ 0 & -2 & 0 \\ 0 & 0 & 0 \end{bmatrix},$$

$$x(t) = Se^{tD}S^{-1}x(0) = \begin{bmatrix} -3e^{-3t} + 2e^{-2t} \\ -e^{-2t} + 3 \\ 3e^{-3t} - 3 \end{bmatrix}$$

or, explicitly, $x_1(t) = -3e^{-3t} + 2e^{-2t}$, $x_2(t) = 3 - e^{-2t}$, $x_3(t) = 3e^{-3t} - 3$, $t \in R$.

Remark. Let $c = {}^t[c_1, \ldots, c_n]$ be an arbitrary constant vector. The solution $x(t) = e^{tA}c$, $t \in R$ of the differential system (5) is called the *general solution*. From it, one may obtain any other solution, by choosing a particular c.

It is quite difficult to compute the exponential matrix and, sometimes, special techniques are used. To find the general solution of the homogeneous linear differential system with constant coefficients, one can go on in the following way. By direct calculation, we notice that $x(t) = he^{\lambda t}$ (h being a column vector with constant coordinates, $t \in R$) is a solution of the homogeneous linear differential system with constant coefficients if and only if h is a proper vector for the matrix A, while λ is the proper value that corresponds to h in the set C of complex numbers. Implicitly, the solutions are sought within the complexification of the vector space $C^\infty(R)$.

Case 1. Let us assume that the proper values $\lambda_1, \ldots, \lambda_n$ of the matrix A are distinct and that $h_1, \ldots, h_n$ are the corresponding proper vectors. For these, we have the corresponding linearly independent solutions

$$x_k = h_k e^{\lambda_k t}, \; t \in R, \; k = 1, \ldots, n.$$

Thus, the general solution of the differential system is

$$x = c_1 x_1 + \cdots + c_n x_n.$$

Obviously, some of λ_k may be complex and thus group in pairs (a complex number and its conjugate). In this case, the real or the imaginary part of x are real general solutions.

Method: One determines the roots of the characteristic equation attached to the matrix A. In the hypothesis that these roots are simple, one searches for solutions of the form $x(t) = he^{\lambda t}$, $t \in R$, where h is a real or complex column vector (depending on what λ is). If λ

is a complex number, then it is not necessary to use the complex conjugate root.

Example. Let there be given the differential system

$$x' = Ax,\ A = \begin{bmatrix} 1 & -1 \\ 1 & 1 \end{bmatrix}.$$

The proper values of the matrix A are $\lambda_{1,2} = 1 \pm i$. Therefore, we search for solutions of the form

$$x(t) = \begin{bmatrix} a + ib \\ c + id \end{bmatrix} \cdot e^{(1+i)t}.$$

Replacing $x(t)$ into the system, by identification one finds $b = c,\ a = -d$. The result

$$x(t) = \begin{bmatrix} a + ib \\ b - ia \end{bmatrix} \cdot e^{(1+i)t}$$

is the general solution. Obviously, $\mathrm{Re}\,x(t)$ or $\mathrm{Im}\,x(t)$ is the real general solution of the given differential system.

Case 2. Let us assume that the characteristic equation has a proper value λ of multiplicity m and that $h_1, \ldots, h_m$ are the vectors attached to λ such that

$$Ah_1 = \lambda h_1,\ Ah_2 = \lambda h_2 + h_1, \ldots, Ah_m = \lambda h_m + h_{m-1}.$$

We form the vector functions

$$P_j(t) = \frac{t^{j-1}}{(j-1)!} h_1 + \frac{t^{j-2}}{(j-2)!} h_2 + \cdots + h_j,\ j = 1, \ldots, m.$$

Let us show that the vector functions defined by $x_j(t) = P_j(t)e^{\lambda t},\ t \in R$, are solutions of the homogeneous linear differential system. Let us first notice that

$$\frac{dP_j}{dt} = P_{j-1},\ AP_j = \lambda P_j + P_{j-1},\ j = 1, \ldots, m.$$

Introducing x_j into $\dfrac{dx}{dt} = Ax$, we get an identity.

In this way, to a proper value of multiplicity m with the corresponding proper vectors $h_1, \ldots, h_m$, there will correspond m linearly independent solutions of the preceding type. The part of the general solution corresponding to these solutions is of the form $x(t) = P(t)e^{\lambda t},\ t \in R$, where $P(t)$ is a column matrix of polynomials of degree $m - 1$.

Method: If λ is a proper value of multiplicity m, then one tries a solution of the form $x(t) = P(t)e^{\lambda t},\ t \in R$, where $P(t)$ is a column matrix whose elements are polynomials of degree $m - 1$ with either real or complex coefficients (depending on λ).

If the general solution we find is complex, then one separates the real or the imaginary part, which we have established are both real general solutions.

Example. To the differential system

$$\frac{dx_1}{dt} = x_2 + x_3, \quad \frac{dx_2}{dt} = x_3 + x_1, \quad \frac{dx_3}{dt} = x_1 + x_2$$

we attach the matrix

$$A = \begin{bmatrix} 0 & 1 & 1 \\ 1 & 0 & 1 \\ 1 & 1 & 0 \end{bmatrix}$$

which has the proper values $\lambda_1 = 2,\ \lambda_{2,3} = -1$.

If $\lambda_1 = 2$, we search for $x_1 = ae^{2t}$, $x_2 = be^{2t}$, $x_3 = ce^{2t}$. Introducing them into the system, it follows that $a = b = c = c_1$. If $\lambda_{2,3} = -1$ we search for $x_1 = (\alpha_1 t + \beta_1)$, $x_2 = (\alpha_2 t + \beta_2)e^{-t}$, $x_3 = (\alpha_3 t + \beta_3)e^{-t}$. Placing them into the system, we find $\alpha_1 = \alpha_2 = \alpha_3 = 0;\ \beta_1 = c_2,\ \beta_2 = c_3,\ \beta_3 = -(c_2 + c_3)$. The general solution of the differential system is

$$x - c_1 \begin{bmatrix} 1 \\ 1 \\ 1 \end{bmatrix} e^{2t} + c_2 \begin{bmatrix} 1 \\ 0 \\ -1 \end{bmatrix} e^{-t} + c_3 \begin{bmatrix} 0 \\ 1 \\ -1 \end{bmatrix} e^{-t}.$$

Remark. If $\operatorname{rank}[a_{ij}] = p$, then the homogeneous linear differential system with constant coefficients

$$\frac{dx_i}{dt} = \sum_{j=1}^{n} a_{ij} x_j, \quad i = 1, \ldots, n,$$

admits $n - p$ linear first integrals. Indeed, one notices that

$$\sum_{i=1}^{n} \lambda_i \frac{dx_i}{dt} = \sum_{j=1}^{n} \left(\sum_{i=-1}^{n} a_{ij} \lambda_i \right) x_j = 0$$

if and only if $\sum_{l-1}^{n} a_{ij} \lambda_i = 0$. This algebraic system admits $n - p$ nonzero solutions λ_i^α, $\alpha = 1, \ldots, n-p$, and the first integrals are $f^\alpha(x) = \sum_{i=1}^{n} \lambda_i^\alpha x_i$.

3.4. RUNGE-KUTTA METHOD

The reasoning presented in 3.3 shows that the field lines of linear vector fields are always defined by quasipolynomials, and the reasoning of 3.1, 3.2 shows that there exist vector fields whose field lines can be expressed by implicit Cartesian equations attached to the first integrals. However, analytic expressions of the field lines cannot be found in the general case. Therefore, we use approximations.

Let $X = (X_1, \dots, X_n)$ be a C^1 vector field on $D \subset R^n$ and let the autonomous differential system

$$\frac{dx_i}{dt} = X_i(x), \ i = 1, \dots, n,$$

generates the field lines of X. The Cauchy problem

$$\frac{dx}{dt} = X(x), \ x(t_0) = x_0$$

has a unique solution $t \to x(t)$, $t \in I$, since the conditions of the Existence and Uniqueness Theorem are satisfied. Finding the exact solution $t \to x(t)$ is possible only in some particular cases. Generally, we only have methods of approximating the exact solution. An example is the Runge-Kutta method that works on the hypothesis that X is at least of class C^2.

Let $h > 0$ and the Taylor Formula

$$x(t+h) = x(t) + hx'(t) + \frac{h^2}{2} x''(t) + O(h^3)$$

or

$$x(t+h) = x(t) + hX(x(t)) + \frac{h^2}{2} X'(x(t))(X(x(t)) + O(h^3),$$

where X' is the Jacobi matrix of X. Denote

$$k_1 = hX(x), \ k_2 = hX(x + \lambda_{21} k_1)$$
$$k_3 = hX(x + \lambda_{31} k_1 + \lambda_{32} k_2), \ k_4 = hX(x + \lambda_{41} k_1 + \lambda_{42} k_2 + \lambda_{43})$$
$$\dots \dots \dots \dots \dots \dots \dots \dots \dots \dots \dots \dots \dots \dots \dots \dots \dots$$

where λ_{ij} are some constants, for the time being undetermined.

The Range-Kutta idea consists of detecting the parameters λ_{ij} and α_i such that the coefficients of the powers of h, from the expression of $x(t+h)$ and from the sum $x + \sum_{i=1}^{s} \alpha_i k_i$, coincide up to some as large as possible powers; that is, we can adopt the approximation $x(t+h) \approx x(t) + \sum_{i=1}^{s} \alpha_i k_i$.

To make them simpler, we will do the calculations for the case $s = 2$. Taking the Taylor Formula into account, we get

$$k_2 = hX(x) + h\lambda_{21} X'(x)(k_1) + \frac{h\lambda_{21}^2}{2} X''(x)(k_2, h_1) + O(k_1^3)$$
$$= hX(x) + h^2 \lambda_{21} X'(x)(X(x)) + \frac{h^3 \lambda_{21}^2}{2} X''(x)(X(x), X(x)) + O(h^4),$$

where $k_1 = hX(x)$. Then

$$x + \alpha_1 k_1 + \alpha_2 k_2 = x + h(\alpha_1 + \alpha_2)X(x) + h^2 \alpha_2 \lambda_{21} X'(x)(X(x))$$
$$+ \frac{h^3 \alpha_2 \lambda_{21}^2}{2} X''(x)(X(x), X(x)) + O(h^4).$$

Comparing this expression with the expression of $x(t+h)$, from the equality of coefficients of h and h^2, we get $\alpha_1 + \alpha_2 = 1$, $\alpha_2 \lambda_{21} = \frac{1}{2}$. Denoting $\alpha_2 = \lambda$, we find

$$\alpha_1 = 1 - \lambda, \ \alpha_2 = \lambda, \ \lambda_{21} = \frac{1}{2\lambda}.$$

These values lead to the system with finite differences

$$x^*_{k+1} = x^*_k + (1-\lambda)k_1 + \lambda k_2, \quad k = 0, 1, \dots, n,$$

where

$$x^*_0 = x_0, \ k_1 = hX(x^*_k), \ k_2 = hX(x^*_k + \frac{1}{2\lambda}k_1),$$

which approximate $x' = X(x)$ with precision up to the second-order term, inclusively, with respect to h. This system was obtained by fixing a division t_0, $t_1 = t_0 + h$, $t_2 = t_0 + 2h, \dots, t_n = t_0 + nh$ of the interval $[t_0, T]$ on which the unknown function x is defined and $x^*_k \approx x(t_k)$.

A case that increases precision is $s = 4$. Then

$$x^*_{k+1} = x^*_k + \frac{1}{6}[k_1 + 2(k_2 + k_3) + k_4], \quad k = 0, 1, \dots, n$$

and

$$k_1 = hX(x^*_k), \ k_2 = hX(x^*_k + \frac{k_1}{2}), \ k_3 = hX(x^*_k + \frac{k_2}{2}), \ k_4 = hX(x^*_k + k_3).$$

For $h \to 0$, the approximating solution in the table

t	t_0	t_1	t_2	...
$x(t)$	$x(t_0) = x_0$	$x(t_1) = x_1$	$x(t_2) = x_2$	...

converges to the exact solution of the Cauchy problem

$$\frac{dx}{dt} = X(x), \ x(t_0) = x_0.$$

Usually, the approximating solution is determined using a computer, rather than manually, as we do here in order to confirm methodology.

Finally, we give the calculation for the case

$$X(x,y) = (x^3 + y, -x + y^3), \ \frac{dx}{dt} = x^3 + y, \ \frac{dy}{dt} = -x + y^3, \ x(0) = x_0 = 1,$$
$$y(0) = y_0 = -1, \ t \in [0; 0,1], \ h = 0,01$$

according to the last Runge-Kutta formulas. Succesively we find

$$(x_0, y_0) = (1; -1),\ k_1 = hX(x_0, y_0) = 0,\ 1(0; -2) = (0; -0{,}2),$$

$$(x_0, y_0) + \frac{k_1}{2} = (1; -1) + (0; -0{,}2) = (1; -1{,}2);$$

$$k_2 = hX[(x_0, y_0) + \frac{k_1}{2}] \approx 0{,}1(-0{,}2; -2{,}7) = (-0{,}02; -0{,}27),$$

$$(x_0, y_0) + \frac{k_2}{2} \approx (1, -1) + (-0{,}01; -0{,}13) = (0{,}99; -1{,}13),$$

$$k_3 = hX[(x_0, y_0) + \frac{k_2}{2}] = 0{,}1(-0, 16; -2{,}43) \approx (-0{,}02; -0{,}24),$$

$$(x_0, y_0) + k_3 = (1, -1) + (-0{,}02; -0{,}24) = (0{,}98; -1{,}24),$$

$$k_4 = hX((x_0, y_0) + k_3) = 0{,}1(-0{,}3; -2{,}88) \approx (-0{,}03; -0{,}29),$$

$$(x_1, y_1) = (x_0, y_0) + \frac{1}{6}(k_1 + 2k_2 + 2k_3 + k_4)$$

$$= (1, -1) + \frac{1}{6}[(0; -0{,}2) + 2(-0{,}02; -0{,}27) + 2(-0{,}02; -0{,}24)$$

$$+ (-0{,}03; -0{,}29)] = (1, -1) + \frac{1}{6}(-0{,}11; -1{,}51) = (0{,}98; -1{,}25).$$

3.5. COMPLETENESS OF VECTOR FIELDS

A C^1 vector field X on a connected open set $D \subset R^n$ is said to be *complete* if for each $x_0 \in D$ the maximal field line of X through x_0 has domain equal to R.

Since it is allowed to reparametrize by translations, in the following we make the problem simpler by considering that the field line of X passes through the point x_0 at the moment $t_0 = 0$.

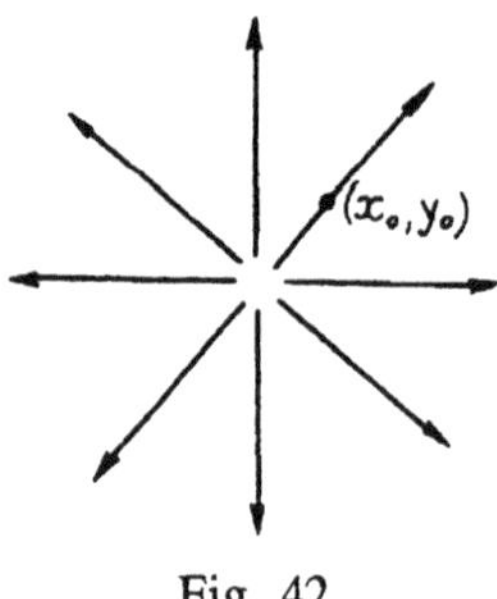

Fig. 42

Examples. 1) Any linear vector field is complete. For example, the vector field $X = (x,y)$ on R^2 admits the field lines $\alpha(t) = (x_0 e^t, y_0 e^t)$, $(x_0, y_0) \in R^2$, defined on R; the zero $(0,0)$ of X generates the equilibrium point (see Fig.42).

In particular, Killing vector fields are complete.

2) A vector field having only closed field lines is complete.

3) The vector fields $X = (y, 0)$, $Y = (0, \frac{x^2}{2})$ are complete, while the bracket $[X, Y]$ is not complete.

4) Newtonian vector fields and electrostatic vector fields with spherical symmetry are complete (see 3.1). The completeness of a vector field may be characterized by either of the following two theorems.

Theorem. *A C^1 vector field X on a connected open set $D \subset R^n$ is complete if and only if there exists a neighborhood I of 0 in R such that any maximal field line of X is defined on I.*

Proof. Necessity is obvious, so it remains to prove sufficiency. We assume there exists an open set I in R with the mentioned property, and we denote by $[-\varepsilon, \varepsilon]$, $\varepsilon > 0$, a closed interval from I and $J(x_0)$ the domain (open interval) of the maximal field line α_{x_0} of X through x_0. By hypothesis, $[-\varepsilon, \varepsilon]$ is included in the domains of all the maximal field lines.

We proceed by reductio ad absurdum. Assume that there exists $x_0 \in D$ such that $J(x_0) \neq R$, a fact that implies existence of the number $\sup J(x_0) = b$ or of the number $\inf J(x_0) = a$. If there exists supremum b, then the field line through $x_1 = \alpha_{x_0}(b-\varepsilon)$ has domain $J(x_1)$ equal to the translation of the open set $J(x_0)$ by $-(b-\varepsilon)$, and then $J(x_1)$ does not contain $[-\varepsilon, \varepsilon]$; a contradiction. If there exists infimum a, then the field line through $x_2 = \alpha_{x_0}(a+\varepsilon)$ has domain $J(x_2)$ equal to the translation of the open set $J(x_0)$ by $-(a+\varepsilon)$ and then $J(x_2)$ does not contain $[-\varepsilon, \varepsilon]$; a contradiction.

Theorem. *A C^1 vector field X on a connected open set $D \subset R^n$ is complete if and only if, for any field line $\alpha : I \to D$ of X, there exists a compact set K (which depends on the field line) such that, for any $\varepsilon > 0$, with $(-\varepsilon, \varepsilon) \subset I$, the image $\alpha(-\varepsilon, \varepsilon)$ remains in K.*

Proof. Necessity being obvious, it remains the prove sufficiency. Let $\alpha : I \to D$ be the maximal field line passing through the point x_0 at the moment $t_0 = 0$, which has the property that $\alpha(-\varepsilon, \varepsilon)$ is included in a compact K for any $(-\varepsilon, \varepsilon) \subset I$. Since X is a continuous function, the restriction of $\|X\|$ to K is bounded.

Let us show that $T = \sup\{\varepsilon \,|\, (-\varepsilon, \varepsilon) \subset I\}$ is ∞. For this goal, we proceed by reductio ad absurdum. We assume that T is finite and consider that

$$\alpha(t) = x_0 + \int_0^t X(\alpha(s))\,ds, \quad t \in [0, T).$$

It follows that

$$\|\alpha(t') - \alpha(t'')\| \leq c|t' - t''| \quad \text{for any} \quad t', t'' \in [0, T)$$

Therefore $\lim_{t \nearrow T} \alpha(t)$ exists (by the Cauchy Criterion) and belongs to K, while $\lim_{t \nearrow T} \frac{dx}{dt}(t)$ exists by the relationship $\frac{dx}{dt} = X(x)$.

Consequently, the restriction of α to $[0, T]$ is a solution for $\frac{dx}{dt} = X(x)$.

We consider the field line $\beta : J \to D$ passing through the point $\lim_{t \nearrow T} \alpha(t)$ at the moment $T \in \text{int}J$. The Existence and Uniqueness Theorem shows that β coincides with α for $t \in [0,T] \cap J$. This implies that α can be extended to the right of T. Analogously one can show that α can be extended to the left of $-T$, which contradicts the definition of T.

Notice. This Hartman Theorem [28] was formulated and proved by Şerban Bolintineanu after an ambiguous statement from [26].

Consequences. *1) If the differential system* $\dfrac{dx}{dt} = X(x)$ *admits a global first integral whose level sets are compact, then the vector field* X *is complete.*

2) If the closure of the set $\{x \in D \mid X(x) \neq 0\} \subset D$ *is compact, then the vector field* X *is complete.*

Proof. 2) Any field line intersecting the set mentioned in the statement is entirely included in this set. Otherwise, the field line reduces to an equilibrium point.

Let us now give other sufficient conditions for the completeness of some vector fields.

Theorem [26]. *Let* X *be a* C^1 *vector field on a connected open set* $D \subset R^n$. *If there exists a* C^1 *function* $g : D \to R$, *a* C^0 *proper function* $h : D \to R$ *and the constants* A, B *such that*

$$|D_X g(x)| \leq A|g(x)|, \quad |h(x)| \leq B|g(x)|, \quad \textit{for any} \quad x \in D,$$

then the vector field X *is complete.*

Proof. We ascertain that the function h is proper if h^{-1} (compact) = compact.

Let $\alpha(t)$, $t \in (-\varepsilon, \varepsilon)$ be a field line of X. Denoting $\varphi(t) = g(\alpha(t))$, $t \in (-\varepsilon, \varepsilon)$, and taking the relation $Dg(\alpha(t)) = \dfrac{d}{dt} g(\alpha(t))$ into account, the first hypothesis-inequality implies

$$\left|\frac{d}{dt}\varphi(t)\right| \leq A|\varphi(t)|, \; \forall t \in (-\varepsilon, \varepsilon),$$

or, in detail,

$$-A\varphi(t)\operatorname{sign}\varphi(t) \leq \frac{d}{dt}\varphi(t) \leq A\varphi(t)\operatorname{sign}\varphi(t) \; \forall t \in (-\varepsilon, \varepsilon),$$

where

$$\operatorname{sign} u = \begin{cases} -1 & \text{for } u < 0 \\ \;\;0 & \text{for } u = 0 \\ \;\;1 & \text{for } u > 0. \end{cases}$$

The function $|\varphi| : (-\varepsilon, \varepsilon) \to R$ is differentiable and $\dfrac{d}{dt}|\varphi(t)| = \dfrac{d\varphi}{dt}(t)\operatorname{sign}\varphi(t)$.

Indeed, the function φ is C^1, the sets

$$\{t|t\in(-\varepsilon,\varepsilon),\ \varphi(t)>0\}\ \text{and}\ \{t|t\in(-\varepsilon,\varepsilon),\ \varphi(t)<0\}$$

are open, while if there exists $t_0\in(-\varepsilon,\varepsilon)$ such that $\varphi(t_0)=0$, then $\frac{d\varphi}{dt}(t_0)=0$ and, consequently, the function $|\varphi|$ is differentiable at the point t_0, with null derivative at this point.

Let $t\in[0,\varepsilon)$. We notice that

$$\frac{d}{dt}e^{-At}|\varphi(t)| = e^{-At}\left(-A|\varphi(t)| + \frac{d\varphi}{dt}(t)\operatorname{sign}\varphi(t)\right) \le 0,\ \forall t\in[0,\varepsilon).$$

It follows that the function $e^{-At}|\varphi(t)|$, $t\in[0,\varepsilon)$, is decreasing and then

$$e^{-At}|\varphi(t)| \le |\varphi(0)| \quad \text{or} \quad |\varphi(t)| \le |\varphi(0)|e^{At},\ t\in[0,\varepsilon).$$

Let $t\in(-\varepsilon,0]$. We notice that

$$\frac{d}{dt}e^{At}|\varphi(t)| = e^{At}\left(A|\varphi(t)| + \frac{d\varphi}{dt}(t)\operatorname{sign}\varphi(t)\right) \ge 0,\ \forall t\in(-\varepsilon,0].$$

It follows that the function $e^{At}|\varphi(t)|$, $t\in(-\varepsilon,0]$, is increasing and then

$$e^{At}|\varphi(t)| \le |\varphi(0)| \quad \text{or} \quad |\varphi(t)| \le |\varphi(0)|e^{-At},\ t\in(\varepsilon,0].$$

Consequently, $|\varphi(t)| \le |\varphi(0)|e^{A|t|}$, for any $t\in(-\varepsilon,\varepsilon)$ or, equivalently, $|g(x(t))| \le |g(x(0))|e^{A|t|}$, for any $t\in(-\varepsilon,\varepsilon)$. From here and from the second hypothesis-inequality, we get $|h(x(t))| \le B|g(x(0)|e^{A|t|}$, for any $t\in(-\varepsilon,\varepsilon)$. Since h is proper, the points $x(t)$ remain in a compact set when t varies on a bounded neighborhood of zero (on which a solution is defined). According to the preceding theorem, X is a complete vector field.

Let X be a C^1 vector field on a connected open set $D\subset R^n$, while $f:D\to R$ is a C^1 scalar field. The field lines of fX are reparametrizations of the field lines of X. Using the preceding theorem we will show that we can fix f to assure, for the field lines of fX, the existence of a parameter that runs along the set of all real numbers.

Consequence. *For any C^1 vector field X on a connected open set $D\subset R^n$, there exists a C^1 scalar field $f:D\to(0,\infty)$ such that the vector field fX is complete.*

Proof. We consider the proper C^∞ function

$$g:D\to[1,\infty),\ g(x) = 1+\sum_{j=1}^{n}x_j^2 .$$

Using X and g, we construct the function $f = \dfrac{2}{1 + (D_X g)^2}$ that is strictly positive and of class C^1 on D. Since $|D_{fX} g(x)| = f(x)|D_X g(x)| \le 1 \le g(x)$, for any $x \in D$, we apply the preceding theorem with $f = g$ and $A = B = 1$. Consequently, fX is a complete vector field.

Applications. 1) Let $X = (X_1, \dots, X_n)$ be a homothetic vector field (see 2.7) on R^n and $f = \frac{1}{2}(X_1^2 + \cdots + X_n^2)$ the energy attached to X. The definition of the homothetic vector field implies $D_X f = \frac{2c}{n} f$, where $c = \operatorname{div} X$ is a constant. If $f: R^n \to R$ is a proper function, then the above theorem, with $g = h = f$, $A = \frac{2|c|}{n}$, $B = 1$ shows that X is a complete vector field.

Notice. The energy of the Killing vector field $(z - y, x - z, y - x)$ is not a proper function since it possesses unbounded level sets. Consequently, there exist homothetic vector fields whose energies are not proper functions.

2) Let $X = (X_1, \dots, X_n)$ be a torse forming vector field (see 2.9) on $D \subset R^n$ and $f = 0{,}5(X_1^2 + \cdots + X_n^2)$ the energy attached to X. The energy f satisfies $D_X f = 2(a + (X, Y))f$. If f is proper and $a + (X, Y)$ is bounded on D, then the preceding theorem, with $g = h = f$, $A = \sup|a + (X, Y)|$, $B = 1$, shows that X is a complete vector field.

3) *Lorenz Equations* [37]

$$\frac{dx}{dt} = -\sigma x + \sigma y, \quad \frac{dy}{dt} = -xz + rx - y, \quad \frac{dz}{dt} = xy - bz$$

are an idealization of the equations of a fluid motion in a stratum of uniform depth, when the difference between the temperatures of the bottom and the surface is maintained constant. The variable x is proportional to the intensity of the convective motion, y is proportional to the difference between the temperatures of the ascending and descending currents, while the similar signs of x and y show that the warm fluid rises and the cold fluid descends. The variable z is proportional to the distortion of profile of the vertical temperature from linearity, a positive value showing that the most powerful gradients appear next to the boundaries. The constant $\sigma = k^{-1}\nu$, is the Prandtl number, k is the thermal dilation coefficient, ν is the viscosity and r is the Rayleigh number.

The vector field $X = (-\sigma x + \sigma y, -xz + rx - y, xy - bz)$ is complete, that is, the solutions of the Lorenz System are defined on the whole real straight line. Indeed, it is sufficient to put $g(x,y,z) = x^2 + y^2 + z^2$, $h(x,y,z) = g(x,y,z)$, $B = 1$, since there is a positive constant A such that

$$-A(x^2 + y^2 + z^2) \le D_X g = 2(-\sigma x^2 - y^2 - bz^2 + (\sigma + r)xy) \le A(x^2 + y^2 + z^2)$$

and the preceding theorem applies.

3.6. COMPLETENESS OF HAMILTONIAN VECTOR FIELDS

A scalar field $H: R^{2n} \to R,\ (x,y) \to H(x,y)$ of class C^2 is called *Hamiltonian*, while the vector field defined on R^{2n} by

$$X = (X_i, X_{n+i}),\ X_i = -\frac{\partial H}{\partial y_i},\ X_{n+i} = \frac{\partial H}{\partial x_i},\ i = 1, \ldots, n,$$

is called a *Hamiltonian vector field*. Hamilton was the first who proved that the functions of the type of H and X play an essential role in the description of some phenomena of the real world (see also 3.2).

If X is a Hamiltonian vector field, then

$$\mathrm{rot}X = \begin{bmatrix} \frac{\partial^2 H}{\partial x_i \partial x_j} - \frac{\partial^2 H}{\partial x_j \partial y_i} & -\frac{\partial^2 H}{\partial x_i \partial x_j} - \frac{\partial^2 H}{\partial y_i \partial y_j} \\ \frac{\partial^2 H}{\partial x_i \partial x_j} + \frac{\partial^2 H}{\partial y_i \partial y_j} & \frac{\partial^2 H}{\partial x_i \partial y_j} - \frac{\partial^2 H}{\partial x_j \partial y_i} \end{bmatrix},\quad \mathrm{div}X = 0.$$

Thus, X is not irrotational in general, but it is solenoidal. One knows that the differential system giving the field lines of a Hamiltonian vector field admits H as a global first integral (see 3.2), while the second theorem of the preceding section shows that if the level sets of H are compact, then the Hamiltonian vector field X is complete.

We illustrate these facts in the following way. Let $TR^n \approx R^{2n}$ be the tangent bundle attached to R^n. The local coordinates in TR^n are (x,y), where $x \in R^n$ and $y \in T_x R^n$. A scalar field $V: R^n \to R$ of class C^2 will be called *potential energy* on R^n. The scalar field $T: R^{2n} \to R,\ T(x,y) = \frac{1}{2}\sum_{i=1}^{n} y_i^2$ is called the *kinetic energy* attached to the Euclidean structure of R^n, while the Hamiltonian

$$H: R^{2n} \to R,\ H = T + V$$

is also called *total energy* on R^{2n}.

Let us give some sufficient conditions for completeness of the Hamiltonian vector field associated to the total energy, different from that mentioned above.

Theorem. *Let $H = T + V$ be the total energy on R^n. The Hamiltonian vector field X is complete if one of the following assertions is true:*

1) V is a proper lower bounded function (for example $V \geq 0$).

2) V is a lower bounded function $(V \geq 0)$.

3) $\|\operatorname{grad} V\|$ *is bounded.*

4) $\|\operatorname{grad} V\| \le k\|\varphi\|$, *where* $x \to \varphi(x)$ *is an isometric embedding of* (R^n, δ_{ij}) into $(R^{n+1}, \delta_{\alpha\beta})$, and k is a constant.

Proof. 1) The function H is proper on R^{2n}, since V is proper on R^n and $V \ge 0$. It satisfies the relation $D_X H = 0$, being a first integral of the system giving the field lines (see 3.2). One can apply the last theorem from the preceding section with $g = h = H$.

Let $\varphi : R^n \to R^{n+1}$, $\varphi(x_1, \dots, x_n) = (x_1, \dots, x_n, 0)$ be the canonical isometric embedding of (R^n, δ_{ij}) into $(R^{n+1}, \delta_{\alpha\beta})$. The Euclidean space R^n is complete. As well, it is a closed submanifold of the Euclidean space R^{n+1}, since it is characterized by the equation $x_{n+1} = 0$. It follows that the real function

$$r^2(x) = \|\varphi(x)\|^2 = x_1^2 + \cdots + x_n^2, \; x = (x_1, \dots, x_n) \in R^n,$$

is proper. This function satisfies the relations

$$|D_X r^2| = 2\left|\sum_{i=1}^{n} x_i y_i\right| \le 2r(x)(2T)^{\frac{1}{2}},$$

where X is the Hamiltonian vector field associated to the total energy.

2) For $g = H + r^2$, one verifies $|D_X g| \le 2|g|$. We add $h = r^2$ or $h = g$ and we apply the last theorem of the above paragraph.

3) + 4) Let $g = h = T + \dfrac{r^2}{2}$. We find

$$|D_X T| = \left|\sum_{i=1}^{n} y_i \frac{\partial V}{\partial x_i}\right| \le (2T)^{\frac{1}{2}} \|\operatorname{grad} V\|,$$

and then

$$\left|\frac{D_X g}{g}\right| \le (2T)^{\frac{1}{2}} \|\varphi\| \frac{1 + \dfrac{\|\operatorname{grad} V\|}{\|\varphi\|}}{T + \dfrac{1}{2}\|\varphi\|^2}.$$

With all these, 4) becomes obvious, while for 3) it is sufficient to choose an embedding for which $\|\varphi\|$ is bounded below by a strictly positive number, for example

$$\varphi(x_1, \dots, x_n) = (x_1, \dots, x_n, 1).$$

The Hamiltonian vector fields appear often from the potential differential systems of order two. By a *potential differential system with n degrees of freedom* one means a physical system depicted by a second-order differential system of the form

$$\frac{d^2 x}{dt^2} + \operatorname{grad} V = 0, \tag{6}$$

where $x = (x_1, \dots, x_n) \in R^n$, while the potential $V: R^n \to R$ has a convenient class. Denoting $\frac{dx}{dt} = -y$, this transfers to the phase space $(x,y) \in R^{2n}$ in a Hamiltonian system,

$$\frac{dx}{dt} = -y, \quad \frac{dy}{dt} = \operatorname{grad} V \quad \text{with} \quad H(x,y) = \frac{1}{2}\sum_{k=1}^{n} y_k^2 + V(x). \tag{6'}$$

The fact that H is a first integral for $(6')$ is established by the fact that the total energy H of the system (6) is conserved. As a consequence, if at the initial moment the total energy is equal to H, then the whole trajectory of (6) is included in the domain characterized by $V(x) \le H$ (the point x always belongs to the interior of the *potential well*).

Remarks. 1) Any potential differential system is a conservative system. The converse is not true.

2) Any conservative differential system with n degrees of freedom can be transferred into the phase space like a Hamiltonian system.

3) All the problems presented until this time, referring to potential systems with one degree of freedom, have been completely solved. We can't say the same thing about conservative systems with at least two degrees of freedom (in this case, there still are open problems [2]).

3.7. FLOWS AND LIOUVILLE'S THEOREM

Let $X = (X_1, \dots, X_n)$ be a C^∞ vector field on R^n. From every point x of R^n begins the (unique) maximal field line $\alpha_x(t)$, $t \in I(x)$, determined by the initial conditions $(0, x)$. The Existence and Uniqueness Theorem and the Differentiability Theorem with respect to the initial conditions (see 3.1) show that, for each $x_0 \in R^n$, there exists a neighborhood U_1 of x_0 in R^n and a neighborhood $I = (-\varepsilon, \varepsilon)$ of 0 in R such that the rule $(t,x) \to \alpha_x(t)$ defines a C^∞ function $T: I \times U_1 \to R^n$ (Fig.43). The partial function $T^t: U_1 \to R^n$, $T^t(x) = \alpha_x(t)$ is then C^∞, too, and $T^0(x) = x$, for any $x \in U_1$. Other theorems from 3.1 show that the set $\{T^t | t \in I\}$ has the group property $T^{r+s} = T^r \circ T^s$ any time when the right-hand side is well-defined. Therefore $T^{-t} = (T^t)^{-1}$, that is $T^t: U \to T^t(U)$, $U \subset U_1$ is a diffeomorphism.

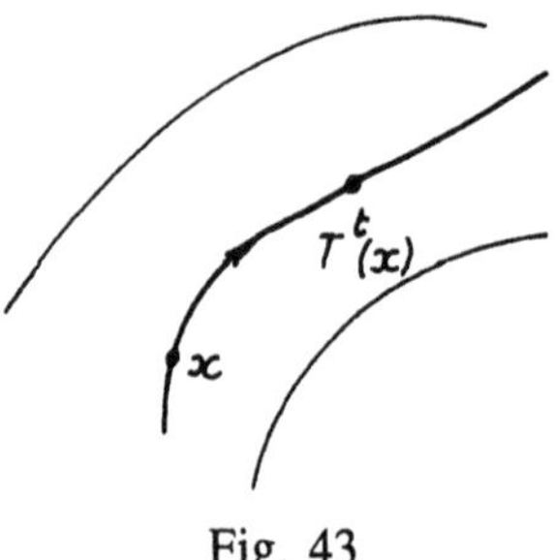

Fig. 43

The set of diffeomorphisms $\{T^t | t \in I, T^t : U \to T^t(U)\}$ is called a *local flow* on $U \subset R^n$ or a *local group with one parameter of diffeomorphisms (transformations)* on U generated by X, the adjective "local" referring to $t \in I \subset R$.

The zeros of the vector field X are the fixed points of the flow.

For t from a neighborhood of 0, one may write

$$T^t(x) = x + tX(x) + O\,(t^2)$$

or

$$x_i' = x_i + tX_i(x) + O_i\;(t^2),\; i = 1, \dots, n.$$

The function defined by $x \to x + tX(x)$ is called the *infinitesimal transformation* associated to X. Obviously, this is the linear approximation of T^t for t sufficiently close to zero.

Any first integral of the system $\dfrac{dx_i}{dt} = X_i(x),\; i = 1, \dots, n$, is an invariant function with respect to the local flow $x \to T^t(x)$ generated by the vector field X. Indeed, taking account of the definition of first integrals, the conservation condition is fulfilled,

$$\frac{d}{dt} f(T^t(x))|_{t=0} = \sum_{i=1}^{n} \frac{\partial f}{\partial x_i'}(x_i') \frac{dx_i'}{dt}|_{t=0} = \sum_{i=1}^{n} X_i(x) \frac{\partial f}{\partial x_i}(x) = D_X f(x) = 0$$

(whatever happens for $t = 0$ also happens for $t = t_0 \in I$, that is $\dfrac{d}{dt} f(T^t(x))|_{t=t_0} = 0$). It follows

$$f(x_1', \dots, x_n') = f(x_1, \dots, x_n).$$

We denote by $D(0)$ an open, connected and bounded set in R^n of volume $v(0)$, included in the domain of definition of T^t. Then $D(t) = T^t(D(0))$ will have the volume $v(t)$.

Liouville's Theorem. *The function* $t \to v(t)$ *has the derivative*

$$\frac{dv}{dt}(t_0) = \int_{D(t_0)} \operatorname{div} \boldsymbol{X}\, dx, \quad \textit{for any} \quad t_0 \in I.$$

Proof. We start from the equality

$$v(t) = \int_{D(t)} dx' = \int_{D(0)} \left| \frac{\partial x_i'}{\partial x_j} \right| dx$$

(see the change of variables in the multiple integral of order n). The relations

$$x_i' = x_i + tX_i(x) + O_i(t^2),$$

$$\frac{\partial x_i'}{\partial x_j} = \delta_{ij} + t\frac{\partial X_j}{\partial x_j} + O_{ij}(t^2), \; i, j = 1, \ldots, n,$$

imply

$$\left| \frac{\partial x_i'}{\partial x_j} \right| = 1 + \operatorname{div}\boldsymbol{X} + O(t^2)$$

and then

$$v(t) = \int_{D(0)} [1 + t\operatorname{div}\boldsymbol{X} + O(t^2)]\, dx.$$

Differentiating at $t = 0 \in I$ we find $\frac{dv}{dt}(0) = \int_{D(0)} \operatorname{div}\boldsymbol{X}\, dx$. The change of 0 into $t_0 \in I$ does not affect the equality; more precisely

$$\frac{dv}{dt}(t_0) = \int_{D(t_0)} \operatorname{div} \boldsymbol{X}\, dx.$$

Consequences. 1) If $\operatorname{div} \boldsymbol{X} = 0$ (that is $\boldsymbol{X}$ is a solenoidal field), then the local flow $\{T^t | t \in I\}$ preserves volumes, that is, $v(t) = v(0)$ for any $t \in I$ (Fig.44).

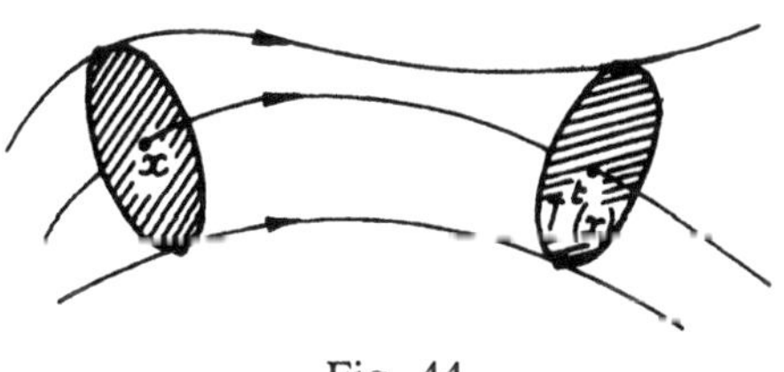

Fig. 44

2) If $\operatorname{div}\boldsymbol{X} \leq 0$, then the local flow generated by $\boldsymbol{X}$ decreases the volume (contraction, see Fig.45).

3) If $\operatorname{div}\boldsymbol{X} \geq 0$, then the local flow associated to $\boldsymbol{X}$ increases the volume (dilation, see Fig. 46).

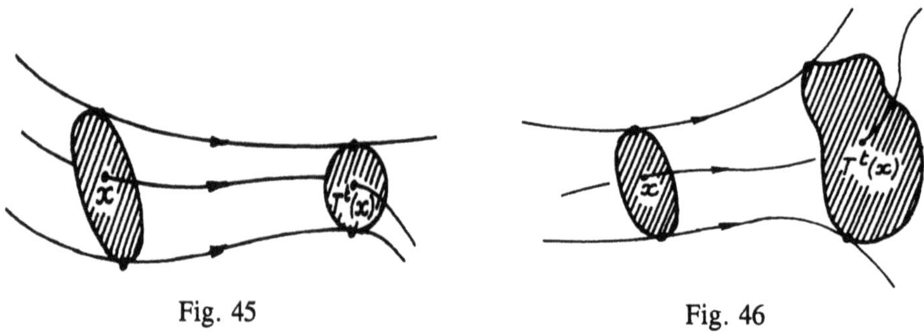

Fig. 45 Fig. 46

Notices. 1) From the Liouville Theorem it follows that the divergence of a vector field defines the *speed of contraction- dilation of volumes* by the corresponding local flow.

2) The local flow generated by X decreases the volume if and only if the local flow generated by $-X$ increases the volume.

3) The inverse of the Jacobi matrix of elements

$$\frac{\partial x_i'}{\partial x_j} = \delta_{ij} + t\frac{\partial X_i}{\partial x_j} + O_{ij}(t^2)$$

is the matrix of elements

$$\frac{\partial x_i}{\partial x_j'} = \delta_{ij} - t\frac{\partial X_i}{\partial x_j'} + O_{ij}(t^2).$$

4) The Liouville Theorem has important applications in statistical mechanics and allows us to study mechanical systems using the methods of Ergodic Theory [14].

Let us assume that X is a complete C^∞ vector field on R^n. In other words, through each point of R^n passes one (and only one) maximal field line of X which is defined on the whole real axis (R^n appears as the disjoint union of the orbits of X). Denoting by $\alpha_x(t)$ the field line given by the initial conditions $(0,x)$, the law $x \to T^x(x) = \alpha_x(t)$ defines a C^∞ diffeomorphism $T^t : R^n \to R^n$; in particular, $T^0(x) = x$, for any $x \in R^n$. The property $T^{r+s} = T^r \circ T^s = T^s \circ T^r$ shows that $\{T^t | t \in R\}$ is an abelian group. The group $\{T^t | t \in R\}$ is called *global flow on* R^n or *(global) group with one parameter of diffeomorphisms (transformations) on* R^n, generated by X.

Remarks. 1) The set R^n can be replaced with any connected open subset.

2) If X is of class C^p, $p \geq 1$, then also the diffeomorphism T^t is of class C^p [1].

3) The set of diffeomorphisms (transformations) on R^n is a group with respect to

the composition of functions. The partial function $t \to T^t(x)$ is a homomorphism from the group R to the transformations group of R^n.

4) Let $f: R^n \to (0,\infty)$. The field lines of the collinear vector fields X and fX are different parametrizations of the same orbits. Therefore, given a vector field X, there exists a scalar field $f: R^n \to (0,\infty)$ such that fX generates a global flow (see also 3.6).

5) A subset S of R^n is called a *(local) invariant set* with respect to the (local) global flow generated by the vector field X if the image of any point of S is also a point of S.

Gronwall's Lemma. *Let* $a > 0$. *If* $f: [0,a] \to R$ *is a continuous function that satisfies*

$$f(t) \leq k + \int_0^t h(s)ds, \quad t \in [0,a],$$

with $k \in R$, $h \in C^0[0,a]$, $h(t) \geq 0$, *then*

$$f(t) \leq k \exp \int_0^t h(s)\,ds.$$

Proof. Let us consider the function

$$\varphi : [0,a] \to R, \quad \varphi(t) = \left(k + \int_0^t h(s)f(s)\,ds \right) \exp\left(-\int_0^t h(s)\,ds \right).$$

Since

$$\frac{d\varphi}{dt} = \left(f(t) - k - \int_0^t h(s)f(s)\,ds \right) h(t) \exp\left(-\int_0^t h(s)\,ds \right) \leq 0,$$

the function φ is decreasing. Therefore $\varphi(t) \leq \varphi(0) = k$, i.e.,

$$k + \int_0^t h(s)f(s)\,ds \leq k \exp \int_0^t h(s)\,ds,$$

which implies the relation in the lemma.

Theorem. *Let* X *be a* C^r *vector field on* R^n *with* $X(0) = 0$. *If* X *satisfies a Lipschitz condition with constant* K, *then the flow* $T_t(x)$ *of* X *is defined on* $R \times R^n$ *and*

$$\|T_t(x) - T_t(y)\| \leq \|x - y\| e^{K|t|}, \quad \forall\, x, y \in R^n.$$

Proof. Let $\alpha : (-\varepsilon, \varepsilon) \to R^n$ be the maximal field line of X which satisfies $\alpha(0) = x \in R^n$. To find a contraction we impose $\varepsilon < \infty$. Then

$$\alpha(t) = x + \int_0^t X(\alpha(s))\,ds.$$

Hence, for $t \geq 0$, we have

$$\|\alpha(t)\| \le \|x\| + \int_0^t \|X(\alpha(s))\|\,ds \le \|x\| + \int_0^t K\|\alpha(s)\|\,ds.$$

Applying Gronwall's lemma, we obtain

$$\|\alpha(t)\| \le \|x\|\, e^{K|t|} \le \|x\|\, e^{K\varepsilon}, \quad \text{for} \quad t \ge 0.$$

Let $t_n \to \varepsilon$. The sequence $\{\alpha(t_n)\}$ is included in the ball with centre at the origin and radius $M = \|x\|\, e^{K\varepsilon}$. Since

$$\alpha(t_n) - \alpha(t_m) = \int_{t_m}^{t_n} X(\alpha(s))\,ds,$$

we find

$$\|\alpha(t_n) - \alpha(t_m)\| \le KM|t_n - t_m|.$$

Thus $\{\alpha(t_n)\}$ is a Cauchy sequence, and so it converges to a point $y \in R^n$. Consequently α can be extended to the right of ε contrary to the initial hypothesis $\varepsilon < \infty$. Thus the flow of X is defined on $R \times R^n$, i.e., X is a complete vector field.

Since

$$T_t(x) - T_t(y) = x - y + \int_0^t [X(T_s(x)) - X(T_s(y))]\,ds,$$

for $t \ge 0$, we get

$$\|T_t(x) - T_t(y)\| \le \|x - y\| + \int_0^t K\|T_s(x) - T_s(y)\|\,ds.$$

Gronwall's lemma gives

$$\|T_t(x) - T_t(y)\| \le \|x - y\|\, e^{K|t|}, \quad \text{for} \quad t \ge 0.$$

For $t \le 0$ we obtain the same estimate by applying the preceding argument to the vector field $-X$. Of course, the hypothesis $X(0) = 0$ is not essential for completeness of X.

Corollary. *Let X be a C^1 vector field on R^n.*

1) The vector field $\dfrac{X}{1 + \|X\|}$ *is complete.*

2) If X has no zero, then the versor field $\dfrac{X}{\|X\|}$ *is complete.*

Applications. 1) **Motion of a charged particle in a stationary electromagnetic field.** Let an electromagnetic field on R^3 be given by the electric field

$$E(x) = (E_1(x), E_2(x), E_3(x))$$

and the magnetic field

$$B(x) = (B_1(x), B_2(x), B_3(x)), \; x = (x_1, x_2, x_3) \in R^3.$$

The motion in this field of a particle of mass m and charge q is described by the Lorentz equation

$$m\frac{dv}{dt} = q(E + v \times B),$$

where v is the field of velocities. Adding the vector equation $\frac{dx}{dt} = v$, we obtain a system of equations in the space of phases $R^6 = \{(x_1, x_2, x_3, v_1, v_2, v_3)\}$, namely the system that gives the field lines of the vector field $X = \left(v, \frac{q}{m}(E + v \times B)\right)$ or, in extenso,

$$X = \left(v_1, v_2, v_3, \frac{q}{m}(E_1 + v_2 B_3 - v_3 B_2), \frac{q}{m}(E_2 + v_3 B_1 - v_1 B_3), \frac{q}{m}(E_3 + v_1 B_2 - v_2 B_1)\right).$$

Since

$$\operatorname{div} X = \frac{\partial X_1}{\partial x_1} + \frac{\partial X_2}{\partial x_2} + \frac{\partial X_3}{\partial x_3} + \frac{\partial X_4}{\partial v_1} + \frac{\partial X_5}{\partial v_2} + \frac{\partial X_6}{\partial v_3} = 0,$$

the local flow generated by X preserves the volume.

2) The stationary magnetic field is described by the intensity vector $B(x) = (B_1(x), B_2(x), B_3(x))$, while the magnetic lines of force are the solutions of the differential system

$$\frac{dx_i}{dt} = B_i(x),\ i = 1, 2, 3.$$

The Maxwell equation $\operatorname{div} B = 0$ ensures the fact that the local flow generated by B preserves the volume.

3) The Biot-Savart-Laplace vector field is solenoidal (see 2.3). Therefore, the local flow generated by it preserves the volume.

4) The local flow generated by a Hamiltonian vector field preserves the volume. Indeed, for

$$X = (X_i, X_{n+i}),\ X_i = -\frac{\partial H}{\partial y_i},\ X_{n+i} = \frac{\partial H}{\partial x_i},\ i = 1, \dots, n,$$

we get

$$\operatorname{div} X = \sum_i \left(-\frac{\partial^2 H}{\partial x_i \partial y_i} + \frac{\partial H}{\partial y_i \partial x_i} \right) = 0,$$

that is, any Hamiltonian field is solenoidal.

5) The Newtonian field $X = (X_1, \dots, X_n),\ X_i(x) = \dfrac{m x_i}{(x_1^2 + \dots + x_n^2)^{\frac{n}{2}}}$ is solenoidal on $R^n \setminus \{0\}$. It is complete as well. It follows that this field generates a global flow on $R^n \setminus \{0\}$ that preserves the volume.

3.8. GLOBAL FLOW GENERATED BY A KILLING OR AFFINE VECTOR FIELD

Let $A = [a_{ij}]$ be a skew-symmetric matrix and

$$X = (X_1, \dots, X_n),\ X_i(x) = \sum_{j=1}^{n} a_{ij} x_j + c_i,\ i = 1, \dots, n,$$

a Killing vector field. The system giving the field lines is $\frac{dx_i}{dt} = \sum_{j=1}^{n} a_{ij} x_j + c_i$ and has the general solution

$$x = e^{At}\left[x_0 + \left(\frac{t}{1!} I - \frac{t^2}{2!} A + \cdots + (-1)^n \frac{t^{n+1}}{(n+1)!} A^n + \cdots\right) c\right],$$

$$t \in R,\ x_0 \in R^n,\ c = {}^t[c_1, \dots, c_n].$$

It follows the global flow on R^n,

$$x = e^{At} y + e^{At}\left[\frac{t}{1!} I - \frac{t^2}{2!} A + \cdots + (-1)^n \frac{t^{n+1}}{(n+1)!} A^n + \cdots\right] c.$$

This flow preserves the volume, since $\operatorname{div} X = \operatorname{trace} A = 0$.

The flow generated by the Killing vector field

$$X_i(x) = \sum_{j=1}^{n} a_{ij} x_j,\ i = 1, \dots, n,$$

that is, $x = e^{At} y,\ t \in R,\ y \in R^n$ is a 1-parameter group of rotations. Indeed, the matrix e^{At} is orthogonal and of determinant 1 [denoting the transpose by *, we get $(e^{At})^* = e^{A^* t} = e^{-At}$, while e^{-At} is the inverse of e^{At}; this means that e^{At} is an orthogonal matrix and then $\det(e^{At}) = \pm 1$, for any $t \in R$; but $e^0 = I$ and $\det I = 1$; we get $\det(e^{At}) = 1$ for any $t \in R$].

If A is nonsingular (it follows that n is even), then the flow generated by the Killing field $Ax + c$ reduces to roto-translations,

$$x = e^{At}(y + A^{-1} c) - A^{-1} c.$$

If A is singular and $Ac = 0$, then the flow generated by the Killing field $Ax + c$ reduces to

$$x = e^{At}(y + tc).$$

A diffeomorphism $F : R^n \to R^n$ is called an *isometry* if it preserves the Euclidean distance.

Theorem. *A vector field X of class C^∞ on R^n is a Killing vector field if and only if the flow generated by X consists of isometries.*

Proof. Let $T^t(x) = x + tX(x) + O(t^2)$ be the global flow generated by the vector field X. It is sufficient to use the conservation condition for the scalar product

$$(dT^t(x)\boldsymbol{u}, dT^t(x)\boldsymbol{v}) = (\boldsymbol{u}, \boldsymbol{v}) = \text{const},$$

where $\boldsymbol{u}$ and $\boldsymbol{v}$ are arbitrary vectors, tangent to R^n at $x \in R^n$.

First, we notice that

$$\frac{d}{dt}(dT^t(x)\boldsymbol{u}, dT^t(x)\boldsymbol{v})\Big|_{t=0} = \frac{d}{dt}\sum_{i=1}^n\left[\sum_{j=1}^n\left(\delta_{ij} + t\frac{\partial X_i}{\partial x_j}(x) + \cdots\right)u_j\right]$$

$$\times\left[\sum_{k=1}^n\left(\delta_{ik} + t\frac{\partial X_i}{\partial x_k}(x) + \cdots\right)v_k\right]\Big|_{t=0} = \frac{d}{dt}\left[(\boldsymbol{u}, \boldsymbol{v}) + t\sum_{j,k}\left(\frac{\partial X_j}{\partial x_k}(x) + \frac{\partial X_k}{\partial x_j}(x)\right)u_j v_k + \cdots\right]\Big|_{t=0}$$

$$= \sum_{j,k}\left(\frac{\partial X_j}{\partial x_k}(x) + \frac{\partial X_k}{\partial x_j}(x)\right)u_j v_k.$$

The condition of preserving the scalar product on R^n,

$$0 = \frac{d}{dt}(dT^t(x)\boldsymbol{u}, dT^t(x)\boldsymbol{v})\Big|_{t=0}, \quad \text{for any} \quad \boldsymbol{u}, \boldsymbol{v},$$

(whatever happens for $t = 0$ happens for $t = t_0$ as well) is equivalent to the Killing equations $\frac{\partial X_j}{\partial x_k} + \frac{\partial X_k}{\partial x_j} = 0$ on R^n.

The global flow generated on R^n by the affine vector field $Ax + c$ (see 2.8) is

$$x = e^{At}y + e^{At}\left[\frac{t}{1!}I - \frac{t^2}{2!}A + \cdots + (-1)^n\frac{t^{n+1}}{(n+1)!}A^n + \cdots\right]c, \; t \in R, \; y \in R^n.$$

For the following theorem, we adopt the definitions:

1) A regular curve $\gamma : I \subset R \to R^n$, $s \to \gamma(s)$, is called a *straight line* if the tangent vector field $\frac{d\gamma}{ds}$ is parallel, i.e., $\frac{d^2\gamma}{ds^2} = 0$;

2) A diffeomorphism $F : R^n \to R^n$ is called an *affine transformation* if $F \circ \gamma$ is a straight line for any straight line γ.

Obviously, an isometry is an affine transformation.

Theorem. *A C^∞ vector field X on R^n is an affine vector field if and only if the flow generated by X consists of affine transformations.*

Proof. For $n \geq 2$, let $\gamma : R \to R^n$, $\gamma(s) = (x_1(s), \dots, x_n(s))$ be an arbitrary (maximal) straight line, that is, $\dfrac{d^2\gamma}{ds^2} = 0$, and $T^t(x) = x + tX(x) + O(t^2)$ the global flow generated by X. We get

$$\frac{d}{ds}(T^t \circ \gamma) = dT^t\left(\frac{d\gamma}{ds}\right), \quad \frac{d^2}{ds^2}(T^t \circ \gamma) = d^2 T^t\left(\frac{d\gamma}{ds}, \frac{d\gamma}{ds}\right)$$

$$= t\sum_{j,k} \frac{\partial^2 X}{\partial x_j \partial x_k}(\gamma(0))\frac{dx_j}{ds}\frac{dx_k}{ds} + O(t^2).$$

It follows that

$$\frac{d}{dt}\frac{d^2}{ds^2}(T^t \circ \gamma)|_{t=0} = \sum_{j,k} \frac{\partial^2 X}{\partial x_j \partial x_k}(\gamma(s))\frac{dx_j}{ds}(s)\frac{dx_k}{ds}(s),$$

which shows that the condition of preserving a straight line, $0 = \dfrac{d}{dt}\dfrac{d^2}{ds^2}(T^t \circ \gamma)|_{t=0}$ (whatever happens for $t = 0$ happens for $t = t_0$ as well) is equivalent to the PDEs $\dfrac{\partial^2 X_i}{\partial x_j \partial x_k} = 0$, $i, j, k = 1, \dots, n$, on R^n.

3.9. LOCAL FLOW GENERATED BY A CONFORMAL VECTOR FIELD

Let us consider the conformal vector field $X = (X_1, \dots, X_n)$,

$$X_i(x) = \frac{1}{2}x_i \sum_{j=1}^{n} c_j x_i - \frac{1}{4}c_i \sum_{j=1}^{n} x_j^2 + \sum_{j=1}^{n} c_{ij} x_j + d_i,$$

$$c_{ij} + c_{ji} = \frac{c}{2}\delta_{ij}, \quad i, j = 1, \dots, n,$$

on R^n, $n \geq 2$. In the case $n = 2$, this is a particular conformal vector field, the most general being an arbitrary holomorphic function on complex numbers C (see 2.7). Denoting $a_{ij} = \dfrac{c_{ij} - c_{ji}}{2}$, we have the equivalent form

$$X_i(x) = \frac{1}{2}x_i \sum_{j=1}^{n} c_j x_j - \frac{1}{4}c_i \sum_{j=1}^{n} x_j^2 + \sum_{j=1}^{n} a_{ij} x_j + \frac{c}{2}x_i + d_i.$$

The global flow generated by the parallel vector field $Y(x) = d$ consists of translations, $x = dt + y$, $t \in R$, $y \in R^n$.

The global flow determined by the concurrent vector field $Z(x) = x$ consists of dilatations, $x = e^t y,\ t \in R,\ y \in R^n$.

The global flow attached to a Killing vector field $V(x) = Ax$ consists of rotations.

Let us find the local flow generated by the vector field

$$W = (W_1, \dots, W_n),\ W_i(x) = \frac{1}{2} x_i \sum_{j=1}^{n} c_j x_j - \frac{1}{4} c_i \sum_{j=1}^{n} x_j^2 .$$

The form of W suggests that the field lines of W could be reparametrized straight lines, $x_i = a_i + b_i s$, where $s = s(t)$. The system $\frac{dx_i}{dt} = W_i(x)$ is satisfied for

$$a_i = 0,\ b_i = \beta c_i,\ \frac{ds}{dt} = \frac{\beta}{4} s^2 \sum_{j=1}^{n} c_j^2$$

and then $s = -\frac{4}{\beta t \Sigma c_j^2}$, that is $x_i = -\frac{4}{t}\frac{c_i}{\Sigma c_j^2}$, $t \neq 0,\ c_i =$ const, $i = 1, \dots, n$, are the field lines of W. Consequently, the local flow generated by W consists of inversions, $x = -\frac{4}{t}\frac{y}{\Sigma y_j^2}$, $t \neq 0,\ y \in R^n \setminus \{0\}$.

Since the set of conformal vector fields is a Lie algebra, while Y, Z, V, W are linearly independent, the local flow generated by the conformal vector field $X = Y + Z + V + W$ on R^n, $n \geq 2$, contains isometries, homotheties and inversions.

A local diffeomorphism $F : D \subset R^n \to R^n$, $n \geq 2$, is called a *conformal transformation* of the Euclidean space R^n if it preserves the measure of angles.

In the case $n \geq 3$, the domain of definition of a conformal transformation is of the form $R^n \setminus A$, where $A = \varnothing$ or $A = \{x_0\}$ or $A =$hyperplane or $A =$ hypersphere. For $n = 2$, these types of domains are only particular cases.

Obviously, an isometry is a conformal transformation. The local flow generated by a conformal vector field on R^n, $n \geq 2$, is a family of conformal transformations.

Theorem. *A C^∞ vector field X on R^n, $n \geq 2$, is a conformal vector field if and only if the local flow generated by X consists of conformal transformations.*

Proof. Let $T^t(x) = x + tX(x) + O(t^2)$, $t \in I$, be the local flow generated by X on $D \subset R^n$, and u, v two arbitrary non-zero vectors tangent to D at $x \in D$. The condition of preserving the measures of angles with the vertex x is

$$\cos\theta(t) = \frac{(dT^t(x)u, dT^t(x)v)}{\|dT^t(x)u\| \|dT^t(x)v)\|} = \frac{(u, v)}{\|u\| \|v\|} = \text{const.}$$

We notice that

$$\frac{d}{dt}\frac{(dT^t(x)u,dT^t(x)v)}{\|dT^t(x)u\|\|dT^t(x)v\|}\Big|_{t=0} = \frac{1}{\|u\|\|v\|}\sum_{j,k}\left(\frac{\partial X_j}{\partial x_k}+\frac{\partial X_k}{\partial x_j}\right)(x)u_j v_k$$

$$-\frac{(u,v)}{\|u\|^2\|v\|^2}\left(\sum_{j,k}\frac{\partial X_j}{\partial x_k}(x)u_j u_k\frac{\|v\|}{\|u\|}+\sum_{j,k}\frac{\partial X_j}{\partial x_k}(x)v_j v_k\frac{\|u\|}{\|v\|}\right).$$

Denoting $\Lambda_{jk} = \frac{\partial X_j}{\partial x_k}+\frac{\partial X_k}{\partial x_j}$ and assuming that u and v are not orthogonal, the condition of preservation $0 = \frac{d}{dt}\cos\theta(t)|_{t=0}$ (whatever happens for $t = 0$ happens for $t = t_0$) is written as by the identity

$$\frac{\sum_{j,k}\Lambda_{jk}u_j v_k}{\sum_{j,k}\delta_{jk}u_j v_k} = \frac{1}{2}\frac{\sum_{j,k}\Lambda_{jk}u_j u_k}{\sum_{j,k}\delta_{jk}u_j u_k}+\frac{1}{2}\frac{\sum_{j,k}\Lambda_{jk}v_j v_k}{\sum_{j,k}\delta_{jk}v_j v_k}$$

with respect to $u = (u_1, \dots, u_n)$, $v = (v_1, \dots, v_n)$. This identity takes place if and only if

$$\frac{\partial X_j}{\partial x_k}+\frac{\partial X_k}{\partial x_j} = \psi\,\delta_{jk}$$

on R^n (Sufficiency is obvious. Necessity: one can differentiate the identity with respect to u_i, then the result with respect to v_l, and contract i and l).

3.10. LOCAL FLOW GENERATED BY A PROJECTIVE VECTOR FIELD

The set of projective vector fields on R^n, $n \geq 2$, is a Lie algebra (see 2.8). Therefore, the local flow generated on R^n, $n \geq 2$, by the projective vector field $X(x) = (c,x)x + Ax + d$, $x \in R^n$, contains the global flow generated by the affine vector field $Ax + d$ (see 3.8), and the local flow generated by the projective vector field $Y(x) = (c,x)x$. The expression $(c,x)x$ suggests that the field lines of $Y(x) = (c,x)x$ are reparametrized straight lines $x = a + bs$, $s = s(t)$. The system $\frac{dx}{dt} = Y(x)$ is satisfied for $a = 0$, b-arbitrary, $\frac{ds}{dt} = (c,b)s^2$. It follows that $s = -\frac{1}{(c,b)t+\alpha}$ and hence $x = -\frac{b}{(c,b)t+\alpha}$, b- an arbitrary vector, α - arbitrary number, c - fixed vector, $(c,b)t + \alpha \neq 0$ are the field lines of $Y = (c,x)x$. Consequently, the local flow generated on R^n by $Y(x) = (c,x)x$ is $x = -\frac{y}{(c,y)t+\alpha}$, $(c,x)t + \alpha \neq 0$.

A local diffeomorphism $F: D \subset R^n \to R^n$ is called a *projective transformation* of the Euclidean space R^n if $F \circ \gamma$ is a reparametrization of a straight line for any straight line $\gamma : I \subset R \to D$.

The domain of definition of a projective transformation is of the form $R^n \setminus A$, where $A = \emptyset$ or $A =$ hyperplane.

Obviously, an affine transformation is a projective one. The local flow generated by a projective vector field is a family of projective transformations of R^n.

Theorem. *A C^∞ vector field X on R^n, $n \geq 2$, is a projective vector field if and only if the local flow generated by X consists of projective transformations.*

Proof. Let $T^t(x) = x + tX(x) + O(t^2)$, $t \in I$, be the local flow defined by X on D and $\gamma : I \to D$, $\gamma(s) = (x_1(s), \dots, x_n(s))$ a straight line. We assume that $T^t \circ \gamma$ is a straight line reparametrized by $s = s(u)$. Then

$$\frac{d}{du}(T^t \circ \gamma \circ s) = dT^t\left(\frac{d\gamma}{ds}\right)\frac{ds}{du},$$

$$\frac{d^2}{du^2}(T^t \circ \gamma \circ s) = d^2 T^t\left(\frac{d\gamma}{ds}, \frac{d\gamma}{ds}\right)\left(\frac{ds}{du}\right)^2 + dT^t\left(\frac{d\gamma}{ds}\right)\frac{d^2 s}{du^2}$$

$$= d^2 T^t\left((dT^t)^{-1}\frac{d}{du}(T^t \circ \gamma \circ s), (dT^t)^{-1}\frac{d}{du}(T^t \circ \gamma \circ s)\right) + \left(\frac{\dfrac{d^2 s}{du^2}}{\dfrac{ds}{du}}\right)\frac{d}{du}(T^t \circ \gamma \circ s)$$

and the condition of conservation of the property of reparametrized straight line, $0 = \frac{d}{dt}\frac{d^2}{du^2}(T^t \circ \gamma \circ s)|_{t=0}$ (whatever happens for $t = 0$ happens for $t = t_0$ as well) is written as

$$\sum_{j,k} \frac{\partial^2 X_i}{\partial x_j' \partial x_k'}\frac{dx_j'}{du}\frac{dx_k'}{du} + \rho\left(\frac{dx'}{du}\right)\frac{dx_i'}{du} = 0.$$

These tensor relations must take place for any $\frac{dx'}{du}$ and, therefore, it is equivalent to the PDEs system

$$\frac{\partial^2 X_i}{\partial x_j \partial x_k} = c_k \delta_{ij} + c_j \delta_{ik}, \; i, j, k = 1, \dots, n.$$

3.11. LOCAL FLOW GENERATED BY AN IRROTATIONAL, SOLENOIDAL OR TORSE FORMING VECTOR FIELD

Let $X = (x_1, \dots, x_n)$ be a C^∞ vector field on R^n. The local flow generated by the vector field X is characterized by the Cauchy problem

$$\frac{d\alpha}{dt} = X(\alpha(t)),\ \alpha(t) = (x_1(t), \dots, x_n(t)) \in R^n,\ \alpha(0) = x.$$

Suppose X is an irrotational vector field, i.e.,

$$\mathrm{rot}X = \left[\frac{\partial X_j}{\partial x_i} - \frac{\partial X_i}{\partial x_j}\right] = 0.$$

A local diffeomorphism $F: D \subset R^n \to R^n$ is called *a local irrotational map* if the differential dF (the Jacobian matrix of F) is symmetric (with respect to the Euclidean metric δ_{ij}, $i, j = 1, \dots, n$).

Theorem. *A vector field $X \in \mathcal{X}(R^n)$ is an irrotationl vector field iff the local flow $T^t(x)$, $t \in (-\varepsilon, \varepsilon)$, $x \in D \subset R^n$ generated by X consists of local irrotational maps* $(n \geq 2)$.

Proof. Let $T^t(x) = x + tX(x) + O(t^2)$ be the local flow generated by the vector field X. It is sufficient to use the conservation condition for the equality

$$(dT^t(x)u, v) = (u, dT^t(x)v), \tag{*}$$

where u and v are arbitrary vectors tangent to R^n at $x \in R^n$.

First we compute

$$\frac{d}{dt}(dT^t(x)u, v)|_{t=0}$$

$$= \frac{d}{dt}\sum_{i=1}^n \left[\left(\sum_{j=1}^n \delta_{ij} + t\frac{\partial X_i}{\partial x_j}(x) + \dots\right) u_j\right] v_i|_{t=0} = \sum_{i,j=1}^n \frac{\partial X_i}{\partial x_j}(x) u_j v_i.$$

Of course, whatever happens for $t = 0$ happens for $t = t_0$ as well. Consequently, the condition of preserving the equality (*) is equivalent to irrotationality of the vector field X, i.e.,

$$\frac{\partial X_i}{\partial x_j} = \frac{\partial X_j}{\partial x_i}$$

on R^n.

Suppose $X = (X_1, \ldots, X_n)$ is a solenoidal vector field, i.e.,

$$\operatorname{div} X = \sum_{i=1}^{n} \frac{\partial X_i}{\partial x_i} = 0.$$

A local diffeomorphism $F : D \subset R^n \to R^n$ is called a *solenoidal map* if the trace of the differential dF (the Jacobian matrix of F) is zero. Of course we may consider that the trace is taken with respect to the Euclidean metric δ_{ij}, $i, j = 1, \ldots, n$.

Theorem. *A vector field $X \in \mathcal{X}(R^n)$ is a solenoidal vector field iff the local flow $T^t(x)$, $t \in (-\varepsilon, \varepsilon)$, $x \in D \subset R^n$ generated by X consists of local solenoidal maps.*

Proof. Starting with the local flow $T^t(x) = x + tX(x) + O(t^2)$ generated by the vector field X, it is enough to use the conservation condition for

$$\operatorname{trace} dT^t(x) = 0.$$

Since

$$(dT^t(x))_{ij} = \delta_{ij} + t \frac{\partial X_i}{\partial x_j}(x) + \cdots$$

$$\frac{d}{dt}(dT^t(x))_{ij}\Big|_{t=0} = \frac{\partial X_i}{\partial x_j}(x),$$

the conservation condition is equivalent to $\operatorname{div} X - 0$.

Suppose $X = (X_1, \ldots, X_n)$ is a torse forming vector field, i.e.,

$$\frac{\partial X_i}{\partial x_j} = a\delta_{ij} + X_i Y_j, \quad i, j = 1, \ldots, n.$$

A local diffeomorphism $F : D \subset R^n \to R^n$ is called a *local torse forming map* with respect to a vector field $X \in \mathcal{X}(R^n)$ if for any $x \in D$ and any $u = (u_1, \ldots, u_n)$ tangent to R^n at x, the image $dF(x)u$ belongs to the plane $\{u, X(x)\}$.

Theorem. *A vector field $X \in \mathcal{X}(R^n)$ is torse forming iff its local flow $T^t(x)$, $t \in (-\varepsilon, \varepsilon)$, $x \in D \subset M$ consists of local torse forming maps with respect to X.*

Proof. Let $T^t(x) = x + tX(x) + O(t^2)$ be the flow generated by the vector field X. Then

$$dT^t(x)u = u + tD_u X + O(t^2)$$

and the conservation condition

$$\frac{d}{dt} dT^t(x)u\Big|_{t=0} = D_u X = a(x)u + b(x, u)X, \ \forall u \subset T_x R^n$$

(whatever happens for $t = 0$ happens for $t = t_0$ as well) is equivalent to

$$\sum_{j=1}^{n} \frac{\partial X_i}{\partial x_j}(x)u_j = a(x)u_i + b(x, u)X_i(x).$$

Since $u = (u_1, \ldots, u_n)$ is arbitrary, it follows that $b(x, u)$ is linear with respect to u, i.e.,

$$b(x,u) = \sum_{j=1}^{n} Y_j(x) u_j .$$

Consequently

$$\frac{\partial X_i}{\partial x_j} = a(x)\,\delta_{ij} + X_i(x)\,Y_j(x),\ \ i,j = 1\,,\,\dots\,,n.$$

3.12. VECTOR FIELDS ATTACHED TO THE LOCAL GROUPS OF DIFFEOMORPHISMS

Let D be an open set of R^n. A family of functions $\{T^t, t \in (-\varepsilon, \varepsilon)\}$ defined on D with values in R^n is called a *local flow* on D or a *local group with one parameter of diffeomorphisms* on D if it satisfies the following conditions:

1) the function $T: (-\varepsilon,\varepsilon) \times D \to R^n$, $(t,x) \to T^t(x)$ is C^∞;

2) for any $t \in (-\varepsilon,\varepsilon)$, the function $T^t : D \to T^t(D)$ is a diffeomorphism;

3) for any $t, s \in (-\varepsilon,\varepsilon)$ such that $t + s \in (-\varepsilon,\varepsilon)$ and $T^s(x) \in D$, we have $T^{t+s}(x) = T^t(T^s(x))$, for any $x \in D$.

The adjective "local" refers to $t \in (-\varepsilon,\varepsilon) \subset R$. If $(-\varepsilon\,,\varepsilon) = R$, then this adjective is replaced by "global." As well, from 3) it follows that $T^0(x) = x$ on D.

To each local group of diffeomorphisms $\{T^t\}$, we attach the velocity $X = \dfrac{dT^t}{dt}(0)$ that is a vector field on $D \subset R^n$. Let us find the vector fields attached to some local groups of diffeomorphisms which present a more special importance.

Let us consider the *group of roto-translations*

$$x_i' = \sum_{j=1}^{n} a_{ij} x_j + a_i ,\ \ \sum_{i=1}^{n} a_{ij} a_{ik} = \delta_{jk},\ \ \det[a_{ij}] = 1$$

on R^n. We assume $a_{ij} = a_{ij}(t)$, $a_i = a_i(t)$, $t \in (-\varepsilon,\varepsilon)$ and $a_{ij}(0) = \delta_{ij}$, $a_i(0) = 0$. It follows that $\sum_{i=1}^{n} a_{ij}(t) a_{ik}(t) = \delta_{jk}$ and then

$$0 = \sum_{i=1}^{n}\left[\frac{da_{ij}}{dt}(0)\,a_{ik}(0) + a_{ij}(0)\,\frac{da_{ik}}{dt}(0)\right] = \sum_{i=1}^{n}\left[\frac{da_{ij}}{dt}(0)\,\delta_{ik} + \delta_{ij}\,\frac{da_{ik}}{dt}(0)\right] = A_{kj} + A_{jk},$$

where $A_{ij} = \dfrac{da_{ij}}{dt}(0)$. Therefore $x_i' = \sum_{j=1}^{n} a_{ij}(t) x_j + a_i(t)$ implies

$$\frac{dx_i'}{dt}(0) = \sum_{j=1}^{n} \frac{da_{ij}}{dt}(0)x_j + \frac{da_i}{dt}(0),$$

this one representing the vector field $X = (X_1, \dots, X_n)$, $X_i = \sum_{j=1}^{n} A_{ij}x_j + A_i$, where $[A_{ij}]$ is a skew-symmetric matrix. Obviously, X is a Killing vector field.

Consider now the *affine group* $x_i' = \sum_{j=1}^{n} a_{ij}x_j + a_i$, $\det[a_{ij}] \neq 0$ on R^n. We assume

$$a_{ij} = a_{ij}(t),\ a_i = a_i(t),\ t \in (-\varepsilon, \varepsilon)$$

and $a_{ij}(0) = \delta_{ij}$, $a(0) = 0$. It follows that

$$\frac{dx_i}{dt}(0) = \sum_{j=1}^{n} \frac{da_{ij}}{dt}(0)x_j + \frac{da_i}{dt}(0),$$

and then

$$X = (X_1, \dots, X_n), \quad X_i = \sum_{j=1}^{n} A_{ij}x_j + A_i,$$

where

$$A_{ij} = \frac{da_{ij}}{dt}(0), \quad A_i = \frac{da_i}{dt}(0)$$

(an affine vector field).

The *Lorentz group* is defined by

$$x_i' = \sum_{j=1}^{4} a_{ij}x_j,\ \det[a_{ij}] \neq 0,\ \sum_{i,k=1}^{4} a_{ij}S_{ik}a_{kl} = S_{jl},\ S_{ij} = \begin{bmatrix} -1 & 0 \\ 0 & \delta_{\alpha\beta} \end{bmatrix},\ \alpha, \beta = 1, 2, 3.$$

We assume $a_{ij} = a_{ij}(t)$, $t \in (-\varepsilon, \varepsilon)$ and $a_{ij}(0) = \delta_{ij}$. From

$$\sum_{i,k=1}^{4} a_{ij}(t)S_{ik}a_{kl}(t) = S_{jl},$$

we find

$$0 = \sum_{i,k=1}^{4} \left(\frac{da_{ij}}{dt}(0)S_{ik}a_{kl}(0) + a_{ij}(0)S_{ik}\frac{da_{kl}}{dt}(0) \right) = \sum_{i,k=1}^{4} (A_{ij}S_{il} + S_{jl}A_{il}), \tag{**}$$

the final notations being obvious. Since $\frac{dx_i'}{dt}(0) = \sum_{j=1}^{4} \frac{da_{ij}}{dt}(0)x_j$, we have the attached vector field $X = (X_1, X_2, X_3, X_4)$, $X_i = \sum_{j=1}^{4} A_{ij}x_j$, where $[A_{ij}]$ is a quadratic matrix of order four whose elements satisfy the relation (**).

Consider the *projective transformation*

$$x_i' = \frac{\sum_{j=1}^{n} a_{ij}x_j + a_i}{\sum_{j=1}^{n} b_j x_j + b}, \quad \det[a_{ij}] \neq 0,$$

defined on the region $D : \sum_{j=1}^{n} b_j x_j + b \neq 0$ from R^n.

The composite of two projective transformations, the identical transformation and the (local) inverse of a projective transformation, are projective transformations on the respective domains of definition. However the set of all projective transformations of R^n is not a group of transformations, since the intersection of their domains of definition is the void set.

We assume $a_{ij} = a_{ij}(t)$, $a_i = a_i(t)$, $b = b(t)$, $t \in (-\varepsilon, \varepsilon)$ and $a_{ij}(0) = \delta_{ij}$, $a_i(0) = 0$, $b_j(0) = 0$, $b(0) = 1$. Since

$$\frac{dx_i'}{dt}(0) = \frac{\left[\sum_{j=1}^{n} \frac{da_{ij}}{dt}(0)x_j + \frac{da_i}{dt}(0)\right]\left[\sum_{j=1}^{n} b_j(0)x_j + b(0)\right]}{\left[\sum_{j=1}^{n} b_j(0)x_j + b(0)\right]^2}$$

$$- \frac{\left[\sum_{j=1}^{n} a_{ij}(0)x_j + a_i(0)\right]\left[\sum_{j=1}^{n} \frac{db_j}{dt}(0)x_j + \frac{db}{dt}(0)\right]}{\left[\sum_{j=1}^{n} b_j(0)x_j + b(0)\right]^2}$$

$$= \sum_{j=1}^{n} \frac{da_{ij}}{dt}(0)x_j + da_i(0) - x_i\left[\sum_{j=1}^{n} \frac{db_j}{dt}(0)x_j + \frac{db}{dt}(0)\right]$$

$$= \sum_{j=1}^{n} A_{ij}x_j + A_i + x_i\left(\sum_{j=1}^{n} B_j x_j + B\right),$$

the final notations being obvious, there follows the projective vector field

$$X = (X_1, \dots, X_n), \; X_i = \sum_{j=1}^{n} (A_{ij} + B\delta_{ij})x_j + x_i \sum_{j=1}^{n} B_j x_j + A_i .$$

Let us consider the matrix

$$\begin{pmatrix} a_{ij} & \vdots & a_{in+1} & a_{i0} \\ \cdots & \vdots & \cdots & \cdots \\ a_{n+1j} & \vdots & a_{n+1n+1} & a_{n+10} \\ a_{0j} & \vdots & a_{0n+1} & a_{00} \end{pmatrix}$$

and the *conformal transformation*

$$x_i' = \frac{\sum_{j=1}^{n} a_{ij} x_j + a_{in+1} \sum_{j=1}^{n} x_j^2 + a_{i0}}{\sum_{j=1}^{n} a_{0j} x_j + a_{0n+1} \sum_{j=1}^{n} x_j^2 + a_{00}}, \quad \det[a_{ij}] \neq 0,$$

$$2 \sum_{i=1}^{n} a_{ij} a_{i\alpha} - a_{0j} a_{n+1\,\alpha} - a_{0\alpha} a_{n+1\,j} = 0, \ \alpha = 0, 1, \dots, n+1; \ j = 1, \dots, n;$$

$$\sum_{i=1}^{n} a_{ij}^2 - a_{0j} a_{n+1\,j} = \rho, \ j = 1, \dots, n;$$

$$2 \sum_{i=1}^{n} a_{i0} a_{in+1} - a_{00} a_{n+1\,n+1} - a_{0\,n+1} a_{n+1\,0} = -\rho,$$

$$\sum_{i=1}^{n} a_{i0}^2 - a_{00} a_{n+1\,0} = 0, \ \sum_{i=1}^{n} a_{i\,n+1}^2 - a_{0\,n+1} a_{n+1\,n+1} = 0$$

defined on the region $D : \sum_{j=1}^{n} a_{0j} x_j + a_{0,n+1} \sum_{j=1}^{n} x_j^2 + a_{00} \neq 0$ from R^n.

The composite of two conformal transformations, the identical transformation and the (local) inverse of a conformal transformation, are conformal transformations on the respective domains of definition. Despite this fact, the set of all conformal transformations of R^n is not a group of transformations, since every conformal transformation is defined on a set of R^n and the intersection of these sets is the void set.

We assume

$$a_{ij} = a_{ij}(t), \ a_{i,n+1} = a_{i,n+1}(t), \ a_{i0} = a_{i0}(t),$$

$$a_{n+1,n+1} = a_{n+1,n+1}(t), \ a_{0j} = a_{0j}(t), \ a_{0,n+1} = a_{0,n+1}(t),$$

$$a_{00} = a_{00}(t), \ t \in (-\varepsilon, \varepsilon),$$

and

$$a_{ij}(0) = \delta_{ij}, \ a_{i\,n+1}(0) = 0, \ a_{i0}(0) = 0,$$

$$a_{n+1,n+1}(0) = 1, \; a_{0j}(0) = 0,$$

$$a_{0,n+1}(0) = 0, \; a_{00}(0) = 1.$$

Taking account of the relations

$$\sum_{i=1}^{n} a_{i\,n+1}^2 - a_{0,n+1}\, a_{n+1,n+1} = 0,$$

we find $\frac{da_{0n+1}}{dt}(0) = 0$. From these relations follows the conformal vector field

$$X = (X_1, \ldots, X_n),$$

$$X_i = \frac{dx_i'}{dt}(0) = \sum_{j=1}^{n} A_{ij} x_j + A_{i,n+1} \sum_{j=1}^{n} x_j^2 + A_{i0} + x_i \left(\sum_{j=1}^{n} A_{0j} x_j + A_{00} \right),$$

the notations being obvious by computing the derivative.

3.13. PROPOSED PROBLEMS

1. Determine a local diffeomorphism that rectifies the vector field $X = (X_1, X_2, X_3)$, $X_1 = x - y + z$, $X_2 = 2y - z$, $X_3 = z$ and control the result by direct calculation.

A. $x' = \frac{x+y}{z}$, $y' = \frac{y-z}{z^2}$, $z' = \ln|z|$, $z \neq 0$.

2. For each of the following vector fields, determine the field lines by the method of first integrals and fix a local rectifying diffeomorphism:

1) $V = xz\boldsymbol{i} + z(2x-y)\boldsymbol{j} - x^2\boldsymbol{k}$,
2) $V = x^2(y+z)\boldsymbol{i} - y^2(z+x)\boldsymbol{j} + z^2(y-x)\boldsymbol{k}$,
3) $V = y^2z^2\boldsymbol{i} + xyz^2\boldsymbol{j} + xy^2z\boldsymbol{k}$,
4) $V = xz\boldsymbol{i} + yz\boldsymbol{j} - (x^2+y^2)\boldsymbol{k}$,
5) $V = (y-z)\boldsymbol{i} + (z-x)\boldsymbol{j} + (x-y)\boldsymbol{k}$,
6) $V = x(y-z)\boldsymbol{i} - y(x-z)\boldsymbol{j} + z(x-y)\boldsymbol{k}$.

Hints.

1) $x^2 + z^2 = c_1$, $x(x-y) = c_2$;
2) $xyz = c_1$, $yz + xz - xy = c_2 xyz$;
3) $y^2 - z^2 = c_1$, $x^2 - y^2 = c_2$;
4) $x = c_1 y$, $x^2 + y^2 + z^2 = c_2$;
5) $x^2 + y^2 + z^2 = c_1$, $x + y + z = c_2$; 6) $xyz = c_1$, $x + y + z = c_2$.

3. (Sequel). The same problem for the vector fields:

1) $V = (x^2 - y^2 - z^2)\boldsymbol{i} + 2xy\boldsymbol{j} + 2xz\boldsymbol{k}$,
2) $V = x\boldsymbol{i} + y\boldsymbol{j} + (z + \sqrt{x^2+y^2+z^2})\boldsymbol{k}$,
3) $V = (x-y)\boldsymbol{i} + (x+y)\boldsymbol{j} + z\boldsymbol{k}$,
4) $V = y(x+y)\boldsymbol{i} - x(x+y)\boldsymbol{j} + (x-y)(2x+2y+z)\boldsymbol{k}$,
5) $V = x\boldsymbol{i} + y\boldsymbol{j} + (z - x^2 - y^2)\boldsymbol{k}$,
6) $V = y\boldsymbol{i} + x\boldsymbol{j} + 2xy\sqrt{a^2 - z^2}\boldsymbol{k}$,
7) $V = (x^2 - yz)\boldsymbol{i} + (y^2 - zx)\boldsymbol{j} + (z^2 - xy)\boldsymbol{k}$,
8) $V = (xy - 2z^2)\boldsymbol{i} + (4xz - y^2)\boldsymbol{j} + (yz - 2x^2)\boldsymbol{k}$.

Hints.

1) $y = c_1 z,\ x^2 + y^2 + z^2 = 2c_2 z;$ 2) $y = c_1 x,\ z = c_2 + \sqrt{x^2 + y^2 + z^2};$

3) $\dfrac{dz}{z} = \dfrac{1}{2}\dfrac{d(x^2+y^2)}{x^2+y^2} = \dfrac{d\left(\dfrac{y}{x}\right)}{1+\left(\dfrac{y}{z}\right)^2};$ 4) $x^2 + y^2 = c_1,\ (x+y)(x+y+z) = c_2;$

5) $y = c_1 x,\ z + x^2 + y^2 = c_2 x;$ 6) $x^2 - y^2 = c_1,\ \dfrac{1}{2}(x^2+y^2) = \arcsin\dfrac{z}{a} + c_2;$

7) $x - y = c_1(y - z),\ xy + yz + zx = c_2;$ 8) $z^2 + xy = c_1,\ x^2 + yz = c_2.$

4. Find the vector fields whose orbits are respectively:

1) $x^2 - yz = c_1,\ y^2 - zx = c_2;$ 2) $x^2 + \dfrac{1}{y^2} = C_1,\ y^2 + \dfrac{1}{z^2} = c_2;$

3) $x + \arcsin\dfrac{y}{z} = c_1,\ y + \arcsin\dfrac{x}{z} = c_2.$

Hint. $X = h\,\mathrm{grad}f \times \mathrm{grad}g.$

5. Solve the linear differential systems $x' = Ax$ in each of the following cases:

1) $A = \begin{bmatrix} 3 & -1 & 1 \\ 2 & 0 & 1 \\ 1 & -1 & 2 \end{bmatrix},\quad x(0) = \begin{bmatrix} 1 \\ -1 \\ 2 \end{bmatrix};$ 2) $A = \begin{bmatrix} 0 & 1 & 0 \\ 0 & 0 & 1 \\ -6 & -11 & -6 \end{bmatrix},\ x(0) = \begin{bmatrix} 1 \\ 0 \\ 0 \end{bmatrix};$

3) $A = \begin{bmatrix} -2 & 2 & -3 \\ 2 & 1 & -6 \\ -1 & -2 & 0 \end{bmatrix},\ x(0) = \begin{bmatrix} 8 \\ 0 \\ 0 \end{bmatrix};$ 4) $A = \begin{bmatrix} 2 & 1 & -1 \\ 1 & 2 & -1 \\ 3 & -3 & -1 \end{bmatrix};$

5) $A = \begin{bmatrix} 3 & 1 & 0 \\ -4 & -1 & 0 \\ 4 & -8 & -2 \end{bmatrix};$ 6) $A = \begin{bmatrix} 5 & -2 & 4 \\ 4 & -1 & 4 \\ 2 & 3 & 1 \end{bmatrix}.$

6. Approximate the solution for each of the following Cauchy problems, by the Runge-Kutta method:

$$\frac{dx}{dt} = xy^2,\ \frac{dy}{dt} = x^2 y,\ x(0) = 1,\ y(0) = -1,\ t \in [0, 1],\ h = 0, 1;$$

$$\frac{dx}{dt} = x(1 - 2y^2),\ \frac{dy}{dt} = -y(1 + 2x^2),\ \frac{dz}{dt} = 2z(x^2 + y^2);$$

$$x(0) = y(0) = z(0) = 1,\ t \in [0, 10],\ h = 0,2.$$

Then check the result using first integrals.

7. Study the completeness of the vector fields from Problems 2 and 3.

8. Consider the Hamiltonian $H(x,y) = \frac{1}{2}\sum_{k=1}^{3} y_k^2 + V(x)$. In each of the following cases, decide the flow generated by the Hamiltonian vector field associated to H:

$$V(x) = x_1 x_2 x_3,\ V(x) = x_1^2 + x_2^2 + x_3^2,\ V(x) = x_1^2 - x_2^2 + x_3.$$

Which of them is a global flow?

9. Determine the motion of an electron in a uniform static electromagnetic field, in which the vector fields $\boldsymbol{E}$ and $\boldsymbol{B}$ are collinear, assuming that the initial speed v_0 of the electron is perpendicular to the direction that is common to the two fields.

Hint. $m\ddot{r} = -q(\boldsymbol{E} + v \times \boldsymbol{B})$, where m is the mass of the electron and $q > 0$ is its charge. It follows that $x = \frac{v_0}{\omega}\sin\omega t$, $y = \frac{v_0}{\omega}(1 - \cos\omega t)$, $z = -\frac{qE}{2m}t^2$, $\omega = \frac{\varepsilon B}{m}$, $t \in R$; hence, the trajectory is a helix of variable step.

10. In each of the following cases, determine the flow generated by the vector field $\boldsymbol{X}$ and show that it preserves the volume:

$$\boldsymbol{X} = (xz, z(2x - y), -x^2),\quad \boldsymbol{X} = (yz, zx, xy),\quad \boldsymbol{X} = (x^2(y + z), -y^2(z + x), z^2(y - x)),$$

$$\boldsymbol{X} = \left(y, x, 4\frac{y^2}{x^2}\right),\ \boldsymbol{X} = (x(y - z), -y(x - z), z(x - y)),\quad \boldsymbol{X} = ((z - y)^2, z, y).$$

Hint. To find the flow, one may use first integrals.

11. In each of the following cases, determine the flow generated by the vector field $\boldsymbol{X}$ and show that it increases the volume:

$$\boldsymbol{X} = (x + y - z, x - y + z, -x + y + z),\ \boldsymbol{X} = (xy^2, x^2y, z(x^2 + y^2)),$$

$$\boldsymbol{X} = (x(y^2 - z^2), -y(x^2 + z^2), z(x^2 + y^2)),\ \boldsymbol{X} = (x(1 - 2y^2), y(1 + 2x^2), 2z(x^2 + y)).$$

Hint. To determine the flow, one may use first integrals.

12. In each of the following cases, determine the flow generated by the vector field $\boldsymbol{X}$ and show that it decreases the volume:

$$\boldsymbol{X} = (x(y^2 - x^2), y(x^2 - y^2), -2z(x^2 + y^2)),$$

$$\boldsymbol{X} = (-x(x^2 + 3y^2), -2y^3, -2y^2z),\quad \boldsymbol{X} = (3xy^2 - x^3, -2y^3, -2y^2z).$$

Hint. In order to determine the flow, one may use first integrals.

13. Write the infinitesimal transformations associated to the vector fields from Problems 10, 11, 12 and for each case, compute the Jacobian of the transformation.

14. Find the curvature and torsion of a field line of $\boldsymbol{X} = (yz, zx, xy)$.

4. STABILITY OF EQUILIBRIUM POINTS

Let us consider a physical system whose states x are described by an evolution differential system $\frac{dx}{dt} = X(x)$. *The fixed points of the flow of the vector field* X, *i.e., the zeros of* X, *are the equilibrium points of the system. If the physical system remains in a neighborhood of the equilibrium point* x_0 *when the evolution starts in a neighborhood of* x_0, *then the point* x_0 *is said to be stable; if not, it is said to be unstable.*

Small oscillations of a plane pendulum and the motion of a rigid solid body are analysed in 4.1 from the point of view of a mathematical definition of the stability of equilibrium points. In 4.2 is presented the stability of equilibrium points generated by the zeros of linear vector fields with application in the Theory of Electric Circuits, while in 4.3 it is shown that equilibrium points in the plane may be: rotation points, attractors, saddle points, etc.

Sometimes, the problem of stability of equilibrium points can be solved by indirect methods. Among these, the most common are the method of linear approximation, which will be applied to differential systems describing biochemical processes or electric circuits (see 4.4) and the method of Lyapunov functions, which is suitable especially for Hamiltonian systems (see 4.5).

In 4.6, some problems concerning stability and classification of equilibrium points are proposed.

4.1. PROBLEM OF STABILITY

Let us consider a physical system whose behaviour in time is described by the autonomous differential system (i.e., does not contain the independent variable explicitly):

$$\frac{dx}{dt} = X(x), \; x = (x_1, \dots, x_n) \in D \subset R^n, \tag{1}$$

$X = (X_1, \dots, X_n)$ being a vector field of convenient class on an open connected set D. The vector field X describes locally the evolution of the system [$X(x)$ gives the velocity of variation].

If a is a point from D for which $X(a) = 0$, then $x(t) = a$ for any $t \in R$, is a solution of the system (1) verifying the initial conditions $x(t_0) = a$. Such a solution is called an *equilibrium point*. From an intuitive point of view, we say that the equilibrium point a is stable if any solution of (1) starting at $t = t_0$ from a point sufficiently close to a remains in a neighborhood of a for $t > t_0$. We assume that X is C^1 on D in order to assure the existence and uniqueness of solutions of the Cauchy problems, and we denote $t \to x(t, x_0)$ the solution of (1) which verifies the initial conditions $x(t_0, x_0) = x_0$.

The equilibrium point a of the system (1) is called (Fig.47):

1) *stable*, if there exists a neighborhood V of the point a such that $x_0 \in V$ implies the existence of the solution $t \to x(t, x_0)$, $t \in [t_0, \infty)$ and if $\lim\limits_{x_0 \to a} x(t, x_0) = a$, uniformly with respect to $t \in [t_0, \infty)$;

2) *asymptotically stable*, if it is stable and there exists a neighborhood $U \subset V$ of *the point a* such that $x_0 \in U$ implies $\lim\limits_{t \to \infty} x(t, x_0) = a$;

3) *unstable*, if it is not stable.

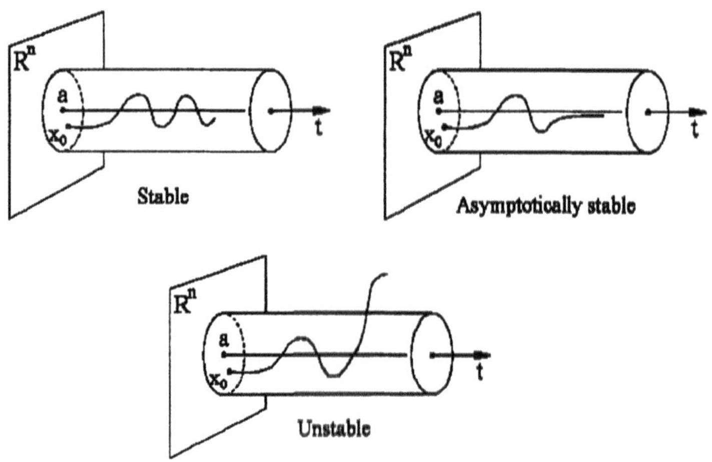

Fig.47. Graph of Solution

We notice that a non-isolated equilibrium point a may be stable, but not asymptotically stable. Indeed, if x_0 is a point of equilibrium different from the point a, then $\lim\limits_{t \to \infty} x(t, x_0) = x_0 \neq a$.

Theorem. *Let X be a C^1 vector field on an open connected set $D \subset R^n$ and $\alpha : [t_0, \infty) \to D$ a field line of X. If there exists $\lim\limits_{t \to \infty} \alpha(t) = x_1 \in D$, then x_1 is a zero of X (a point of equilibrium of the differential system (1)).*

Proof. From the hypothesis and from $\alpha(t) = \alpha(t_0) + \int_{t_0}^{t} X(\alpha(t))\,dt$ it follows that

$x_1 = \alpha(t_0) + \int_{t_0}^{\infty} X(\alpha(t))dt$. The convergence of the integral and the existence of $\lim_{t\to\infty} X(\alpha(t)) = X(x_1)$ imply $X(x_1) = 0$.

Applications. 1) *The small oscillations of a plane pendulum* (Fig.48). The autonomous system $\frac{dx}{dt} = y$, $\frac{dy}{dt} = -x$ admits the equilibrium point $(0,0)$. Differentiating the first equation with respect to t and taking account of the second equation, we obtain $\frac{d^2x}{dt^2} + x = 0$ (the equation of small oscillations of the pendulum about the inferior equilibrium position) with the general solution $x(t) = c_1 \cos t + c_2 \sin t$, $t \in R$. It follows that $y(t) = c_2 \cos t - c_1 \sin t$, $t \in R$.

Let us have the initial conditions $t = 0$, $x(0) = x_0$, $y(0) = y_0$, $(x_0, y_0) \in R^2$. The field line satisfying them is the circle

$$x(t) = x_0 \cos t + y_0 \sin t,\ y(t) = y_0 \cos t - x_0 \sin t,\ t \in R.$$

The equilibrium point $(0,0)$ is stable, since

$$\lim_{\substack{x_0 \to 0 \\ y_0 \to 0}} x(t) = 0 = \lim_{\substack{x_0 \to 0 \\ y_0 \to 0}} y(t) \quad \text{for any} \quad t \in [0, \infty).$$

It is not asymptotically stable, since $\lim_{t\to\infty} x(t)$ does not exist.

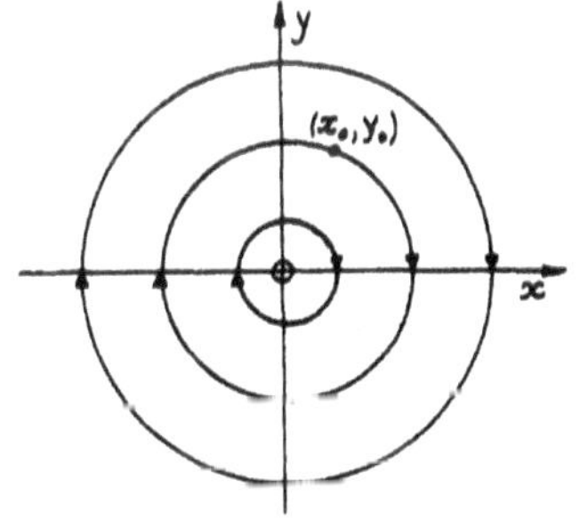

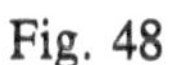
Fig. 48

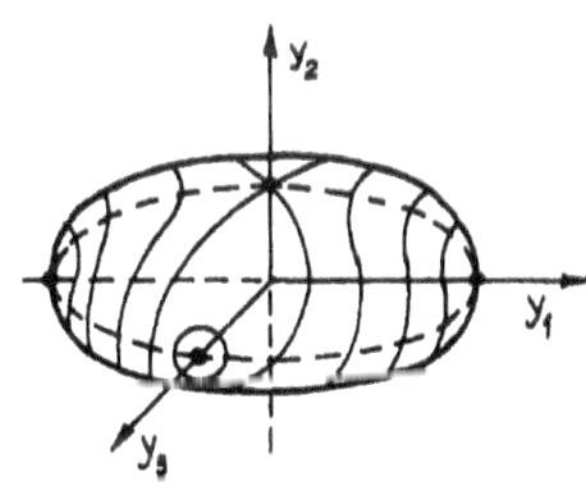

Fig. 49

2) *The motion of a rigid solid body around a fix point* O (arbitrary rotation!) is characterized by Euler Equations

$$I_1 \frac{dx_1}{dt} = (I_2 - I_3)x_2 x_3, \; I_2 \frac{dx_2}{dt} = (I_3 - I_1)x_3 x_1, \; I_3 \frac{dx_3}{dt} = (I_1 - I_2)x_1 x_2,$$

where (x_1, x_2, x_3) are the components of the angular velocity, while I_1, I_2, I_3 are the principal moments of inertia with respect to the point O. The Cartesian axes Ox_1, Ox_2, Ox_3 coincide with the principal axes of inertia with respect to O. They consist of equilibrium points of the preceding differential system.

The system admits global first integrals $I_1 x_1^2 + I_2 x_2^2 + I_3 x_3^2$ (energy), $I_1^2 x_1^2 + I_2^2 x_2^2 + I_3^2 x_3^2$ (angular moment) and, consequently, the general solution $I_1 x_1^2 + I_2 x_2^2 + I_3 x_3^2 = c_1$, $I_1^2 x_1^2 + I_2^2 x_2^2 + I_3^2 x_3^2 = c_2$ (defined with respect to time t on the whole real axis).

To comment on the orbits, we use the diffeomorphism

$$y_1 = I_1 x_1, \; y_2 = I_2 x_2, \; y_3 = I_3 x_3$$

that transfers the preceding families of ellipsoids into a family of ellipsoids

$$\frac{y_1^2}{I_1} + \frac{y_2^2}{I_2} + \frac{y_3^2}{I_3} = c_1 = 2E$$

and a family of spheres

$$y_1^2 + y_2^2 + y_3^2 = c_2 = \|y\|^2,$$

where $y = (y_1, y_2, y_3)$ is the kinetic momentum vector of the solid body with respect to O. We assume $I_3 < I_2 < I_1$, fix $E > 0$, and make the radius $\|y\|$ of the sphere vary (Fig.49). The semiaxes of the ellipsoid are $\sqrt{2EI_3} < \sqrt{2EI_2} < \sqrt{2EI_1}$. If $\|y\| < \sqrt{2EI_1}$, then the intersection is void and hence there are no motions with such values of E and $\|y\|$. If $\|y\| = \sqrt{2EI_3}$, then the intersection reduces to two points (equilibrium points), while for $\sqrt{2EI_2} < \|y\| < \sqrt{2EI_1}$ one finds two closed curves about these endpoints. For $\|y\| = \sqrt{2EI_2}$, the intersection consists of two circles passing through the endpoints of the middle axis (equilibrium points).

The equilibrium points $(a,0,0)$ or $(0,0,c)$ are stable, since for a small deviation of the initial condition from the point $(a,0,0)$ or $(0,0,c)$, the trajectory will be a closed curve in a small neighborhood of the respective equilibrium position. The equilibrium point $(0,b,0)$, $b \neq 0$, is unstable, since a small deviation from this point determines closed orbits which do not lie entirely in a small neighborhood of the equilibrium point (see Fig.49 giving the orbits of Euler equations on a surface of constant level of the energy).

4.2. STABILITY OF ZEROS OF LINEAR VECTOR FIELDS

Let us consider the homogeneous linear differential system with constant coefficients

$$\frac{dx}{dt} = Ax, \tag{2}$$

where A is an $n\times n$ matrix of real elements, while x is a column vector. The equilibrium points of this system are generated by the solutions of the algebraic system $Ax = 0$ (a homogeneous linear system of n equations with n unknowns). Obviously, among these there is also the point $x(t) = 0,\ t \in R$, whose stability will be our next aim. The study of stability for any other equilibrium point reduces to that of $x = 0$ by a translation. The equilibrium point $x = 0$ is isolated if and only if $\det A \neq 0$.

Theorem. *Let $x(t) = 0,\ t \in R$ be an equilibrium point.*

1) If all the proper values of the matrix A have strictly negative real part, then the equilibrium point is stable and asymptotically stable.

2) We assume that all the proper values of the matrix A have negative real part, and each purely imaginary proper value (if it exists) has the property that the dimension of the attached proper space is equal to the multiplicity of the proper value. If among the proper values of A there is a purely imaginary one, then the equilibrium point is stable, but not asymptotically stable.

3) If a proper value of the matrix A has strictly positive real part, or if there exists a purely imaginary proper value such that the dimension of the attached proper subspace is less than the multiplicity of the proper value, then the equilibrium point is not stable.

Proof. The general solution of a homogeneous linear system with constant coefficients can be written as (see 3.4)

$$x(t) = \varphi(t; c_1, \dots, c_n) = c_1 x_1(t) + \cdots + c_n x_n(t) = w(t)c,\ t \in R,$$

where $x_1(t), \dots, x_n(t)$ are linearly independent solutions, $w(t) = [x_1(t), \dots, x_n(t)]$ is the Wronski matrix and $c = {}^t[c_1, \dots, c_n]$. From this we get the solution that satisfies the initial condition $x(t_0) = x_0$ and then $w(t_0)c = x_0$. Since $w(t_0) \neq 0$ (the particular solutions are linearly independent), the matrix x_0 tends to the zero matrix if and only if the matrix c tends to the zero matrix.

The elements of the column matrix $x(t)$ are *quasipolynomials*.

1) Each term of the general solution contains factors of type $e^{\alpha t}$, $\alpha < 0$. The relation $\lim_{t\to\infty} e^{\alpha t} = 0$ implies

$$\lim_{c\to 0} \varphi(t; c) = 0 \text{ (the zero matrix), for any } t \in [t_0, \infty), \tag{*}$$

$$\lim_{t\to\infty} \varphi(t; c) = 0 \text{ (the zero matrix).} \tag{**}$$

(the limit of a matrix is the matrix of limits!) Thus, the equilibrium point is stable and asymptotically stable.

2) We assume that the matrix A also has purely imaginary values. The relation (*) holds in this case, too. But $\varphi(t;c)$ also contains terms of type $C_j \sin\beta t$, while $\lim_{t\to\infty} \sin\beta t$ does not exist. Therefore, the relation (**) is not fulfilled. In other words, the equilibrium point is stable, but not asymptotically stable.

3) There exist factors of type $e^{\alpha t}$, $\alpha > 0$, and $\lim_{t\to\infty} e^{\alpha t} = \infty$ or unbounded factors of type $t\sin t$ and $\lim_{t\to\infty} (t\sin t)$ does not exist. Therefore, the relation (*) cannot take place (due to uniform limits with respect to t).

Comment. The study of stability for the equilibrium point $x = 0$ can be made starting from the fact that the solution of the Cauchy problem $\frac{dx}{dt} = Ax$, $x(0) = x_0$ is $x(t) = e^{tA}x_0$, $t \in R$. But then the theorems regarding the exponential matrix and some lemmas such as the following are necessary.

Lemma. *If all the proper values, in the set of complex numbers* C, *of the real quadratic matrix* A *have strictly negative real parts, then there exist constants* $M > 0$ *and* $a > 0$ *such that* $\|e^{tA}\| \le Me^{-at}$, $t \in [0,\infty)$.

Proof. Each element of the matrix e^{tA} is a quasipolynomial, which is a finite linear combination of functions of the form $P(t)e^{\lambda t}$, where $P(t) = \sum_{k=0}^{m} c_k t^k$, while λ is a proper value of the matrix A.

Let $\alpha > 0$. From $e^{\alpha t} = \sum_{k=0}^{\infty} \frac{(\alpha t)^k}{k!}$, $t \in [0,\infty)$ we infer $t^k < \frac{k!}{\alpha^k} e^{\alpha t}$, $t \in [0,\infty)$. Imposing $0 < \alpha < -Re\lambda$ and denoting $\gamma = -Re\lambda - \alpha > 0$, we get

$$t^k e^{tRe\lambda} < \frac{k!}{\alpha^k} e^{-t\gamma},\ t \in [0,\infty).$$

Consequently, for $t \in [0,\infty)$ we obtain

$$|P(t)e^{\lambda t}| \le e^{tRe\lambda} \sum_{k=0}^{m} |c_k| t^k \le e^{-\gamma t} \sum_{k=0}^{m} |c_k| \frac{k!}{\alpha^k}$$

and thus the lemma becomes obvious.

The proper values of a real skew-symmetric matrix A are purely imaginary and each purely imaginary proper value has the property that the dimension of the associated proper subspace is equal to the multiplicity of the proper value. Therefore, the zeros of the Killing vector fields Ax are stable, but not asymptotically stable.

In order to be more effective in applications of the preceding theorem, we need to establish if the roots of the characteristic polynomial of the matrix A have strictly negative real part, without really computing these roots. In this sense, we can use either the fact that a polynomial with real coefficients whose roots in C have strictly negative real parts must have strictly positive coefficients, or the

Hurwitz Criterion. *The roots of the polynomial*

$$f(z) = a_0 z^n + a_1 z^{n-1} + \cdots + a_{n-1} z + a_n,\ a_i \in R,\ a_0 > 0,\ a_n \neq 0,\ z \in C,$$

have strictly negative real part if and only if $a_i > 0$ *and the matrix*

$$\begin{bmatrix} a_1 & a_0 & 0 & \dots & \dots & 0 \\ a_3 & a_2 & a_1 & a_0 & \dots & 0 \\ \dots & \dots & \dots & \dots & \dots & \dots \\ a_{2n-1} & a_{2n-2} & \dots & \dots & \dots & a_n \end{bmatrix}, \quad \text{where } a_s = 0 \text{ for } s > n,$$

has all the principal minors strictly positive.

Examples. We assume $a_0 = 1$. If $n = 2$, that is $f(z) = z^2 + a_1 z + a_2$, the Hurwitz conditions $a_1 > 0$, $\begin{vmatrix} a_1 & 1 \\ 0 & a_2 \end{vmatrix} > 0$ are equivalent to $a_1 > 0,\ a_2 > 0$. Therefore, the region of stability of the trivial solution of the differential system (respectively, differential equation) for which $z^2 + a_1 z + a_2$ is a characteristic polynomial, coincides with the first (open) quadrant from the plane $a_1 O a_2$.

If $n = 3$, that is, $f(z) = z^3 + a_1 z^2 + a_2 z + a_3$, the Hurwitz conditions are $a_1 > 0$, $\begin{vmatrix} a_1 & 1 \\ a_3 & a_2 \end{vmatrix} > 0$, $\begin{vmatrix} a_1 & 1 & 0 \\ a_3 & a_2 & a_1 \\ 0 & 0 & a_3 \end{vmatrix} > 0$. Taking into account that $a_2 > 0,\ a_3 > 0$, these reduce to $a_3 < a_1 a_2,\ a_1 > 0,\ a_2 > 0,\ a_3 > 0$, that is the region of the first octant of the Cartesian frame $Oa_1 a_2 a_3$ situated between the plane $a_3 = 0$ and the saddle $a_3 = a_1 a_2$ (Fig.50).

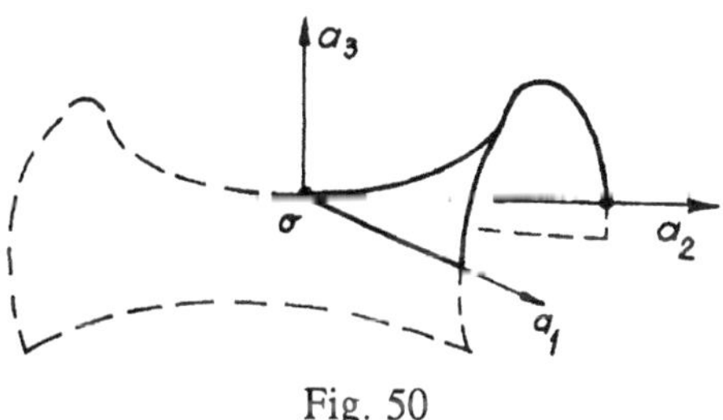

Fig. 50

Applications. 1) Study the stability of the equilibrium points of the linear differential systems

$$\begin{cases} \dfrac{dx}{dt} = 3x + y, \\ \dfrac{dx}{dt} = -2x + y, \end{cases} \qquad \begin{cases} \dfrac{dx}{dt} = -2x - y \\ \dfrac{dy}{dt} = 3x - y, \end{cases} \qquad \begin{cases} \dfrac{dx}{dt} = -x + z \\ \dfrac{dy}{dt} = -2y - z \\ \dfrac{dz}{dt} = y - z. \end{cases}$$

Solution. 1) The matrix $A = \begin{bmatrix} 3 & 1 \\ -2 & 1 \end{bmatrix}$ has the proper values $2 \pm i$, with strictly positive real parts. Therefore, the equilibrium point $x = 0,\ y = 0$ is not stable.

2) The matrix $A = \begin{bmatrix} -2 & -1 \\ 3 & -1 \end{bmatrix}$ has the proper values $-\dfrac{5}{2},\ -\dfrac{1}{2}$, that are strictly negative. Therefore, the equilibrium point $(0, 0)$ is asymptotically stable.

3) The matrix $A = \begin{bmatrix} -1 & 0 & 1 \\ 0 & -2 & -1 \\ 0 & 1 & -1 \end{bmatrix}$ has the proper values $-1,\ \dfrac{-3 \pm 3i}{2}$, with strictly negative real parts. Therefore, $(0, 0, 0)$ is asymptotically stable.

2) The stability of an electric circuit with negative resistance [11].

Let us study the stability of a circuit consisting of a series resistance R with inductance L, having also a resistance r and a capacity C in derivation (Fig.51). L, C, R, r are interpreted as real parameters, while the states of the physical system are characterized by the linear differential system

$$\frac{di_L}{dt} = -\frac{R}{L} i_L + \frac{1}{CL} q, \quad \frac{dq}{dt} = i_L - \frac{1}{Cr} q.$$

The matrix $A = \begin{bmatrix} -\dfrac{R}{L} & \dfrac{1}{CL} \\ -1 & -\dfrac{1}{Cr} \end{bmatrix}$ has the characteristic equation

$$\lambda^2 + \left(\frac{R}{L} + \frac{1}{Cr}\right)\lambda + \frac{1}{LC}\left(\frac{R}{r} + 1\right) = 0.$$

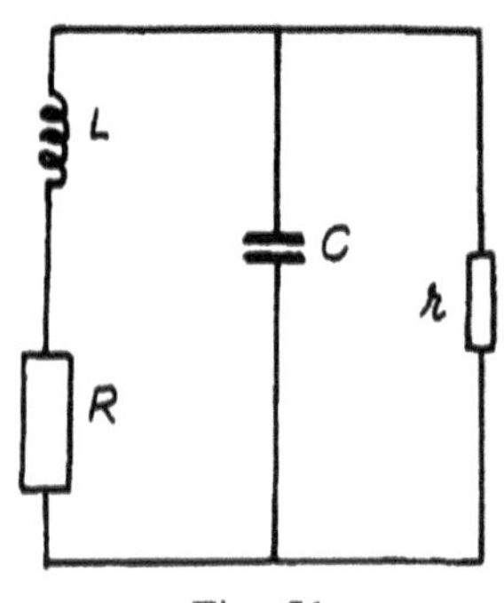

Fig. 51

The point $(0,0)$ is asymptotically stable if and only if

$$\frac{R}{L}+\frac{1}{Cr}>0,\ \frac{1}{LC}\left(\frac{R}{r}+1\right)>0.$$

Assuming $L>0,\ C>0$, the asymptotic stability conditions reduce to $R+\frac{L}{Cr}>0,\ 1+\frac{R}{r}>0$. The last ones are examined within two hypotheses:

(1) $R<0$, the case of negative resistance due to electronic devices with S type - characteristic (e.g., the unloading tubes in gas);

(2) $r<0$, the case of negative resistance due to electronic devices with N type - characteristic (e.g., some grid screens tubes).

4.3. CLASSIFICATION OF EQUILIBRIUM POINTS IN THE PLANE

Let there be the C^1 vector field $X=(X_1,X_2)$ on R^2 and the differential system

$$\frac{dx}{dt}=X(x),\ x=(x_1,x_2),$$

giving the field lines. We assume that $x=0$ is an isolated zero of the vector field X and hence the solution of the system verifying the conditions $x(0)=0$ is the equilibrium point $x(t)=0,\ t\in R$ (This means that no solution $x(t)\neq 0$ tends to zero within a finite interval of time).

If any neighborhood of $x=0$ contains closed orbits around $x=0$, then the equilibrium point $x(t)=0,\ t\in R$, is called a *rotation point*. The rotation point $x=0$ with the property that every orbit from a neighborhood of $x=0$, different from $x(t)=0,\ t\in R$, is closed is called a *centre* (Fig.52).

The equilibrium point $x(t)=0,\ t\in R$, is called an *attractor* for $t=\infty$ (or $t=-\infty$) if all the solutions $x(t,x_0)$ of the problems $x'=X(x),\ x(0)=x_0$, with $\|x\|<\varepsilon$, can be prolonged to $t\in[0,\infty)$ (respectively, to $t\in[0,-\infty)$) and $\lim_{t\to\infty}x(t,x_0)=0$ (respectively, $\lim_{t\to-\infty}x(t,x_0)=0$).

Let us be given the field line $x(t,x_0)=(x_1(t,x_0),x_2(t,x_0))$ and $\theta(t)$ a continuous determination of the polar angle $\mathrm{Arc\,tan}\,\frac{x_2(t,x_0)}{x_1(t,x_0)}$. The attractor $x(t)=0,\ t\in R$, for $t=\infty$ is called (Fig.52):

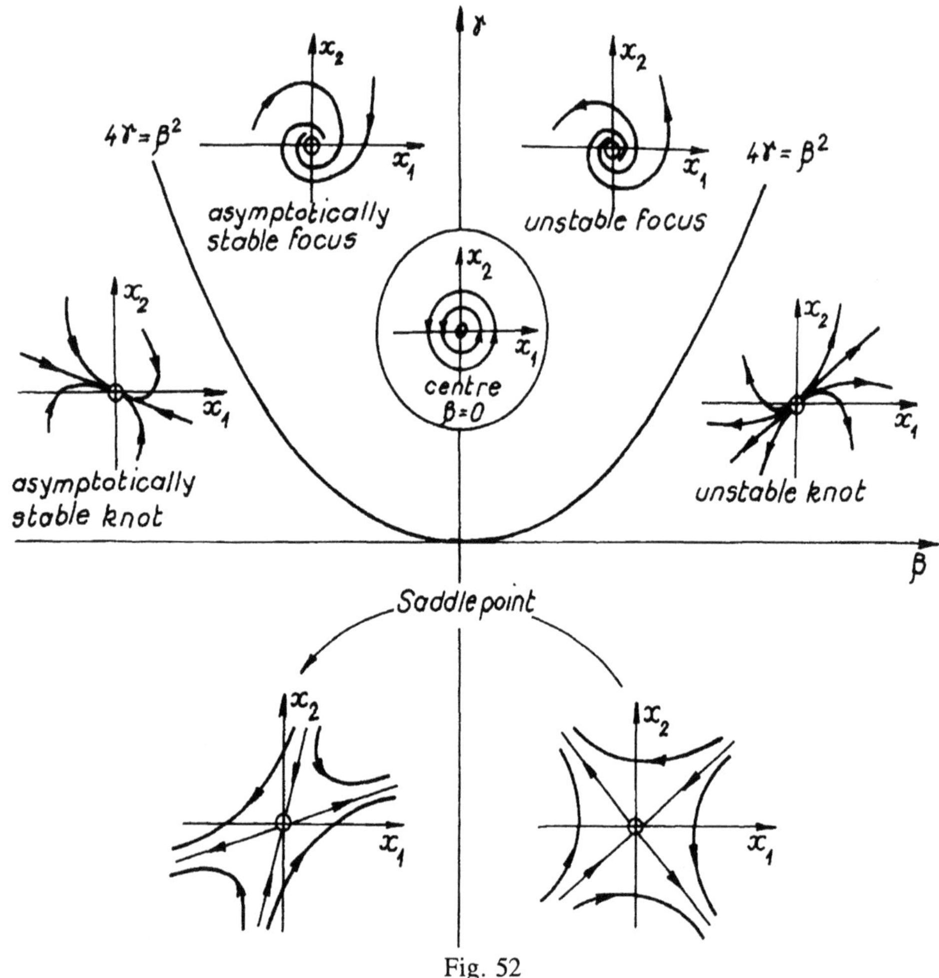

Fig. 52

1) *focus,* if every field line $x(t,x_0) \not\equiv 0$ is a spiral around the origin, that is, a curve with the property $\lim\limits_{t\to\infty} \theta(t) = \pm\infty$;

2) *knot,* if for any field line $x(t,x_0) \not\equiv 0$ it holds that $\lim\limits_{t\to\infty} \theta(t) = \theta_0$ (finite); the limit slope $\tan\theta_0$ together with the asymptotic point $x = 0$ of the field line determine a straight line representing the limit of the tangent to the field line.

The knot $x(t) = 0$, $t \in R$, for $t = \infty$ is called a *proper knot* if for any $\theta_0 (\bmod 2\pi)$

there exists a single field line $x(t,x_0)$ such that $\lim_{t\to\infty} \theta(t) = \theta_0$; otherwise, that knot is called *improper*.

Analogously we can classify the attractors for $t = -\infty$.

There exist some attractors that are neither focuses, nor knots.

The simplest point that is not an attractor is the *saddle point*. This is an equilibrium point $x(t) = 0$, $t \in R$, with the property that only finitely many solutions $x(t,x_0)$ tend to 0 when $t \to \infty$ or $t \to -\infty$ (Fig.52).

We illustrate the preceding ideas by a linear system

$$\frac{dx}{dt} = Ax,\ A = \begin{bmatrix} a_{11} & a_{12} \\ a_{21} & a_{22} \end{bmatrix},\ \det A \neq 0,\ a_{ij} \in R.$$

One notices that $x(t) = 0$, $t \in R$ is the single equilibrium point. The proper values λ_1, λ_2 of the matrix A are the solutions of the equation with real coefficients

$$\lambda^2 - \beta\lambda + \gamma = 0,\ \beta = a_{11} + a_{22},\ \gamma = a_{11}a_{22} - a_{12}a_{21},$$

$$\text{that is } \lambda_1 = \frac{\beta + \sqrt{\beta^2 - 4\gamma}}{2},\ \lambda_2 = \frac{\beta - \sqrt{\beta^2 - 4\gamma}}{2}.$$

Let $\beta^2 - 4\gamma = 0$, i. e., $\lambda_1 = \lambda_2 = \lambda$. If there exist two linearly independent proper vectors u_1, u_2 (which takes place iff $a_{11} = a_{22} \neq 0$, $a_{12} = a_{21} = 0$), then the general solution of the system is $x(t) = (C_1u_1 + C_2u_2)e^{\lambda t}$, $t \in R$. If there exist a single proper vector u and a principal vector v, then the general solution of the system is $x(t) = [(C_1 + C_2t)u + C_2v]e^{\lambda t}$, $t \in R$. As a result the following assertions are true (Fig.52):

1) $x(t) = 0$, $t \in R$, is a centre if and only if $Re\lambda_1 = Re\lambda_2 = 0$;

2) $x(t) = 0$, $t \in R$, is an attractor for $t = \infty$ (or $t = -\infty$) if and only if $Re\lambda_k < 0$ (or > 0), $k = 1, 2$;

- the attractor $x(t) = 0$, $t \in R$, is a focus if and only if λ_1, λ_2 are complex conjugates but not real or purely imaginary;

- the attractor $x(t) = 0$, $t \in R$, is a proper knot if $\lambda_1 = \lambda_2$ and there exist two proper vectors;

- the attractor $x(t) = 0$, $t \in R$, is an improper knot if $\lambda_1, \lambda_2 > 0$ or $\lambda_1, \lambda_2 < 0$ and $\lambda_1 \neq \lambda_2$ or $\lambda_1 = \lambda_2$ with a single proper vector;

3) $x(t) = 0$, $t \in R$, is a saddle point if $\lambda_1\lambda_2 < 0$.

The classification from the point of view of stability (with respect to λ_1, λ_2; see 4.2) is obvious. Its illustration in the plane $\beta O\gamma$ is very interesting (Fig.52):

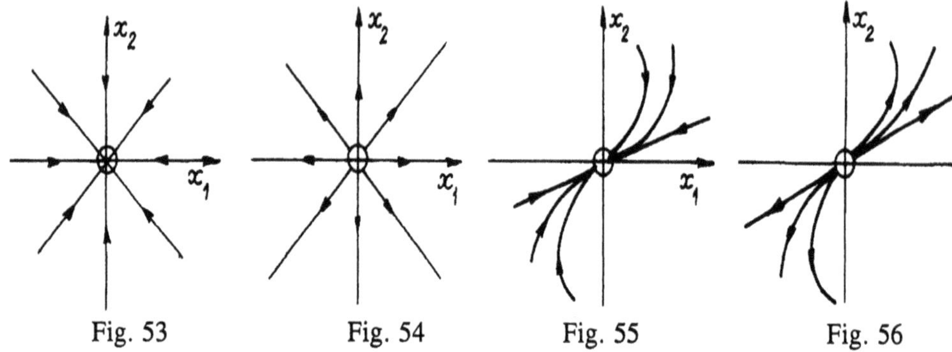

Fig. 53 Fig. 54 Fig. 55 Fig. 56

1) if $\beta = 0,\ \gamma > 0$, then the origin is a *centre (neutral stable point)*;

2) if $\beta > 0,\ \gamma > 0,\ \gamma > \frac{\beta^2}{4}$, then the origin is an *unstable focus*;

3) if $\beta < 0,\ \gamma > 0,\ \gamma > \frac{\beta^2}{4}$, then the origin is a *(stable and) asymptotically stable focus*;

4) if $\beta > 0,\ \gamma > 0,\ \gamma < \frac{\beta^2}{4}$, then the origin is an *unstable knot*;

5) $\beta < 0,\ \gamma > 0,\ \gamma < \frac{\beta^2}{4}$: the origin is a *(stable and) asymptotically stable knot*;

6) if $\gamma < 0,\ \gamma \neq \frac{\beta^2}{4}$, then the origin is a *saddle point*; any saddle point is unstable.

If $\beta^2 - 4\gamma = 0$ and there exist two proper vectors, then: (1) for $\lambda = \frac{\beta}{2} < 0$ the origin is a *(stable and) asymptotically stable knot* (Fig.53); (2) for $\lambda = \frac{\beta}{2} > 0$ the origin is an *unstable proper knot* (Fig. 54).

If $\beta^2 - 4\gamma = 0$ and there exists a single proper vector, then: (1) for $\lambda = \frac{\beta}{2} < 0$ the origin is a *(stable and) asymptotically stable improper knot* (Fig.55); (2) for $\lambda = \frac{\beta}{2} > 0$ the origin is an *unstable improper knot* (fig.56).

Application. The mechanical vibrations with one degree of freedom [57] and the behaviour of the autonomous electric circuits [11] are described by differential equations of type $\frac{d^2x}{dt^2} = \varphi\left(x, \frac{dx}{dt}\right)$. Denoting the velocity $\frac{dx}{dt}$ by y, we get the system

$$\frac{dx}{dt} = y, \quad \frac{dy}{dt} = \varphi(x, y).$$

The equilibrium points of this system verify $y = 0$, $\varphi(x,0) = 0$, that is, they are points on the axis Ox from the plane xOy. The classification of these equilibrium points in the above manner gives us topological information concerning the states of vibration and, respectively, the states of circuits.

4.4. STABILITY BY LINEAR APPROXIMATION

We consider the autonomous differential system

$$\frac{dx_i}{dt} = X_i(x_1, \dots, x_n),\ i = 1, \dots, n.$$

From the physical point of view such a differential system is interpreted as the local law of evolution of a process. The points at which $X = (X_1, \dots, X_n)$ vanishes generate the equilibrium points of the differential system. Their stability is most useful for concrete problems.

The case of a homogeneous linear differential system with constant coefficients was already discussed in 4.2. This case is important in itself, but also for the fact that more general situations are often reduced to it.

Suppose $X = (X_1, \dots, X_n)$ is a C^2 vector field on $D \subset R^n$ and $x = 0$ is an equilibrium point (the study of any other equilibrium point is reduced to the case $x = 0$ by a translation). The conditions $X_i(0) = 0$ and the differentiability of X imply

$$X_i(x) = \sum_{j=1}^{n} \frac{\partial X_i}{\partial x_j}(0)x_j + \|x\| F_i(x),\ \lim_{x \to 0} F_i(x) = 0.$$

Assume that $A = \left[\frac{\partial X_i}{\partial x_j}(0)\right]$ is not the zero matrix and we use the matrix language. To the differential system

$$\frac{dx}{dt} = Ax + \|x\| F(x) \tag{3}$$

one attaches the homogeneous linear differential system with constant coefficients

$$\frac{dx}{dt} = Ax,$$

called the *linear approximation* of (3).

The next theorem shows that the perturbation $\|x\| F(x)$ does not destroy the asymptotic stability of the equilibrium point $x = 0$, if this asymptotic stability is stated for the linear approximation.

Theorem. *1) If all the proper values of the matrix A have strictly negative real parts, then the equilibrium point $x = 0$ of the differential system (3) is asymptotically stable (and therefore stable).*

2) If the matrix A has a proper value whose real part is strictly positive, then the equilibrium point $x = 0$ of the differential system (3) is unstable.

Proof. Since the vector field X is of class C^2, the solution $x(t, x_0)$ of the differential system (3) is of class C^1 with respect to the point $x_0 = x(t_0, x_0)$.

1) For simplification of the expression we suppose $t_0 = 0$, and instead of $x(t, x_0)$ we shall write $x(t)$. The solution $x(t)$ of the differential system (3) verifies the integral equation

$$x(t) = e^{tA} x_0 + \int_0^t e^{(t-s)A} \|x(s)\| F(x(s))\, ds.$$

As all proper values of the matrix A, in the set C of complex numbers, have strictly negative real parts, by the lemma in 4.2, there exist $k > 0$, $\alpha > 0$ such that

$$\| e^{tA} x_0 \| \le K \|x_0\| e^{-\alpha t}, \quad \| e^{(t-s)A} \| \le K e^{-\alpha(t-s)}.$$

On the other hand, the fact that $\lim\limits_{x \to 0} F(x) = 0$ is equivalent to: $\forall\, \varepsilon > 0$, $\exists\, \delta > 0$, such that $\|x\| < \delta$ to imply $\|F(x)\| < \varepsilon$. Consequently

$$\| x(t) \| \le K e^{-\alpha t} \|x_0\| + K \varepsilon \int_0^t e^{-\alpha(t-s)} \| x(s) \|\, ds.$$

We fix $\varepsilon = \dfrac{\alpha}{2k}$, multiply by $e^{\alpha t}$ and denote

$$f(t) = e^{\alpha t} \| x(t) \|, \quad k = K \|x_0\|, \quad h(t) = K\varepsilon.$$

Then we have the conditions of Gronwall's lemma (see 3.7) and therefore

$$e^{\alpha t} \| x(t) \| \le K \|x_0\| e^{\frac{\alpha}{2} t}.$$

For $\|x_0\|$ sufficiently small, it follows that

$$\| x(t) \| \le K \|x_0\| e^{-\frac{\alpha}{2} t}, \quad \forall\, t \in [0, \infty),$$

a relation that implies stability and asymptotic stability.

2) We refer the reader to [1], [4], [27], [28] since the proof is too complicated to reproduce here.

Remarks. 1) Let $x = 0$ be an equilibrium point of the differential system (1). If $\det \left[\dfrac{\partial X_i}{\partial x_j}(0) \right] \ne 0$, then $x = 0$ is an isolated equilibrium point. The converse is true only if the vector field X is a linear field.

2) Finding the equilibrium point of the differential system (1) is reduced to solving the algebraic system

$$X_1(x_1, \ldots, x_n) = 0, \; \ldots, \; X_n(x_1, \ldots, x_n) = 0. \tag{4}$$

We build the energy (see chapter 9)

$$f(x) = \frac{1}{2} \| X(x) \|^2 = \frac{1}{2} \sum_{i=1}^{n} X_i^2(x).$$

Obviously $f(x) = 0$ if and only if $X(x) = 0$. Also we remark that critical points of the energy f are given as solutions of the system

$$\frac{\partial f}{\partial x_1}(x) = X_1(x)\frac{\partial X_1}{\partial x_1}(x) + \cdots + X_n(x)\frac{\partial X_n}{\partial x_1}(x) = 0$$

$$\cdots\cdots\cdots\cdots\cdots\cdots\cdots\cdots\cdots\cdots\cdots\cdots\cdots\cdots\cdots\cdots\cdots\cdots\cdots$$

$$\frac{\partial f}{\partial x_n}(x) = X_1(x)\frac{\partial X_1}{\partial x_n}(x) + \cdots + X_n(x)\frac{\partial X_n}{\partial x_n}(x) = 0.$$

Suppose $\det\left[\frac{\partial X_i}{\partial x_j}(x)\right] \neq 0$, excepting a finite number of points eliminated from the argument. In other words, we assume that the functions X_i, $i = 1, \ldots, n$, are functionally independent. Under this condition the solutions of the algebraic system (4) are isolated (if they exist), and the set of these solutions coincides with the set of global minimum points of the energy f. Thus finding the isolated solutions of the algebraic system (4) is reduced to finding the minimum points of the function f. A specific numerical method for solving such problems is the gradient method.

Example. Find the zeros of the vector field

$$\boldsymbol{X} = (X_1, X_2),\ X_1(x,y) = x^3 + y^3 - 2,\ X_2(x,y) = x - y$$

using the gradient method.

Solution. One remarks that $\boldsymbol{X}(1,1) = (0,0)$. Since

$$\frac{D(X_1, X_2)}{D(x,y)} = -3(x^2 + y^2) = 0$$

if and only if $x = y = 0$, the origin is excluded from the argument.

We build the energy function

$$2f(x,y) = (x-y)^2 + (x^3 + y^3 - 2)^2$$

whose gradient is

$$\operatorname{grad} f = [(x-y) + 3x^2(x^3+y^3-2)]\boldsymbol{i} + [-(x-y) + 3y^2(x^3+y^3-2)]\boldsymbol{j}.$$

Choose the initial point $x_1 = \frac{1}{2}$, $y_1 = \frac{1}{2}$. Since

$$\operatorname{grad} f\left(\frac{1}{2}, \frac{1}{2}\right) = -\frac{21}{16}\boldsymbol{i} - \frac{21}{16}\boldsymbol{j} \neq 0$$

we can set

$$x_2 = x_1 - \alpha_1 \frac{\partial f}{\partial x}(x_1, y_1) = \frac{1}{2} + \frac{21}{16}\alpha_1$$

$$y_2 = y_1 - \alpha_1 \frac{\partial f}{\partial x}(x_1, y_1) = \frac{1}{2} + \frac{21}{16}\alpha_1,\ \alpha_1 > 0.$$

We form the function

$$\varphi(\alpha_1) = (x_2, y_2) = 2\left[\left(\frac{1}{2} + \frac{21}{16}\alpha_1\right)^3 - 1\right]^2,\ \alpha_1 > 0$$

whose minimum point is $\alpha_1 = \frac{8}{21}$. It follows that $x_2 = y_2 = 1$. Since $\mathrm{grad}f(1,1) = 0$, the point $x_2 = y_2 = 1$ is a critical point of f. Furthermore it is a minimum point of f and therefore a solution of the system

$$x^3 + y^3 - 2 = 0, \; x - y = 0.$$

Applications. 1) Some biochemical processes with negative feedback can be modeled by the Goodwin differential system [59]

$$\frac{dx}{dt} = \frac{1}{1+z^n} - ax, \; \frac{dy}{dt} = x - by, \; \frac{dz}{dt} = y - cz,$$

where a, b, c are strictly positive real parameters, n is a fixed natural number, and x, y, z are functions of concentration.

First, let us show that significant solutions for biology have images in a closed bounded region in the concentration space $x \geq 0,\; y \geq 0,\; z \geq 0$. Particularly we shall describe an invariant set with respect to the flow attached to the Goodwin differential system.

Since x, y, z are concentration functions, the initial conditions $x(0) \geq 0,\; y(0) \geq 0,\; z(0) \geq 0$ are perfectly suited for biological applications. These initial conditions and the positiveness of derivatives $\frac{dx}{dt}, \frac{dy}{dt}, \frac{dz}{dt}$ for $x = y = z = 0$ show that

$$x(t) \geq 0,\; y(t) \geq 0,\; z(t) \geq 0,\; \forall\, t > 0.$$

The inequality $z \geq 0$ implies

$$\frac{dx}{dt} = \frac{1}{1+z^n} - ax \leq 1 - ax$$

and consequently: 1) if $x(0) \leq \frac{1}{a}$, then $x(t) \leq \frac{1}{a}$, $\forall\, t > 0$; 2) if $x(0) > \frac{1}{a}$, then the derivative $\frac{dx}{dt}$ is negative as long as $x(t) > \frac{1}{a}$ and hence $x(t)$ will decrease, becoming after a while at most $\frac{1}{a}$. In conclusion

$$0 \leq x(t) \leq \max\left\{x(0), \frac{1}{a}\right\},\; \forall\, t > 0.$$

The inequality $x(t) < \frac{1}{a}$ implies

$$\frac{dy}{dt} = x - by \leq \frac{1}{a} - by$$

and arguments similar to the preceding ones show that

$$0 \leq y(t) \leq \max\left\{y(0), \frac{1}{ab}\right\},\; \forall\, t > 0.$$

Analogously,

$$0 \le z(t) \le \max\left\{z(0), \frac{1}{abc}\right\}, \quad \forall t > 0.$$

Implicitly we have shown that the parallelepiped

$$\bar{D} = \left\{(x,y,z) \mid 0 \le x \le \frac{1}{a}, 0 \le y \le \frac{1}{ab}, 0 \le z \le \frac{1}{abc}\right\} \subset R^3_+$$

is an invariant set (the orbits determined by initial points in $\bar{D}$ are included in $\bar{D}$). This result is completed by the remark that the divergence of the Goodwin vector field

$$X = (X_1, X_2, X_3),$$

$$X_1(x,y,z) = \frac{1}{1+z^n} - ax, \quad X_2(x,y,z) = x - by, \quad X_3(x,y,z) = y - cz$$

is strictly negative, $\operatorname{div} \boldsymbol{X} = -a - b - c$, and hence the flow generated by $\boldsymbol{X}$ decreases the volumes.

Let us show that the Goodwin differential system admits a single equilibrium point belonging to the parallelepiped $\bar{D}$. For this we consider the algebraic system

$$\frac{1}{1+z^n} - ax = 0, \; x - by = 0, \; y - cz = 0, \; x, y, x \ge 0$$

whose solutions generate the equilibrium points. Eliminating x and y, we obtain the equation

$$\frac{1}{1+z^n} = abcz$$

which has a single strictly positive root z_0. Thus there exists a single equilibrium point $(x_0 = bcz_0, y_0 = cz_0, z_0)$. Since $\psi(z) = 1 - abcz(1+z^n)$ satisfies

$$\psi(0) = 1 > 0, \; \psi\left(\frac{1}{abc}\right) < 0$$

it follows that

$$0 < z_0 < \frac{1}{abc}, \; 0 < y_0 < \frac{1}{ab}, \; 0 < x_0 < \frac{1}{a}.$$

Let us analyse the stability of equilibrium point (x_0, y_0, z_0) using linear approximation with the matrix

$$A = \left[\frac{\partial X_i}{\partial x}, \frac{\partial X_i}{\partial y}, \frac{\partial X_i}{\partial z}\right](x_0, y_0, z_0) = \begin{bmatrix} -a & 0 & \dfrac{-nz_0^{n-1}}{1+z_0^n} \\ 1 & -b & 0 \\ 0 & 1 & -c \end{bmatrix}.$$

The characteristic equation of the matrix A is

$$(\lambda + a)(\lambda + b)(\lambda + c) + \frac{nz_0^{n-1}}{1+z_0^n} = 0.$$

This equation has surely a real root λ_1 (as an equation of degree 3), and necessarily $\lambda_1 < 0$ (since all the coefficients of the equation are strictly positive). As the preceding equation can be written

$$\lambda^3 + (a+b+c)\lambda^2 + (ab+ac+bc)\lambda + abc + \frac{n z_0^{n-1}}{1+z_0^n} = 0,$$

the Hurwitz criterion shows that all the roots of this equation have strictly negative real parts if and only if

$$(a+b+c)(ab+ac+bc) - abc - \frac{n z_0^{n-1}}{1+z_0^n} > 0.$$

In this hypothesis the equilibrium point (x_0, y_0, z_0) is asymptotically stable.

2) By analogy there exist biochemical processes with positive feedback described mathematically by the differential system [59]

$$\frac{dx}{dt} = \frac{1+z^n}{k+z^n} - ax, \quad \frac{dy}{dt} = x - by, \quad \frac{dz}{dt} = y - cz,$$

where a, b, c are strictly positive real parameters, k is a supraunitary real parameter, n is a fixed natural number, and x, y, z are functions of concentration. The function

$$\varphi : [0,\infty) \to R, \ \varphi(z) = \frac{1+z^n}{k+z^n}$$

admits the derivative

$$\varphi'(z) = \frac{n z^{n-1}(k-1)}{(k+z^n)^2} > 0,$$

and hence it is strictly increasing. Since

$$\varphi(0) = \frac{1}{k}, \ \lim_{z\to\infty} \varphi(z) = 1, \ \lim_{z\to 0} \varphi'(z) = 0, \ \lim_{z\to\infty} \varphi'(z) = 0,$$

the graph of the function φ has the shape in Fig.57.

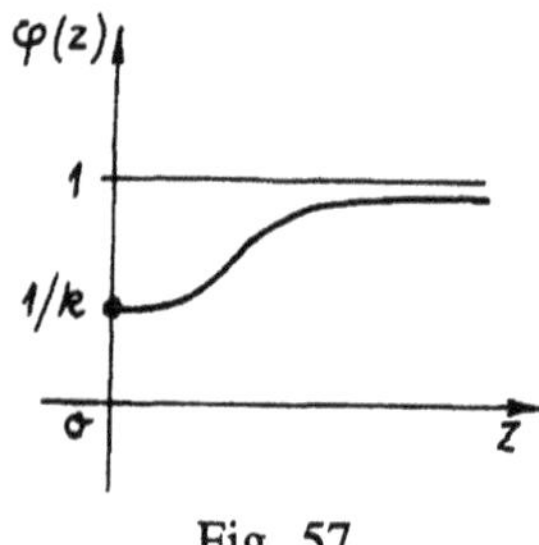

Fig. 57

The inequalities

$$\frac{dx}{dt} = \frac{1+z^n}{k+z^n} - ax \le 1 - ax, \ z \ge 0, \ x \ge 0$$

together with arguments similar to those used in the preceding application lead to

$$0 \le x(t) \le \max\left\{x(0), \frac{1}{a}\right\}, \ \forall t > 0.$$

Then we deduce

$$0 \le y(t) \le \max\left\{y(0), \frac{1}{ab}\right\}, \ 0 \le z(t) \le \max\left\{z(0), \frac{1}{abc}\right\}, \ \forall t > 0.$$

Consequently the parallelepiped

$$\bar{D} = \left\{(x,y,z) | 0 \le x \le \frac{1}{a}, \ 0 \le y \le \frac{1}{ab}, \ 0 \le z \le \frac{1}{abc}\right\}$$

is an invariant set, in the sense that the orbits determined by initial points in $\bar{D}$ are included in $\bar{D}$.

The divergence of the vector field

$$X(X_1, X_2, X_3),$$

$$X_1(x,y,z) = \frac{1+z^n}{k+z^n} - ax, \quad X_2(x,y,z) = x - by, \quad X_3(x,y,z) = y - cz$$

is strictly negative, $\operatorname{div} X = -a-b-c$. Therefore the flow generated by X decreases the volumes.

The preceding differential system has at least one equilibrium point in $\bar{D}$. Indeed, from

$$\frac{1+z^n}{k+z^n} - ax = 0, \ x - by = 0, \ y - cz = 0$$

we deduce the equation

$$\frac{1+z^n}{k+z^n} = abcz$$

which has at least a positive root z_0. We obtain the equilibrium point $(x_0 = bcz_0, y_0 = cz_0, z_0)$ which belongs to $\bar{D}$. The matrix of the corresponding linear approximation is

$$A = \begin{bmatrix} -a & 0 & \varphi'(z_0) \\ 1 & -b & 0 \\ 0 & 1 & -c \end{bmatrix}$$

and has the characteristic equation

$$\lambda^3 + (a+b+c)\lambda^2 + (ab+ac+bc)\lambda + abc - \varphi'(z_0) = 0.$$

The Hurwitz criterion shows that all the roots of this equation have strictly negative real parts if and only if

$$(a+b+c)(ab+ac+bc) - abc + \varphi'(z_0) > 0, \ abc - \varphi'(z_0) > 0.$$

In these conditions the equilibrium point (x_0, y_0, z_0) is asymptotically stable.

3) Stability of an electrical circuit [11] (Fig.58).

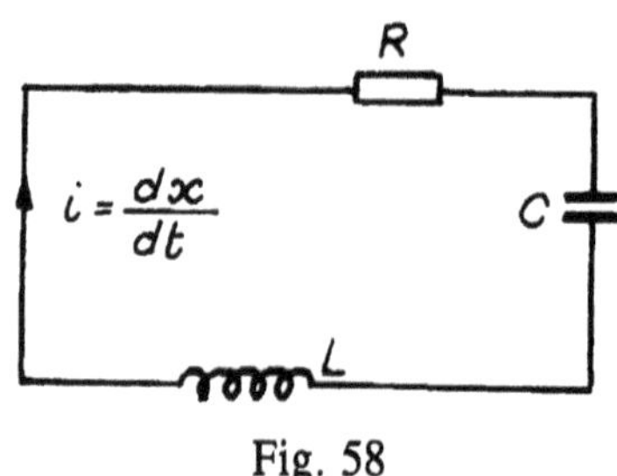

Fig. 58

Denote by x the electric charge of a capacitor, with $\frac{dx}{dt}$ the current in the circuit and with

$$f(x, \frac{dx}{dt}),\ f(0,0) = 0,$$

the nonlinear term having a Taylor expansion around $(0,0)$ of order greater than 2. Then

$$L\frac{d^2x}{dt^2} + R\frac{dx}{dt} + \frac{1}{C}x + f(x, \frac{dx}{dt}) = 0,$$

where L, R, C are strictly positive real parameters. This differential equation of order two is equivalent to the nonlinear differential system

$$\frac{dx}{dt} = y,\ \frac{dy}{dt} = -\frac{1}{LC}x - \frac{R}{L}y - \frac{1}{L}f(x,y)$$

for which $(0,0)$ is an equilibrium point. The matrix of the linear approximation

$$\frac{dx}{dt} = y,\ \frac{dy}{dt} = -\frac{1}{LC}x - \frac{R}{L}y$$

has the characteristic equation

$$\lambda^2 + \frac{R}{L}\lambda + \frac{1}{LC} = 0.$$

If $R^2 \neq \frac{4L}{C}$, then the equilibrium point $(0,0)$ is asymptotically stable. This result is a consequence of physical reasons: if the Ohm resistance is positive, then the current ceases inevitably by disappearing in time.

4.5. STABILITY BY LYAPUNOV FUNCTIONS

Let $X = (X_1, \dots, X_n)$ be a C^1 vector field on an open and connected set $D \subset R^n$ such that $x = 0$ is a zero of X. In vectorial notations, the differential system that describes the field lines of X is

$$\frac{dx}{dt} = X(x). \tag{5}$$

The second method of Lyapunov for analysing the stability of the equilibrium point $x(t) = 0$, $\forall t \in R$ is based on the use of Lyapunov functions.

To explain the technique proposed by Lyapunov, we denote with $x(t, x_0)$ the solution of the differential system (5) determined by the initial conditions (t_0, x_0), in the hypothesis that x_0 belongs to a neighborhood V of the origin. If $f: V \to R$ is a C^1 scalar field on V, then $D_X f(x) = (X(x), \text{grad} f(x))$. Also, for any solution $x(t)$, $t \in I$, of the differential system (5), we have

$$D_X f(x(t)) = (X(x(t)), \text{grad} f(x(t)) = \sum_{i=1}^{n} X_i(x(t)) \frac{\partial f}{\partial x_i}(x(t))$$

$$= \sum_{i=1}^{n} \frac{\partial f}{\partial x_i}(x(t)) \frac{dx_i}{dt}(t) = \frac{d}{dt} f(x(t)),$$

and consequently D_X is a derivative operator along the field lines of X.

A C^0 function $f: V \to R$, with $f(0) = 0$, is called

1) *positive (negative) definite*, if $f(x) > 0 (< 0)$, $\forall x \in V - \{0\}$;

2) *positive (negative) semidefinite*, if $f(x) \geq 0 (\leq 0)$ $\forall x \in V$.

Example. If $X(x) = 0 \Leftrightarrow x = 0$, then the energy $f = \frac{1}{2} \| X \|^2$ is positive definite.

Let $f: V \to R$ be a positive (negative) definite function. Since f is continuous, and $f(0) = 0$ if and only if $x = 0$, it follows that the assertions $x \to 0$ and $f(x) \to 0$ are equivalent. Also, we can prove that the constant level sets $M_c : f(x) = c$, for sufficiently small c, are continuous deformations of the sphere containing the origin in its interior. Particularly, $M_0 = \{0\}$.

Theorem. *If there exists a* C^1 *positive definite function* $f: V \to R$ *such that the function* $D_X f$ *is negative semidefinite on* V, *then the equilibrium point* $x(t) = 0$, $t \in R$, *of the differential system (5) is stable.*

Proof. Let $\varepsilon > 0$ be so small that the sphere $\|x\| = \varepsilon$ is included in V. Define $m = \min_{\|x\| = \varepsilon} f(x)$. Since f is positive definite it follows that $m > 0$. Also there exists $\delta < \varepsilon$ such that $\| x\| < \delta$ to imply $f(x) < m$.

We consider a solution $x(t,x_0)$ of the differential system (5) with $\|x_0\| < \delta$. Let us show that $\|x(t,x_0)\| < \varepsilon$ for $t \geq t_0$, in the hypothesis that the solution $x(t,x_0)$ has a boundless extension in the future. Contrary, there exists $T > 0$ such that $\|x(T,x_0)\| = \varepsilon$, but $\|x(t,x_0)\| < \varepsilon$ for $t \in [t_0, T)$. On the other hand, the relation

$$\frac{d}{dt} f(x(t,x_0)) = D_X f(x(t,x_0)) \leq 0$$

shows that $f(x(t,x_0))$ is a decreasing function of t for $t \in [t_0, T)$. Since $f(x_0) < m$ by the definition of δ, it follows that $f(x(T,x_0)) \leq f(x_0) < m$, but this result contradicts the definitions of T and m. Thus, under the condition that the solution $x(t,x_0)$ can be extended, we have proved that: $\forall\, \varepsilon > 0$, $\exists\, \delta > 0$ such that $\|x_0\| < \delta$ implies $\|x(t,x_0)\| < \varepsilon$, $\forall\, t \geq t_0$, i.e., the origin is a stable equilibrium point (Fig.47).

Let us show that the solution $x(t,x_0)$ can be extended boundlessly in the future. For that reason we consider the compact cylinder

$$A = \{(x,t) \mid 0 \leq f(x) \leq m,\ t \in [t_0, T]\}$$

in R^{n+1} and a solution $x(t,x_0)$ with the property $f(x_0) \leq m$. According to the extension theorem (see 3.1), the solution $x(t,x_0)$ can be extended in the future up to the boundary ∂A. But the relation $(x(t,x_0), t) \in A$ implies $D_X f(x(t,x_0)) \leq 0$. For that reason the solution $x(t,x_0)$ cannot reach the lateral surface of the cylinder A, where $f(x) = m$, and hence it can be extended till the cap $t = T$. Since T is arbitrary (and does not depend on m), the solution $x(t,x_0)$ can be extended without bound in the future and $f(x(t,x_0)) < m$, $\forall\, t \in [t_0, \infty)$.

Remarks. 1) The preceding theorem can be formulated in the following fashion: if there exists a C^1 negative definite function f on V and $D_X f$ is positive semidefinite on V, then the point $x = 0$ is a stable equilibrium point for the differential system (5).

2) There are no general methods for finding the functions $f: V \to R$ such that f and $D_X f$ satisfy the conditions imposed in the preceding theorem. But it is natural to start with the energy $f = \frac{1}{2}\|X\|^2$ or with first integrals of the differential system (5). Indeed, if f is a first integral of (5) defined in a neighborhood of the origin, then without loss of generality we can accept the condition $f(0) = 0$, and $D_X f = 0$ is automatically (positive, negative) semidefinite. If the first integral f is (negative, positive) definite, then the equilibrium point $x(t) = 0$, $\forall\, t \in R$ is stable.

The Hamiltonian differential systems

$$\frac{dx_i}{dt} = -\frac{\partial H}{\partial y_i}, \quad \frac{dy_i}{dt} = \frac{\partial H}{\partial x_i}, \quad i = 1, \dots, n$$

are examples, where $H: R^{2n} \to R$ is a global first integral. In particular cases, the properties of the function H can decide the stability of equilibrium points.

3) By the preceding theorem, a field line of X starting in the interior of the closed level set (sometimes, hypersurface) $M_c : f(x) = c$ cannot go outside the boundary (Fig.59). Indeed,

$$D_X f(x(t)) = \left(\text{grad} f(x(t)), \frac{dx}{dt} \right) \le 0$$

if and only if $\frac{\pi}{2} \le \theta \le \frac{3\pi}{2}$.

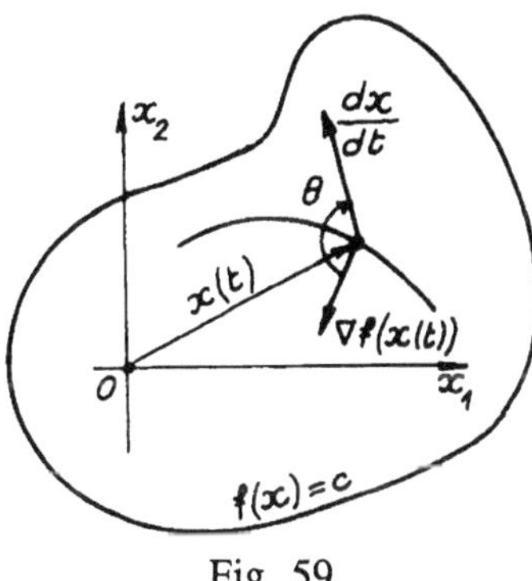

Fig. 59

Theorem. *Suppose there exists a* C^1 *positive definite function* $f: V \to R$ *such that* $D_X f$ *is negative semidefinite on* V. *If* $M_0 = \{x | x \in V, D_X f(x) = 0\}$ *does contain not completely any nonconstant orbit of the differential system (5), then the equilibrium point* $x = 0$ *is asymptotically stable (Fig.47).*

Proof. The preceding theorem shows that the equilibrium point $x(t) = 0,\ t \in R$ is stable, i.e., there exists $\delta > 0$ such that $\|x_0\| < \delta$ to imply the existence of the solution $x(t, x_0),\ t \in [t_0, \infty)$ and

$$\lim_{x_0 \to 0} x(t, x_0) = 0,\ \forall\, t \in [t_0, \infty).$$

Therefore it is sufficient to prove that there exists $\delta_1 \in (0, \delta)$ such that $\|x_0\| < \delta_1$ to imply $\lim_{t \to \infty} \|x(t, x_0)\| = 0$.

By the hypothesis $D_X f(x) \le 0,\ \forall\, x \in V$, the function $t \mapsto f(x(t, x_0))$ is decreasing. On the other hand, the positivity of f shows that if we would have $\lim_{t \to \infty} x(t, x_0) \neq 0$, then

$\lim_{t \to \infty} f(x(t,x_0)) = l > 0$, and so

$$0 < \lambda < \|x(t,x_0)\| < \varepsilon, \ \forall t \geq t_0 .$$

Suppose $\lim_{t \to \infty} f(x(t,x_0)) = l > 0$. Let x_* be a limit point of the field line $t \to x(t,x_0)$.

Obviously, $x_* \neq 0$. Since $f(x_*) = l > 0$ and the orbit $x(t,x_*)$ is not included in M_0, follows the existence of T satisfying $f(x(T,x_*)) < l$. Since the differential system we refer to is autonomous, the continuity of the function $x_0 \to x(t,x_0)$ implies the existence of t_* such that $f(x(t_*, x_0)) < l$. The property of decreasing of the function $t \to f(x(t,x_0))$ implies $f(x(t,x_0)) < l, \ \forall t \geq t_*$, contradicting $\lim_{t \to \infty} f(x(t,x_0)) = l > 0$. Thus $\lim_{t \to \infty} f(x(t,x_0)) = 0$ and therefore $\lim_{t \to \infty} \|x(t,x_0)\| = 0$.

Application. Let us consider the linear differential equation of order two

$$\frac{d^2 x}{dt^2} + \varphi(x) \frac{dx}{dt} + \psi(x) = 0, \tag{6}$$

where $\varphi, \psi : (-a,a) \to R$ are C^1 functions and $\psi(0) = 0$, $\varphi(x) > 0$, $x\psi(x) > 0$, $\forall x \neq 0$. In the phase space $\{(x,\dot{x}) = (x,y)\}$ there corresponds the differential system

$$\frac{dx}{dt} = y, \ \frac{dy}{dt} = -\varphi(x)y - \psi(x). \tag{7}$$

The solution $x(t) = 0$, $t \in R$ of the equation (6) is called *stable, asymptotically stable or unstable* if the equilibrium position of the differential system (7) has such a quality.

Denote $\boldsymbol{X}(x,y) = (y, -\varphi(x)y - \psi(x))$. The function

$$f(x,y) = \frac{1}{2} y^2 + \int_0^x \psi(x)dx$$

is positive definite, and $D_{\boldsymbol{X}} f = -\varphi(x)y^2$ is negative definite on a neighborhood of the origin; the set M_0 is the interval $(-a, a)$, and the differential equation $x = y$ shows that the nontrivial orbits cut this interval. According to the preceding theorem, the equilibrium point $x = 0$, $y = 0$ of the differential system (7) is asymptotically stable, and hence the solution $x(t_0) = 0$, $t \in R$ of the differential equation (6) is asymptotically stable.

Let us speak now about instability. If $f: V \to R$, $f(0) = 0$ is a C^1 function, then we denote by V^+ any open connected subset of the open set

$$\{x | f(x) > 0, \ \|x\| < \delta\}$$

with the property that ∂V^+ contains the origin.

Theorem. *If there exists* V^+ *on which* $D_X f > 0$, *then the equilibrium point* $x(t) = 0$, $t \in R$, *of the differential system (5) is unstable (Fig.47).*

Proof. Let $0 < \delta_1 < \delta$ and the solution $x(t,x_0)$ exist with the initial point $x_0 \in V^+$, $\|x_0\| < \delta_1$. Since $0 \in \partial V^+$, it is sufficient to show that for any solution there exists a moment T such that $\|x(T,x_0)\| = \delta_1$.

Suppose the opposite: $\exists\, x(t,x_*)$, $x_* \in V^+$, $\|x_*\| < \delta_1$ such that $\|x(t,x_*)\| < \delta_1$, for $\forall t \geq t_0$. Since $D_X f > 0$ on V^+, the function $t \to f(x(t,x_*))$ is strictly increasing and $x(t,x_*) \in V^+$. That is why, $f(x(t,x_*)) > f(x_*) > 0$, $\forall\, t > t_0$. This, with the fact that $f(x)$, $\|x\| < \delta_1$ vanishes only at $0 \in \partial V^+$, imply

$$\frac{d}{dt} f(x(t,x_*)) = D_X f(x(t,x_*)) \geq l > 0, \ \forall\, t \in t_0.$$

By integrating on $[t_0, t]$, we obtain

$$f(x(t,x_*)) \geq f(x_*) + l(t - t_0)$$

and hence $\lim\limits_{t \to \infty} f(x(t,x_*)) = \infty$. This result contradicts the boundedness of the function $x \to f(x)$, $\|x\| < \delta_1$.

The functions $f: V \to R$ in the preceding theorems are called *Lyapunov functions* associated to the vector field X on V.

Application. We shall consider a *potential differential system* of order two ($\Rightarrow$ a conservative system)

$$\frac{d^2 x}{dt^2} + \operatorname{grad} F(x) = 0, \tag{8}$$

where $F: R^n \to R$ is an analytic scalar field in a neighborhood of the origin. Without loss of generality we can suppose $F(0) = 0$. To this differential system of order two we attach, in the phase space $\left(x, \dfrac{dx}{dt}\right) \in R^{2n}$, a Hamiltonian differential system

$$\frac{dx_k}{dt} = -y_k, \quad \frac{dy_k}{dt} = \frac{\partial F}{\partial x_k}, \ k = 1, \dots, n \tag{9}$$

with the Hamiltonian

$$H(x,y) = \frac{1}{2} \sum_{k=1}^{n} y_k^2 + F(x),$$

which verifies $H(0,0)=0$. Introducing the Hamiltonian vector field $X=\left(-y_k, \frac{\partial F}{\partial x_k}\right)$ we remark that $D_X H = 0$, i.e., H is a first integral of the differential system (9).

Sometimes, the Hamiltonian H is a Lyapunov function attached to the vector field X. For example, we assume that $x=0$ is a minimum point of the function F. Then $x=0$, $y=0$ is a minimum point of H, and $H(x,y)>0$ for $(x,y)\neq(0,0)$ in a neighborhood of $(0,0)$. The first theorem shows that the equilibrium point $(0,0)$ of the differential system (9) is stable and hence the equilibrium point $x(t)=0$, $t\in R$ of the differential system (8) is stable. This result is known in Analytical Mechanics as the *Lagrange Theorem*.

Let us suppose that $x=0$ is a maximum point of F. It follows that $\operatorname{grad} F(x)=0$ and representing F in the Taylor series form

$$F(x)=\sum_{j=m}^{\infty} F^{(j)}(x),\ m\geq 2,$$

where $F^{(j)}$ is a homogeneous form of order j, necessarily $F^{(m)}$ must be negative definite. Here one can use $g(x,y)=-\sum_{k=1}^{n} x_k y_k$ like a Lyapunov function. Indeed

$$D_X g = -\sum_{k=1}^{n} y_k \frac{\partial g}{\partial x_k}+\sum_{k=1}^{n} \frac{\partial F}{\partial x_k}\frac{\partial g}{\partial y_k}=\sum_{k=1}^{n} y_k^2-\sum_{k=1}^{n} x_k \frac{\partial F}{\partial x_k}=\sum_{k=1}^{n} y_k^2 - mF^{(m)}+\cdots,$$

where the unwritten terms are homogeneous polynomials in $(x_1,\dots,x_n)$ of degree greater then m. Thus $D_X g$ is positive definite on a neighborhood of the origin. Particularly, it is also positive definite on the connected component V^+, containing the point $(a,\dots,a)$, $a>0$, of the point set on which g is strictly positive. According to the last theorem, the equilibrium point $(0,0)$ of the differential system (9) is unstable, and therefore the maximum point $x=0$ of F generates an unstable equilibrium point of the differential system (8).

4.6. PROPOSED PROBLEMS

1. Study the stability of the equilibrium points for the following differential systems

1) $\frac{dx}{dt}=-x+\alpha y,\ \frac{dy}{dt}=\beta x-y+\alpha z,\ \frac{dz}{dt}=\beta y-z;$

2) $\frac{dx}{dt}=-x+\alpha y+\beta z,\ \frac{dy}{dt}=-\alpha x-y+\alpha z,\ \frac{dz}{dt}=-\beta x-\alpha y-z,$

where α, β are real parameters.

2. Classify the equilibrium points of the following differential systems

1) $\dfrac{dx}{dt} = -ax + (a-1)y, \ \dfrac{dy}{dt} = x;$

2) $\dfrac{dx}{dt} = -x + ay, \ \dfrac{dy}{dt} = bx - y;$

3) $\dfrac{dx}{dt} = -a^2x + ay, \ \dfrac{dy}{dt} = x - y;$

4) $\dfrac{dx}{dt} = y + ax(x^2+y^2), \ \dfrac{dy}{dt} = -x + ay(x^2+y^2),$

where a and b are real parameters.

3. Using linear approximation, test the stability of the equilibrium points of the following differential systems:

1) $\dfrac{dx}{dt} = \ln(e+ax) - e^y, \ \dfrac{dy}{dt} = bx + \mathrm{tg}y;$

2) $\dfrac{dx}{dt} = 2e^{-x} - \sqrt{4+ay}, \ \dfrac{dy}{dt} = \ln(1+9x+ay);$

3) $\dfrac{dx}{dt} = e^{x+2y} - \cos 3x, \ \dfrac{dy}{dt} = \sqrt{4+8x} - 2e^y.$

4. Study the stability of equilibrium points of the following differential systems, taking suitable homogeneous polynomials as Lyapunov functions:

1) $\dfrac{dx}{dt} = y + x^3, \ \dfrac{dy}{dt} = -x + y^3;$

2) $\dfrac{dx}{dt} = -y - \dfrac{x}{2} - \dfrac{x^3}{4}, \ \dfrac{dy}{dt} = x - \dfrac{y}{2} - \dfrac{y^3}{4};$

3) $\dfrac{dx}{dt} = 2y^3 - x^5, \ \dfrac{dy}{dt} = -x - y^3 + y^5.$

Hint. 1) $f(x,y) = x^2 + y^2$, unstable; 2) $f(x,y) = x^2 + y^2$, asymptotically stable; 3) stable.

5. Study the stability of the equilibrium point $(0,0)$ of the differential system

$$\frac{dx}{dt} = y - ax(x^2+y^2), \ \frac{dx}{dt} = -x - ay(x^2+y^2).$$

Hint. $f(x,y) = x^2 + y^2$ is a Lyapunov function.

6. The same problem for the following differential systems

$$\begin{cases} \dfrac{dx}{dt} = y \\ \dfrac{dy}{dt} = -xe^{-x^2} - ye^{-y^2}x^2e^{-2x^2}, \end{cases} \qquad \begin{cases} \dfrac{dx}{dt} = x^2 - y^2 \\ \dfrac{dy}{dt} = -2xy. \end{cases}$$

Hint. $f(x,y) = -x^3 + 3xy^2$ can be used like a Lyapunov function.

7. Consider the differential system

$$\frac{dx}{dt} = Ax, \quad A = \begin{bmatrix} 0 & 0 & -1 \\ 0 & 2 & 0 \\ 4 & 0 & -3 \end{bmatrix}.$$

1) Build a Lyapunov function f for which $D_{Ax} f = -\|x\|^2$ and show that the equilibrium point $x = 0$ is unstable.

2) Show that $f(x_0) < 0$ implies $\lim_{t\to\infty} \|x(t,x_0)\| = \infty$.

3) Does the hypothesis $f(x_0) > 0$ imply $\lim_{t\to\infty} \|x(t,x_0)\| = \infty$?

8. Let X be a C^1 vector field on R^n with the property $(x, X(x)) \le 0,\ \forall x \in R^n$. Show that $X(0) = 0$, the equilibrium point $x = 0$ of the differential system $\frac{dx}{dt} = X(x)$ is stable and the field lines of X are bounded.

Hint. $f(x) = \|x\|^2$ is a Lyapunov function.

9. A mechanical system with one degree of freedom, with the mass m, driven by a harmonic perturbation force has the elastic characteristic

$$f(x) = \begin{cases} k_1 & \text{if} \quad -a \le x \le a \\ k_2 x + (k_1 - k_2) a & \text{if} \quad x \ge a \\ k_2 x - (k_1 - k_2) a & \text{if} \quad x \le -a. \end{cases}$$

Study the stability of the movement of the mechanical system.

Hint. $m\ddot{x} + f(x) = F_0 \cos(\omega t + \varphi)$. Denoting $y = b\sin(\omega t + \varphi)$, we find:

$\ddot{x} = -\frac{1}{m} f(x) + \frac{F_0}{b\omega}\dot{y},\ \ddot{y} = -\omega^2 y$. Set $x = x_1,\ \dot{x}_1 = x_2,\ y = x_3,\ \dot{y} = x_4$.

10. Prove that for any Hamiltonian differential system there are no asymptotically stable equilibrium points or asymptotically stable limit cycles (in the phase space).

Hint. One can use linear approximation.

11. Rolling of a circular disk on a horizontal plane is described by the differential system [137]

$$\frac{d\theta}{dt} = p,\ (\gamma + 1)\frac{dr}{dt} = pq$$

$$(\alpha + 1)\frac{dp}{dt} = -qr(\gamma + 1) + \alpha q \operatorname{ctg}\theta - \frac{g}{a}\cos\theta,\ \alpha\frac{dq}{dt} = -p(\alpha q \operatorname{ctg}\theta - \gamma r),$$

where g is the gravitational acceleration, and α, γ, a are real parameters. Study the stability of equilibrium points.

5. POTENTIAL DIFFERENTIAL SYSTEMS OF ORDER ONE AND CATASTROPHE THEORY

The nonconstant gradient lines of a scalar field f cannot be closed curves. These are trajectories orthogonal to constant level hypersurfaces of the scalar field f, and curves of maximal local increase of f. If the potential f is a subharmonic (respectively harmonic or supraharmonic) function, i.e., $\Delta f \geq 0$ (respectively $\Delta f = 0$ or $\Delta f \leq 0$), then the flow generated by $\operatorname{grad} f$ *increases (respectively preserves or decreases) the volume (see 5.1).*

The classification of potentials with at most four parameters implies a classification of the corresponding differential potential systems. Also notions from the theory of elementary catastrophes reveal new possibilities regarding the study of gradient lines (see 5.2).

The gradient lines of the fold (see 5.3), the cusp (see 5.4), the swallowtail (see 5.5) and the butterfly (see 5.6) are respectively solutions of some ordinary differential equations with separable variables,

$$\frac{dx}{dt} = P(x),$$

where $P(x)$ is respectively a polynomial function of degree two, three, four, and five. If x_0 is not an equilibrium point, then the solution determined by the initial condition (t_0, x_0) is of the type

$$t - t_0 = \int_{x_0}^{x} \frac{du}{P(u)} .$$

If the interval $[x_0, \infty]$ does not contain zeros of P, then the integral

$$\int_{x_0}^{\infty} \frac{du}{P(u)}$$

is convergent. In problems of motion, this fact shows that the particle moves to infinity in a finite time (in the future) or comes from infinity in a finite time (in the past).

If on the interval $[x_0, b]$ there exists a zero of P, then

$$\int_{x_0}^{b} \frac{du}{P(u)}$$

is a divergent improper integral of the second kind; in concrete problems this integral can be used as such or with its principal value.

The equilibrium points of the elliptic umbilic (see 5.7), the hyperbolic umbilic (see 5.8) and the parabolic umbilic (see 5.9) can be attractors, proper knots, improper knots and saddle points, either asymptotically stable or unstable.

The problems proposed in 5.10 refer to the steepest crescent direction, to the flows generated by potential vector fields and the stability of equilibrium points of the potential systems.

The mathematical ideas presented in Chapters 5 and 7 have applications in cosmology, gravitational collapse of stars, thermodynamics, theory of elastic structures [25], nonlinear resonance of mechanical systems, instability of electrical networks, instability of hydrodynamic systems, laser physics, crystallography, navigation, biology and ecology, psychology, formation of cyclones, economic crises, problems of social modeling, etc.

5.1. CRITICAL POINTS AND GRADIENT LINES

Let D be an open set in R^n, and $x = (x_1, \dots, x_n)$ be a point in D. To the C^1 scalar field $f: D \to R$ we can attach the gradient vector field $\nabla f(x) = \left(\frac{\partial f}{\partial x_1}(x), \dots, \frac{\partial f}{\partial x_n}(x) \right)$. Zeros of ∇f, i.e., the solutions of the system

$$\frac{\partial f}{\partial x_1}(x) = 0, \dots, \frac{\partial f}{\partial x_n} = 0, \; x \in D \tag{1}$$

are called the *critical points* of the function f. If x_0 is a critical point of f, then the number $f(x_0)$ is called the *critical value* of f. In order to have a geometrical image around the critical points of the function f, we use either the shape of the graph of f in a neighborhood of such a point or the shape of the constant level sets of f. The hyperplane tangent to the graph of f at the point $(x_0, f(x_0))$, x_0 being a critical point, is horizontal.

Fermat's Theorem. *If $f: D \to R$ is a C^1 scalar field and $x_0 \in D$ is a point of local extremum, then $\nabla f(x_0) = 0$, i.e., x_0 is a critical point of f.*

Proof. Let v be a vector tangent to D at the point x_0. We fix $r > 0$ such that $f(x) - f(x_0)$ has constant sign on the ball $B_r(x_0)$. The function $g: (-r, r) \to R$, $g(t) = f(x_0 + tv)$ is of class C^1 and the difference $g(t) - g(0)$ has constant sign on $(-r, r)$. Thus $t = 0$ is a point of local extremum of g and consequently (Fermat's Theorem for real functions of a real variable)

$$0 = g'(0) = (\nabla f(x_0), v).$$

Since v is arbitrary, $\nabla f(x_0) = 0$.

Corollary. *A C^1 scalar field on a compact set attains its bounds (minimum and maximum) either at a critical point or at a boundary point.*

The next theorem gives a sufficient condition for the existence of the global extrema.

Theorem. *Let D be an open and convex set in R^n, and $f: D \to R$ be a C^1 convex (concave) scalar field on D. If x_0 is a critical point, then x_0 is a global minimum (maximum) point.*

Proof. Since D is convex, f is convex and differentiable at $x_0 \in D$, and we have

$$f(x_0) + (\nabla f(x_0), x - x_0) \le f(x), \; \forall x \in D.$$

If x_0 is a critical point, i.e., $\nabla f(x_0) = 0$, then

$$f(x_0) \le f(x), \ \forall x \in D$$

and therefore x_0 is a global minimum point on D.

Now, what happens from a local point of view?

Theorem. *Let D be an open set in R^n and $f: D \to R$ be a C^p, $p \ge 2$, scalar field.*

1) If $x_0 \in D$ is a point of local extremum of f, then $d^2 f(x_0)$ is (positive or negative) semidefinite.

2) Let x_0 be a critical point of f. If $d^2 f(x_0)$ is positive (negative) definite, then x_0 is a point of local minimum (maximum) of f.

Proof. For both parts of the theorem we use the Taylor formula

$$f(x) = f(x_0) + df(x_0)(x - x_0) + \frac{1}{2} d^2 f(x_0 + \tau(x - x_0))(x - x_0, x - x_0), \ \tau \in (0,1).$$

1) Suppose that x_0 is a point of local minimum, i.e., $f(x) \ge f(x_0)$, for any x in a neighborhood of x_0. By the Fermat theorem, x_0 is a critical point of f, i.e., $df(x_0) = 0$. From the Taylor formula and by the continuity of the second differential it follows that $d^2 f(x_0)$ is positive semidefinite.

An immediate consequence of this part of the theorem is: if $d^2 f(x_0)$ does not preserve constant sign, then x_0 cannot be a local extremum.

2) By continuity, $d^2 f$ will be positive definite in a neighborhood of x_0. That is why Taylor formula gives $f(x) > f(x_0)$ for any $x \ne x_0$ in a neighborhood of x_0, i.e., x_0 is the unique point of local minimum.

Let $f: D \to R$ be a C^2 scalar field and $x_0 \in D$ be a critical point of f. If the quadratic form $d^2 f(x_0)$ is nondegenerate, i.e.,

$$\det \left[\frac{\partial^2 f}{\partial x_i \partial x_j}(x_0) \right] \ne 0,$$

then x_0 is called a *nondegenerate critical point*. Otherwise x_0 is called a *degenerate critical point*. The nondegenerate critical points are isolated, and the diffeomorphisms of class C^2 preserve the quality of degenerate or nondegenerate critical points.

Examples. In the case $n = 2$, the origin is a critical point for each of the C^∞ scalar fields defined respectively by

$$x^2 + y^2, \quad -x^2 - y^2, \quad x^2 - y^2, \quad x^3 - 3xy^2, \quad x^2, \quad x^2 y^2.$$

The usual denominations for these types of critical points are respectively *minimum point* (Fig.1), *maximum point*, *saddle point* (Fig.2), *monkey saddle* (Fig.3), *pig-through* (Fig.4) and *crossed pig-through* (Fig.5). The critical points of the functions

$$x^2 + y^2, \quad -x^2 - y^2, \quad x^2 - y^2, \quad x^3 - 3xy^2$$

are isolated critical points, while the critical points of the functions

$$x^2, \quad x^2y^2$$

are respectively nonisolated. Also, minimum, maximum, and saddle points are nondegenerate critical points. The monkey saddle, pig-through, and crossed pig-through points are degenerate.

Let $X = (X_1, \dots, X_n)$ be a C^1 vector field on D, which we attach the differential system

$$\frac{dx_1}{dt} = X_1(x), \dots, \frac{dx_n}{dt} = X_n(x). \tag{2}$$

If X is a potential vector field on D, then the differential system (2) is called *potential*. The potential $f: D \to R$ of the vector field X is a called the *potential* of the differential system (2). Since $X = \text{grad} f$, the potential differential system is written as

$$\frac{dx_1}{dt} = \frac{\partial f}{\partial x_1}(x), \dots, \frac{dx_n}{dt} = \frac{\partial f}{\partial x_n}(x). \tag{3}$$

The solutions of the potential differential system (3) are called *gradient lines* of the scalar field f. The following theorem shows that the nonconstant gradient lines cannot be closed curves.

The set of equilibrium points (constant gradient lines) of the potential differential system (3) coincides to the set of critical points of f, being described by the algebraic system (1).

Let us consider the Cauchy problem

$$\frac{d\alpha}{dt} = \text{grad} f(\alpha), \quad \alpha(0) = x$$

whose solution is called the *gradient line of the function f through the point x*. Since $\text{grad} f$ is of class C^1, this Cauchy problem has a unique maximal solution

$$\alpha_x : (\omega_-(x), \omega_+(x)) \to D, \quad \omega_-(x) < 0 < \omega_+(x)$$

and the gradient flow is defined by $T_t(x) = \alpha_x(t)$.

Theorem. *Let $I = (\omega_-(x), \omega_+(x))$ and $\alpha : I \to D$ be a gradient line of f through the point x.*

1) α is a curve of maximal local increase of f; consequently there exist the limits

$$\lim_{t \searrow \omega_-(x)} f(T_t(x)), \quad \lim_{t \nearrow \omega_+(x)} f(T_t(x)).$$

2) α is a closed curve only in the case it is reduced to an equilibrium point (critical point of f).

3) If $\omega_+(x)$ is finite, then

$$\lim_{t \nearrow \omega_+(x)} f(T_t(x)) = \infty.$$

4) If $\omega_+(x) = \infty$ *and there exists* $\lim_{t\to\infty} \alpha(t) = x_0$, *then* x_0 *is a critical point of the real function* f.

Proof. 1) According to the chain rule, it results that

$$\frac{d}{dt} f(\alpha(t)) = df(\alpha(t)\left(\frac{d\alpha}{dt}(t)\right) = \|\operatorname{grad} f(\alpha(t)\|^2 \geq 0, \ \forall t \in I.$$

So either $f(\alpha(t)) = f(x)$ for all $t \in I$, or $f \circ \alpha$ is increasing and consequently the limits in the theorem exist.

Let us show that for each $t_0 \in I$, the function f is increasing faster along α at $\alpha(t_0)$, than along any other curve passing through $\alpha(t_0)$ with the same speed. Indeed, if $\alpha : (a,b) \to D$ is a gradient line of f and $\beta : (c,d) \to D$ is any other curve of class C^1 such that

$$\beta(s_0) = \alpha(t_0), \ \|\beta'(s_0)\| = \|\alpha'(t_0)\|, \ s_0 \in (c,d), \ t_0 \in (a,b),$$

then

$$\frac{d(f\circ\beta)}{ds}(s_0) = df(\beta(s_0))(\beta'(s_0)) \leq \|\nabla f(\alpha(t_0))\|^2$$

$$= df(\alpha(t_0))(\alpha'(t_0)) = \frac{d(f\circ\alpha)}{dt}(t_0).$$

2) Let $[a,b] \subset I$ and $\alpha : [a,b] \to D$ be a closed gradient line of f, i.e., $\alpha(a) = \alpha(b)$. If $\alpha(a) = \alpha(b)$ is not an equilibrium point, then we find the contradiction

$$0 = f(\alpha(b)) - f(\alpha(a)) = \int_a^b df(\alpha(t))(\alpha'(t))\,dt = \int_a^b \|\operatorname{grad} f(\alpha(t))\|^2\,dt > 0.$$

3) The relation

$$\frac{d}{dt} f(\alpha(t)) = \|\operatorname{grad} f(\alpha(t))\|^2, \ \forall t \in I$$

implies

$$f(\alpha(t)) = f(\alpha(s)) + \int_s^t \|\operatorname{grad} f(\alpha(r))\|^2\,dr, \ \omega_-(x) < s \leq t < \omega_+(x).$$

For $0 \leq s \leq t < \omega_+(x)$, the definition of the Euclidean distance d on D, the Cauchy-Schwarz inequality and the preceding relation imply

$$d(\alpha(t), \alpha(s)) \leq \int_s^t \|\operatorname{grad} f(\alpha(r))\|\,dr \leq (t-s)^{\frac{1}{2}} \left(\int_s^t \|\operatorname{grad} f(\alpha(r))\|^2\,dr\right)^{\frac{1}{2}}$$

$$= (t-s)^{\frac{1}{2}} (f(\alpha(t)) - f(\alpha(s)))^{\frac{1}{2}}.$$

Since $\omega_+(x) < \infty$, $\alpha(t)$ has no limit when $t \to \omega_+(x)$, and therefore α does not verify the corresponding Cauchy condition. Since $f \circ \alpha$ is increasing, the above inequality implies that

$$\lim_{t \nearrow \omega_+(x)} f(\alpha(t)) = \infty.$$

4) Obviously $\lim_{t\to\infty} f(\alpha(t)) = f(x_0)$. Then

$$f(x_0) - f(\alpha(t_0)) = \lim_{t\to\infty} (f(\alpha(t)) - f(\alpha(t_0))) = \lim_{t\to\infty} \int_{t_0}^{t} df(\alpha(r))(\alpha'(r))dr$$

$$= \lim_{t\to\infty} \int_{t_0}^{t} \|\operatorname{grad} f(\alpha(r))\|^2 dr = \int_{t_0}^{\infty} \|\operatorname{grad} f(\alpha(r))\|^2 dr.$$

The convergence of this integral and $\lim_{t\to\infty} \operatorname{grad} f(\alpha(t)) = \operatorname{grad} f(x_0)$ imply $\|\operatorname{grad} f(x_0)\| = 0$ and therefore x_0 is a critical point of f.

Remark. There exist irrotational vector fields that have nonconstant closed field lines. For example, the field lines of the irrotational vector field

$$X(x,y) = \left(\frac{y}{x^2+y^2}, \frac{-x}{x^2+y^2}\right), \quad (x,y) \in R^2 \setminus \{0,0\}$$

are circles with the centre at the origin. This result shows the existence of irrotational vector fields that are not globally equivalent to potential vector fields.

Theorem. *If the potential $f: D \to R$ is a C^2 convex function, then the gradient flow of f increases the volume.*

Proof. By hypothesis $d^2 f(x)$ is positive semidefinite for every $x \in D$. It follows $\operatorname{div}(\operatorname{grad} f) = \operatorname{trace} d^2 f \geq 0$ and hence the gradient flow of f is a dilatation (see 3.7).

Let x_0 be an equilibrium point of the potential differential system (3). The differentiability of the partial derivatives $\dfrac{\partial f}{\partial x_i}$ imply

$$\frac{\partial f}{\partial x_i}(x) = \frac{\partial f}{\partial x_i}(x_0) + \sum_{j=1}^{n} \frac{\partial^2 f}{\partial x_i \partial x_j}(x_0)(x_j - x_{j0}) + \|x - x_0\| F_i(x), \quad \lim_{x\to x_0} F_i(x) = 0.$$

Thus the linear approximation of the nonlinear differential system (3) is

$$\frac{dx_i}{dt} = \sum_{j=1}^{n} \frac{\partial^2 f}{\partial x_i \partial x_j}(x_0)(x_j - x_{j0}), \quad i = 1, \dots, n. \tag{3'}$$

The matrix $\left[\dfrac{\partial^2 f}{\partial x_i \partial x_j}(x_0)\right]$ has real proper values, being a real symmetric matrix. These proper values are strictly negative if and only if $d^2 f(x_0)$ is negative definite (it follows that x_0 is a strictly local maximum point of the function f). Consequently, if $d^2 f(x_0)$ is negative definite, then the equilibrium point x_0 is asymptotically stable and hence stable. These results can be proved without the stability theory.

Theorem. *Let* $D \subset R^n$ *be an open set,* $f: D \to R$ *be a* C^2 *function and* $x_0 \in D$ *be a critical point of* f *for which* $d^2 f(x_0)$ *is negative definite. If* $r > 0$ *is sufficiently small and* x_1 *belongs to the ball* $B_r(x_0)$, *then the gradient line* α *of* f *starting from* x_1 *at the time* t_1 *is defined on* $[t_1, \infty)$ *and* $\lim_{t\to\infty} \alpha(t) = x_0$.

Proof. Let

$$h(t) = \frac{1}{2}\|\alpha(t) - x_0\|^2, \quad t \in [t_1, \infty).$$

It follows that

$$\begin{aligned} h'(t) &= (\alpha'(t), \alpha(t) - x_0) = (\operatorname{grad} f(\alpha(t)), \alpha(t) - x_0) = df(\alpha(t))(\alpha(t) - x_0) \\ &= (df(\alpha(t)) - df(x_0))(\alpha(t) - x_0) = d^2 f(x_1)(\alpha(t) - x_0, \alpha(t) - x_0) \\ &\le -m\|\alpha(t) - x_0\|^2, \quad m > 0. \end{aligned}$$

In other words

$$h'(t) \le -m\, h(t) \quad \text{or} \quad \ln h(t) - \ln h(t_1) \le -m(t - t_1).$$

The relations

$$0 \le h(t) \le h(t_1)\exp(-m(t - t_1)), \quad t \in [t_1, \infty)$$

imply

$$\lim_{t\to\infty} h(t) = 0, \quad \text{i.e.,} \quad \lim_{t\to\infty} \alpha(t) = x_0.$$

It remains to prove that the solution $\alpha(t, x_1)$, $x_1 \in B_r(x_0)$ is extended without bound in the future. For this we consider the compact set (cylinder)

$$A = B_r(x_0) \times [t_1, T] \subset R^{n+1}.$$

According to the extension theorem (see 3.1), the solution $\alpha(t, x_1)$ can be extended in the future up to the boundary ∂A. The solution cannot reach $\partial B_r(x_0)$ since $h: [t_1, T] \to R$ is a decreasing function; it results that $\alpha(t, x_1)$ can be extended till the cap $t = T$, which is arbitrary and independent of $B_r(x_0)$

The preceding explanations refer to the field lines of $\operatorname{grad} f$. From these or directly from the definition follow analogous properties for the field lines of $-\operatorname{grad} f$.

Theorem. *Let* $f: R^n \to R$ *be a* C^2 *function. If* f *admits a unique critical point* x_* *that is a minimum point of* f, *and* $\|\operatorname{grad} f(x)\| > m > 0$ *on* $\operatorname{Ext} B_r(x_0)$ *with* $r \to \infty$, *then for any* $x_1 \in R^n \setminus \{x_*\}$, *the solution* α *of the Cauchy problem*

$$\frac{d\alpha}{dt} = -\frac{\operatorname{grad} f}{\|\operatorname{grad} f\|}(\alpha(t)), \quad \alpha(t_1) = x_1$$

has the property

$$\lim_{t \to \infty} \alpha(t) = x_* .$$

Proof. Suppose that x_* is found. Let $\alpha(t, t_1)$ be the solution of the preceding Cauchy problem. We shall show that for any $\varepsilon > 0$ and $x_1 \in R^n \setminus \{x_*\}$ there exists $T(\varepsilon, x_1)$ such that $t \geq T(\varepsilon, x_1)$ implies $\| \alpha(t, x_1) - x_* \| < \varepsilon$.

The function $V(x) = f(x) - f(x_*)$ is positive definite, and

$$\frac{dV}{dt} = - \| \mathrm{grad} f(x) \|,$$

and $\mathrm{grad} f$ vanishes only at x_*. Having conditions similar to those in the theorem of asymptotic stability (see 4.5), for any $\varepsilon > 0$ there exists $\delta(\varepsilon) > 0$ such that $\| x_1 - x_* \| < \delta(\varepsilon)$ implies

$$\| \alpha(t, x_1) - x_* \| < \varepsilon, \ \forall t \geq 0,$$

$$\| \alpha(t, x_1) - x_* \| \to 0 \quad \text{for} \quad t \to \infty.$$

We have two cases: either there exists $T(x_1)$ such that $\| \alpha(t, x_1) - x_* \| < \delta$ or $T(x_1)$ does not exist. In the first case we have

$$\| \alpha(t, x_1) - x_* \| < \varepsilon, \ \forall t > T(x_1).$$

In the second case, we must have

$$\| \alpha(t, x_1) - x_* \| > \delta_1,$$

and from $\| \mathrm{grad} f \| > m > 0$ it follows

$$\frac{dV}{dt} < -m, \ \forall t \geq 0,$$

i.e., $V(\alpha(t)) \leq V(x_1) - mt$, which shows that $V(\alpha(t))$ decreases indefinitely along the field line α, a contradiction. This solves only the first case.

Examples. In the case $n = 2$, the types of equilibrium points for the potential differential system can be *receiver* (Fig.60, *minimum point*), *source* (Fig.61, *maximum point*), *saddle* (Fig.62), *monkey saddle* (Fig.63), and *dipole* (Fig.64). The equilibrium points of potential differential systems cannot be points of rotation.

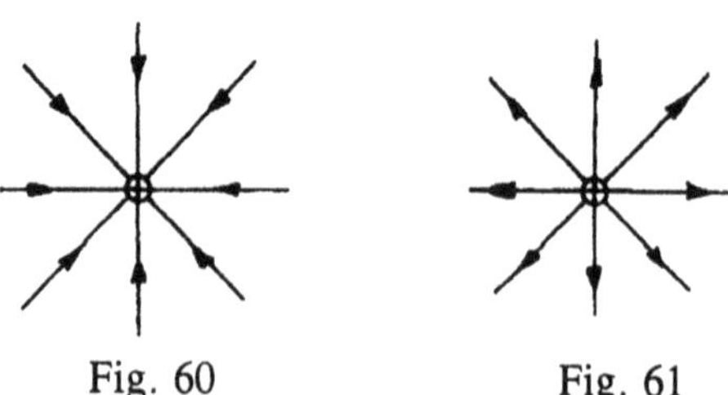

Fig. 60 Fig. 61

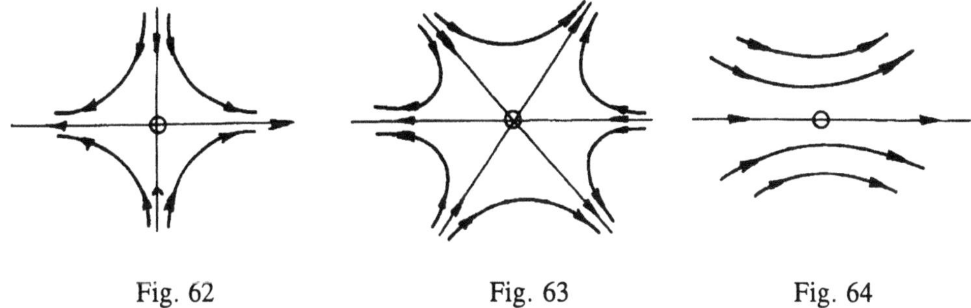

Fig. 62 Fig. 63 Fig. 64

Remarks. 1) If $\text{grad}f$ is not a complete vector field, then one can use one of the following complete vector fields:

a) $\dfrac{\text{grad}f}{\|\text{grad}f\|}$ if f has no critical point,

b) $\dfrac{\text{grad}f}{1 + \|\text{grad}f\|^2}$

which have the same orbits as $\text{grad}f$.

2) Suppose $n = 1$. The potential differential system (3) is reduced to the differential equation with separable variables $\dfrac{dx}{dt} = f'(x)$. The gradient lines of f viewed as orbits are oriented intervals of increase of the function f or zeros of f'; special parametrizations of the intervals of increasing or equilibrium points are viewed as functions. If x_0 is not an equilibrium point, then the solution fixed by the conditions (t_0, x_0) is $t - t_0 = \displaystyle\int_{x_0}^{x} \frac{du}{f'(x)}$. Hence there follows a method of establishing the monotony intervals of a C^1 function: zeros of f' lie between the finite extremities, and the sense of increasing or decreasing on every interval can be fixed by at least two values of the primitive (obtained by exact methods or by numerical methods). If x_0 is an equilibrium point of the differential equation $\dfrac{dx}{dt} = f'(x)$, then the associated linear differential equation is $\dfrac{dx}{dt} = (x - x_0)f''(x_0)$.

Application. Suppose that the motion of a particle in R^3 is described by the potential differential system

$$\frac{dx}{dt} = yz, \quad \frac{dy}{dt} = zx, \quad \frac{dz}{dt} = xy.$$

Show that:

1) If two of the numbers $x(0), y(0), z(0)$ are zero, then the particle does not move;

2) if $x(0) = y(0) = 1$, $z(0) = 0$, then the trajectory of the motion has the parametric equations

$$x = \sec t,\ y = \sec t,\ z = \tan t,\ t \neq (2k+1)\frac{\pi}{2},\ k \in Z;$$

3) if $x(0) = y(0) = 1,\ z(0) = -1$, then the trajectory of the motion has the parametric equations

$$x = \frac{1}{1+t},\ y = \frac{1}{1+t},\ z = -\frac{1}{1+t},\ t \neq -1;$$

4) if at least two of the values $x(0), y(0), z(0)$ are different from zero, then either the particle moves to infinity in a finite time (in the future) or comes from infinity in a finite time (in the past).

Solution. One observes that the vector field $X(x,y,z) = (yz, zx, xy)$ admits the global potential $f: R^3 \to R$, $f(x,y,z) = xyz$. The surfaces of nonzero constant level attached to f are Ţiţeica surfaces.

The relations $\mathrm{rot}X = 0$, $\mathrm{div}X = 0$ imply $\Delta X = 0$ and therefore X is a harmonic vector field.

1) The axes Ox, Oy, Oz consist of equilibrium points.

2); 3) From

$$\frac{dx}{yz} = \frac{dy}{zx} = \frac{dz}{xy}$$

we find the Cartesian implicit equations of the family of trajectories,

$$x^2 - y^2 = k_1,\ x^2 - z^2 = k_2.$$

The initial conditions determine the constants k_1, k_2 and then the proposed parametrizations are verified.

4) From $xx' = yy' = zz'$ it follows that $x^2 - c_1 = y^2 - c_2 = z^2 - c_3$. Suppose $c_1 \geq c_2 \geq c_3 = 0$. Hence $z^2 \leq y^2 \leq x^2$ and

$$z^2 = x^2 - c_1 = y^2 - c_2;\ c_1, c_2 \geq 0;\ \frac{dz}{dt} = \pm\sqrt{(z^2+c_1)(z^2+c_2)}.$$

For simplicity we suppose $z(0) \geq 0$ and

$$\frac{dz}{dt} = \sqrt{(z^2+c_1)(z^2+c_2)}.$$

It follows that

$$t(z) = \int_{z(0)}^{z} \frac{du}{\sqrt{(u^2 + c_1)(u^2 + c_2)}}$$

and

$$\lim_{z \to \infty} t(z) = \int_{z(0)}^{z} \frac{du}{\sqrt{(u^2 + c_1)(u^2 + c_2)}}$$

is finite (since the integral is convergent).

5.2. POTENTIAL DIFFERENTIAL SYSTEMS AND ELEMENTARY CATASTROPHES

Let x be a point of R^n, let c be a point of R^m, and let

$$f : R^n \times R^m \to R, \ (x, c) \to f(x, c)$$

be a C^∞ function. The set R^n is called the *state space* and the set R^m is called the *control space*.

The restriction of f to $R^n \times \{c\}$, i.e., the partial function $x \to f_c(x)$ is denoted by f_c and is called a *potential*. Thus, f can be thought as a family of potentials.

To the potential f_c one attaches the potential differential system

$$\frac{dx_1}{dt} = \frac{\partial f_c}{\partial x_1}(x), \ldots, \frac{dx_n}{dt} = \frac{\partial f_c}{\partial x_n}(x). \tag{4}$$

The set M of equilibrium points of the differential system (4) coincides with the set of critical points of potentials family f_c and as a subset of $R^n \times R^m$ it is described by

$$\frac{\partial f_c}{\partial x_1}(x) = 0, \ldots, \frac{\partial f_c}{\partial x_n}(x) = 0, \ x = (x_1, \ldots, x_n) \in R^n, \ c \in R^m.$$

This subset is called the *catastrophe manifold* associated to the potentials f, or the *equilibrium set* of the differential system (4). The set M is a submanifold of dimension m of $R^n \times R^m$ only if f has certain properties verified in some particular cases (e.g., it is sufficient that conditions from the implicit function theorem be verified).

Let $\pi : R^n \times R^m \to R^m$ be the natural projection defined by $\pi(x, c) = c$. The restriction of π to M is denoted by χ and is called the *catastrophe map*.

The subset S of M consisting of singular (critical) points of the catastrophe map

$\chi : M \to R^m$, i.e., the points at which the rank of the Jacobian matrix $J(\chi)$ is less than m, is called the *singularity set*. The image $B = \chi(S) \subset R^m$ is called the *bifurcation set*. This is directly observable, for it lies in the control space.

Having in mind the Jacobian of χ it comes out that S is in fact the set of points $(x, c) \in M$ that are degenerate critical points of the function $x \to f_c(x)$. In other words

$$S : \frac{\partial f_c}{\partial x_1}(x) = 0 \, , \dots , \frac{\partial f_c}{\partial x_n}(x) = 0, \quad \det\left[\frac{\partial^2 f_c}{\partial x_i \partial x_j}(x)\right] = 0.$$

It follows that B is the set on which the number and the nature of the critical points of $x \to f_c(x)$, or of equilibrium points of the differential system (4), change. The theory of structural stability of Morse functions shows that such a change for $x \to f_c(x)$ can only occur by passing through a degenerate critical point. To the degenerate critical points of the function $x \to f_c(x)$ there correspond points of the graph of the function at which the Gauss-Kronecker curvature

$$K = \frac{\det\left[\dfrac{\partial^2 f_c}{\partial x_i \partial x_j}\right]}{(1 + \|\nabla f_c\|^2)^{1 + \frac{n}{2}}}$$

vanishes.

The term catastrophe is used sometimes as a synonym for "point of S" to suggest that a smooth variation in the control space determines a discontinuous change (a jump) in the state space. The jump means the passing from a minimum to a maximum point (or conversely) of the function $x \to f_c(x)$ or the passing from one solution of the differential system (4) to another which is not topologically equivalent to the first. We specify that the potential differential systems never oscillate, and the only jumps which can appear for such systems are those associated to a change of the number of equilibrium points.

The general theory shows that the families of functions can be classified such that the structure of critical points is not affected qualitatively by suitable changing of coordinates. Particularly, almost all the families of real C^∞ functions on R^n, with $m \le 4$ parameters, are structurally stable, and are equivalents, in a neighborhood of each point, to one of the following forms [92]:

1) **not catastrophic functions**

noncritical, x_1,

Morse l-saddle, $x_1^2 + \cdots + x_l^2 - x_{l+1}^2 - \cdots - x_n^2$, $0 \le l \le n$.

(These two types are not catastrophic forms, since they have no degenerate critical points and rest unchanged under variations in the control space. All the followings have degenerate critical points, depend on control variables and therefore are catastrophic forms).

2) **cuspidal catastrophes**

fold, $\frac{1}{3}x_1^3 + c_1 x_1 + (M)$,

cusp, $\pm\left(\frac{1}{4}x_1^4 + \frac{1}{2}c_1 x_1^2 + c_2 x_1\right) + (M)$,

swallowtail, $\frac{1}{5}x_1^5 + \frac{c_1}{3}x_1^3 + \frac{c_2}{2}x_1^2 + c_3 x_1 + (M)$,

butterfly, $\pm\left(\frac{1}{6}x_1^6 + \frac{c_1}{4}x_1^4 + \frac{c_2}{3}x_1^3 + \frac{c_2}{2}x_1^2 + c_4 x_1\right) + (M)$;

3) **umbilic catastrophes**

elliptic umbilic, $x_1^3 - 3x_1 x_2^2 + c_1(x_1^2 + x_2^2) + c_2 x_1 + c_3 x_2 + (N)$,
hyperbolic umbilic, $x_1^3 + x_2^3 + c_1 x_1 x_2 + c_2 x_1 + c_3 x_2 + (N)$,
parabolic umbilic, $\pm(x_1^2 x_2 + x_2^4 + c_1 x_1^2 + c_2 x_2^2 + c_3 x_1 + c_4 x_2) + (N)$,

where $(x_1, \ldots, x_n) \in R^n$, $(c_1, \ldots, c_m) \in R^m$, $m \le 4$, and *(M)* indicates a Morse function of the form

$$x_2^2 + \cdots + x_l^2 - x_{l+1}^2 - \cdots - x_n^2, \; 1 \le l \le n,$$

and (N) indicates a Morse function of the form

$$x_3^2 + \cdots + x_l^2 - x_{l+1}^2 - \cdots - x_n^2, \; 2 \le l \le n.$$

The preceding names have been suggested by the geometry of every family of functions and are used both for the family of functions and for the corresponding degenerate critical points. The signs $\pm$ give dual possibilities and are left aside since the geometry of the two situations is essentially the same. Leaving aside the functions 1) and the terms (M), and (N), we obtain seven types of families of functions called in short *elementary catastrophes*. These contain *subcatastrophes*, the subordination diagram as follows:

butterfly ➔ swallowtail ➔ cusp ➔ fold ➔ (Morse)
parabolic umbilic ➔ swallowtail
parabolic umbilic ➔ elliptic umbilic ➔ cusp
parabolic umbilic ➔ hyperbolic umbilic ➔ cusp.

5.3. GRADIENT LINES OF THE FOLD

The standard *fold potential* is

$$x \to f_a(x) = \frac{1}{3}x^3 + ax,$$

where a is a real parameter. The gradient lines of this potential are given by the differential equation with separable variables

$$\frac{dx}{dt} = x^2 + a. \tag{5}$$

Viewed as orbits, the gradient lines of f_a are either oriented intervals on which f_a increases or solutions of the equation $x^2 + a = 0$. From this follows the equilibrium set

$$M : x^2 + a = 0 \text{ (parabola)},$$

which can be viewed as the image of the chart $\alpha : x = t,\ a = -t^2,\ t \in R$. We deduce that the expression in coordinates of the catastrophe application is

$$\chi \circ \alpha(t) = -t^2,$$

with one critical point $t = 0$. Thus χ has the critical point $(0, 0)$ and therefore $S = \{(0,0)\}$ is the singularities set, and $B = \chi(S) = \{0\}$ is the bifurcation set.

Let $a > 0$. Then the differential equation (5) does not admit equilibrium points, and the general solution is

$$x = \sqrt{a}\tan\sqrt{a}\,(t + c),\ t \in R \setminus \left\{ \frac{(2k+1)\pi}{2\sqrt{a}} - c,\ k \in Z \right\}.$$

The solution fixed by the initial conditions (t_0, x_0) is determined by

$$c = \frac{1}{\sqrt{a}}\arctan\frac{x_0}{\sqrt{a}} - t_0,$$

and it has the graph in Fig.65.

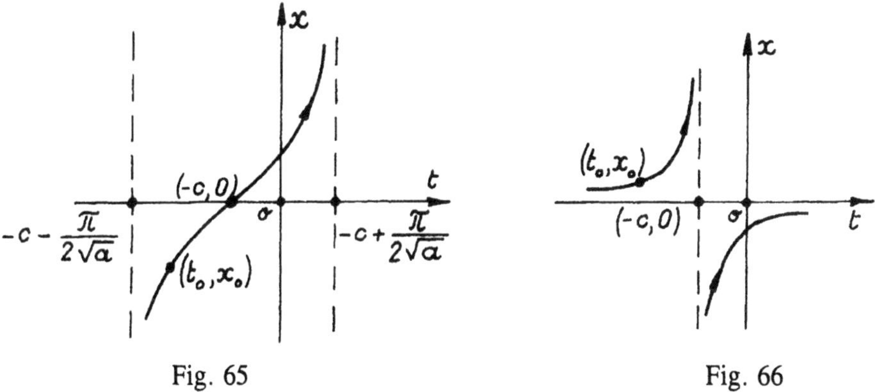

Fig. 65 Fig. 66

Let $a = 0$. Then $x = 0$ is the single equilibrium point and

$$x = \frac{-1}{t+c}, \quad t \in R \setminus \{-c\}$$

is the general solution. Obviously the equilibrium point cannot be an initial value of a solution obtained from the general solution. For Fig.66 the constant c is fixed by the initial conditions (t_0, x_0) and hence $c = -\frac{1}{x_0} - t_0$. Denote

$$x(t,x_0) = \frac{-1}{t - t_0 - \frac{1}{x_0}};$$

the equilibrium point $x_0 = 0$ is stable and asymptotically stable since

$$\lim_{x_0 \to 0} x(t,x_0) = 0, \ \forall\, t \in [t_0, \infty) \quad \text{and} \quad \lim_{t \to \infty} x(t,x_0) = 0.$$

Let $a < 0$. Then the differential equation (5) admits two equilibrium points $x = \pm\sqrt{a}$, and the general solution is

$$x = -\sqrt{-a}\coth\sqrt{-a}(t+c_1) \quad \text{for} \quad x \in (-\infty, -\sqrt{-a}) \cup (\sqrt{-a}, \infty)$$

and

$$x = -\sqrt{-a}\tanh\sqrt{-a}(t+c_2) \quad \text{for} \quad x \in (-\sqrt{-a}, \sqrt{-a}).$$

Giving the initial conditions (t_0, x_0) which determine the solution $x(t)$ of the differential equation (5), we arrive at the following conclusions: if x_0 is an equilibrium point, then $x(t) = x_0$, $\forall\, t \in R$; if $x_0 \in (-\infty, -\sqrt{-a}) \cup (\sqrt{-a}, \infty)$, then the solution $x(t)$ has the behavior of of the hyperbolic cotangent (Fig.67), $c_1 = \frac{1}{\sqrt{-a}} \operatorname{argcoth} \frac{x_0}{-\sqrt{-a}} - t_0$; if $x_0 \in (-\sqrt{-a}, \sqrt{a})$, then the solution $x(t)$ has the behavior of the hyperbolic tangent (Fig.68), $c_2 = \frac{1}{\sqrt{-a}} \operatorname{argtanh} \frac{x_0}{-\sqrt{-a}} - t_0$.

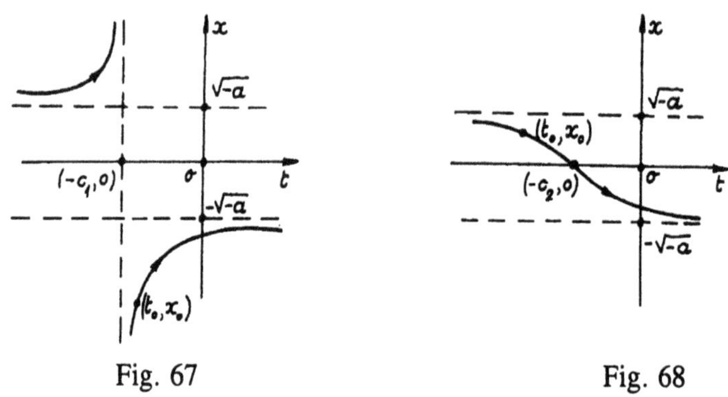

Fig. 67 Fig. 68

The equilibrium point $x = -\sqrt{-a}$, $a \neq 0$, is asymptotically stable, since (see 5.1)

$$\frac{d^2 f_a}{dx^2}(-\sqrt{-a}) = -2\sqrt{-a} < 0.$$

Also, we remark that

$$\lim_{x_0 \to \sqrt{-a}} x(t, x_0) = \sqrt{-a}, \ \forall t \in (-\infty, t_0],$$

$$\lim_{t \to -\infty} x(t, x_0) = \sqrt{-a}$$

(a fact that would correspond to a stability in the past).

The catastrophe takes place at the passing through $a = 0$, since at this moment the number of equilibrium points is changed.

The arrows of Figs.65-68 show the sense on the graphs of gradient lines, and hence the sense of increasing of f_a. Projecting the graphs on the Ox-axis, we find the orbits (segments of a straight line) and an increasing sense of f_a along these orbits. Obviously, these results can be read directly from the graph of f_a whose tracing does not raise any problem (Fig.69).

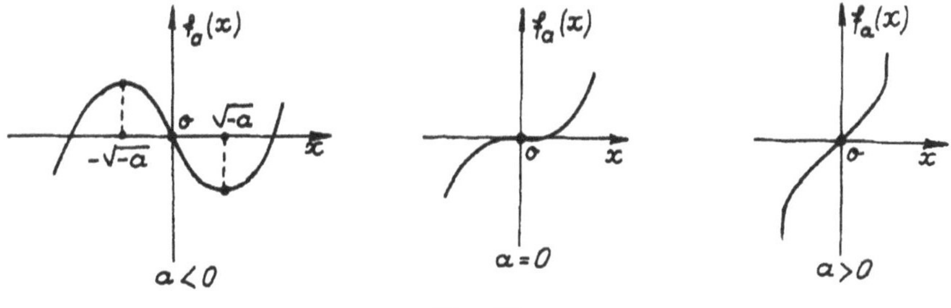

Fig. 69

5.4. GRADIENT LINES OF THE CUSP

The standard *cusp potential* is

$$x \to f_{ab}(x) = \frac{1}{4}x^4 + \frac{1}{2}ax^2 + bx,$$

where a, b are real parameters. The gradient lines of the cusp are the solutions of the differential equation with separable variables

$$\frac{dx}{dt} = x^3 + ax + b. \tag{6}$$

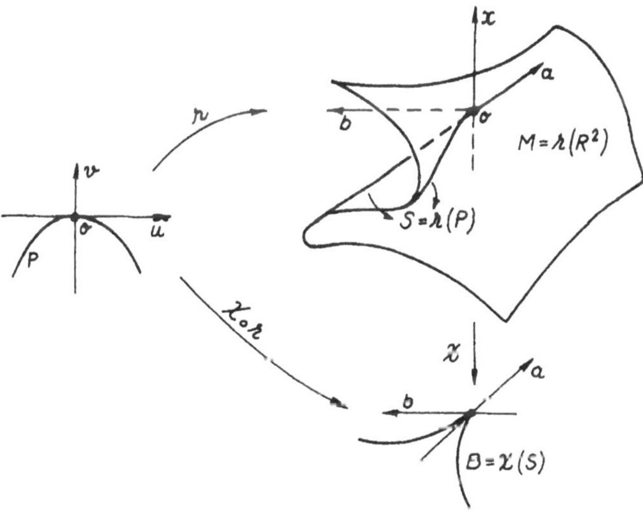

Fig. 70

The equilibrium set (Fig.70)

$$M : x^3 + ax + b = 0,$$

which coincides with the image of the Monge chart

$$r : x = u, \ a = v, \ b = -u^3 - vu, \ (u,v) \in R^2,$$

is a ruled surface in R^3. The expression in coordinates of the catastrophe application is

$$\chi \circ r(u,v) = (v, -u^3 - vu)$$

and has the Jacobian

$$\begin{vmatrix} 0 & 1 \\ -3u^2 - v & -u \end{vmatrix} = 3u^2 + v = \frac{d^2 f_{ab}}{dx^2}\Big|_{x=u,\, a=v}.$$

Thus the points of the parabola

$$P : 3u^2 + v = 0$$

in the plane uOv are singular points of $\chi \circ r$, and the singularities set S is characterized by the parametric equations

$$x = u, \ a = v, \ b = -u^3 - vu, \ 3u^2 + v = 0.$$

We remark that S is a twist cubic (fold-type cubic) of parametric equations

$$x = u, \ a = -3u^2, \ b = 2u^3.$$

Correspondingly the bifurcation set B has the parametrization

$$\chi(u, -3u^2, 2u^3) = (-3u^2, 2u^3).$$

In other words, B is the semicubic parabola of Cartesian implicit equation (Fig.70)

$$4a^3 + 27b^2 = 0.$$

Let us analyse the number of equilibrium points and the general solution of the differential equation (6) as functions of the parameters a and b. The equation

$$x^3 + ax + b = 0$$

has always a real solution (being an equation of order three) and the nature of its roots is given by the discriminant

$$D = 4a^3 + 27b^2.$$

It will follow that the number of equilibrium points is changed at passing through the bifurcation set.

If $D < 0$, i.e., (a,b) belong to the region I of Fig.71, then the differential equation (6) admits three equilibrium points, let us say $x_1 = \alpha$, $x_2 = \beta$, $x_3 = \gamma$. The general solution is defined by

$$|x-\alpha|^{\gamma-\beta}|x-\beta|^{\alpha-\gamma}|x-\gamma|^{\beta-\alpha} = c\exp[(\alpha-\beta)(\beta-\gamma)(\gamma-\alpha)t],\ t \in R,$$

where c is an arbitrary constant.

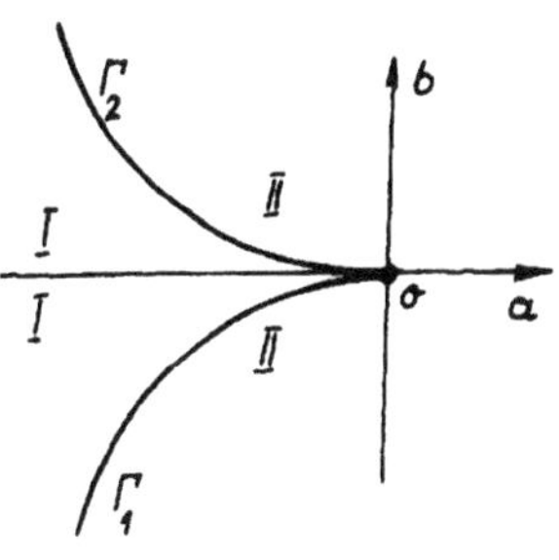

Fig. 71

Let $D = 0$, and $a \neq 0$ or $b \neq 0$, i.e., $(a,b) \in \Gamma_1 \cup \Gamma_2 \setminus \{(0,0)\}$. The equation $x^3 + ax + b = 0$ has three real roots, one being double; the differential equation (6) admits two equilibrium points $x_1 = x_3 = \alpha$, $x_2 = \beta$, and its general solution is defined by

$$-\frac{1}{\alpha-\beta}\frac{1}{x-\alpha} - \frac{1}{(\alpha-\beta)^2}\ln|x-\alpha| + \frac{1}{(\alpha-\beta)^2}\ln|x-\beta| = t + c,\ t \in R,$$

where c is an arbitrary constant.

If $D = 0$, and $a = 0$, $b = 0$, then $x = 0$ is a triple equilibrium point, and the general solution of the differential equation (6) is defined by

$$-\frac{1}{2x^2} = t + c,\ t \in R \setminus \{-c\},$$

where c is an arbitrary constant.

For $D > 0$, i.e., for (a,b) belonging to the region II of Fig.71, the differential equation (6) has a unique equilibrium point $x_1 = \alpha$. Since

$$x^3 + ax + b = (x-\alpha)(x^2 + \alpha x + \alpha^2 + a),\ 3\alpha^2 + 4a > 0,$$

the general solution is defined by

$$\frac{1}{3\alpha^2 + a}\ln|x-\alpha| - \frac{1}{2(3\alpha^2+a)}$$

$$\times\left[\ln(\alpha^2 + \alpha x + \alpha^2 + a) + \frac{3\alpha}{\sqrt{3\alpha^2+4a}}\operatorname{argtan}\frac{2x+\alpha}{\sqrt{3\alpha^2+4a}}\right] = t + c,$$

where c is an arbitrary constant.

The orbits (in the sense of oriented intervals on which f_{ab} increases) can be read directly on the sketch of the graph of f_{ab} (Fig.72).

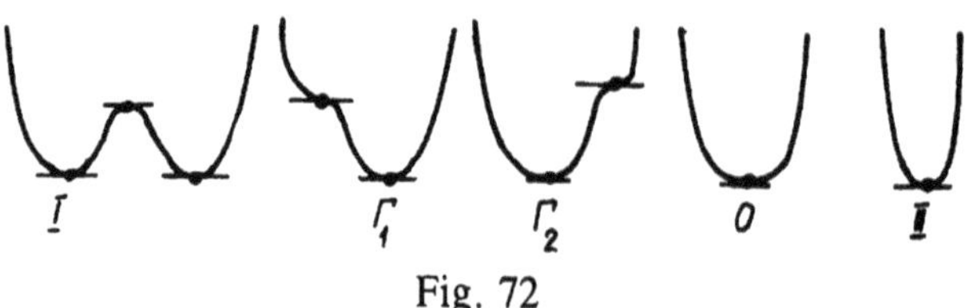

Fig. 72

Let x_0 be an equilibrium point. Since

$$\frac{d^2}{dx^2} f_{ab}(x) = 3x^2 + a,$$

the hypothesis $3x_0^2 + a < 0$ implies asymptotic stability and therefore stability of the equilibrium point x_0 (see 5.1 and Fig.70).

5.5. EQUILIBRIUM POINTS OF GRADIENT OF SWALLOWTAIL

The standard *swallowtail potential* is

$$x \to f_{abc}(x) = \frac{1}{5}x^5 + \frac{a}{3}x^3 + \frac{b}{2}x^2 + cx,$$

where a, b, c are real parameters. The gradient lines of the swallowtail are solutions of the differential equation with separable variables

$$\frac{dx}{dt} = x^4 + ax^2 + bx + c. \tag{7}$$

The equilibrium set

$$M : x^4 + ax^2 + bx + c = 0$$

coincides to the image of the Monge chart

$$r : x = u, \ a = v, \ b = w, \ c = -u^4 - vu^2 - wu, \ (u, v, w) \in R^3$$

and it is a ruled hypersurface of R^4. Denoting by χ the catastrophe application, the function $\chi \circ r$ is defined by

$$\chi \circ r(u, v, w) = (v, w, -u^4 - vu^2 - wu).$$

The Jacobian of $\chi \circ r$ is

$$\begin{vmatrix} 0 & 1 & 0 \\ 0 & 0 & 1 \\ -4u^3 - 2vu - w & -u^2 & -u \end{vmatrix} = -(4u^3 + 2vu + w) = -\frac{d^2 f_{abc}}{dx^2}\Big|_{x=u,\, a=v,\, b=w}.$$

This expression shows that the points of ruled surface

$$\Sigma : 4u^3 + 2vu + w = 0$$

of the space $Ouvw$ are singular points of $\chi \circ r$. The shape of Σ is the same as the shape of the catastrophe manifold represented in Fig.70.

The set S of singularities has the equations

$$x = u,\ a = v,\ b = w,\ c = -u^4 - vu^2 - wu,\ 4u^2 + 2vu + w = 0,$$

i.e., S is a ruled surface (2-dimensional manifold) in R^4 of parametric equations

$$x = u,\ a = v,\ b = -4u^3 - 2vu,\ c = 3u^4 + vu^2.$$

The bifurcation set B is the image of the application

$$a = v,\ b = -4u^3 - 2vu,\ c = 3u^4 + vu^2,\ (u, v) \in R^2.$$

Since the rank of the Jacobian matrix attached to this map is 1 if and only if $6u^2 + v = 0$, otherwise being 2, it follows that

$$(-6u^2, 8u^3, -3u^4),\ u \in R,$$

are the singular points of B, and

$$B \setminus \{(-6u^2, 8u^3, -3u^4), u \in R\}$$

is a ruled surface of R^3.

The discussion of number of equilibrium points and the finding of a general solution of differential equation (7), as functions of the parameters a, b, c, are clear from the theoretical point of view, but difficult from the point of view of analytical calculus. That is why Fig.73 refers to some Runge-Kutta approximations of gradient lines realized via a PC program of plotting (a=1, b=2, c=0; t=0; x∈{1;1.1;1.2;1.3}).

The number of equilibrium points is changed at passing through the bifurcation set.

Let x_0 be an equilibrium point and

$$\frac{d^2 f_{abc}}{dx^2}(x_0) = 4x_0^3 + 2ax_0 + b.$$

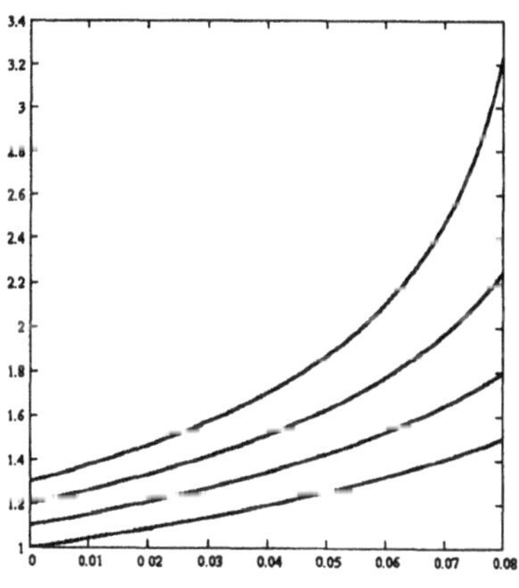

Fig. 73

If $4x_0^3 + 2ax_0 + b < 0$, then the equilibrium point x_0 is asymptotically stable.

5.6. EQUILIBRIUM POINTS OF GRADIENT OF BUTTERFLY

The standard *butterfly potential* is

$$x \to f_{abcd}(x) = \frac{1}{6}x^6 + \frac{a}{4}x^4 + \frac{b}{3}x^3 + \frac{c}{2}x^2 + dx,$$

where a, b, c, d are real parameters. Consequently, the gradient lines of the butterfly are solutions of the differential equation with separable variables

$$\frac{dx}{dt} = x^5 + ax^3 + bx^2 + cx + d. \tag{8}$$

The equilibrium set

$$M : x^5 + ax^3 + bx^2 + cx + d = 0$$

is a ruled surface in R^5. The Monge chart whose image covers M is

$$r(x,a,b,c) = (x,\ a,\ b,\ c,\ -x^5 - ax^3 - bx^2 - cx).$$

If χ is the catastrophe map, then

$$\chi \circ r(x,a,b,c) = (a,\ b,\ c,\ -x^5 - ax^3 - bx^2 - cx).$$

This last function has the Jacobian

$$\begin{vmatrix} 0 & 1 & 0 & 0 \\ 0 & 0 & 1 & 0 \\ 0 & 0 & 0 & 1 \\ -5x^4 - 3ax^2 - 2bx - c & -x^3 & -x^2 & -x \end{vmatrix} = 5x^4 + 3ax^2 + 2bx + c = \frac{d^2}{dx^2} f_{abcd}(x).$$

It follows the set of singularities

$$S : x^5 + ax^3 + bx^2 + cx + d = 0,\ 5x^4 + 3ax^2 + 2bx + c = 0$$

(ruled manifold of dimension 3 in R^5), and the bifurcation set

$$B : c = -5x^4 - 3ax^2 - 2bx,\ d = 4x^5 + 2ax^3 + bx^2.$$

To the map $(x,a,b) \to (c,d)$ we can attach the Jacobian matrix

$$J = \begin{bmatrix} -20x^3 - 6ax - 2b & -3x^2 & -2x \\ 20x^4 + 6ax^2 + 2bx & 2x^3 & x^2 \end{bmatrix}$$

having

$$\operatorname{rank} J = \begin{cases} 0 & \text{for } x = 0 \quad \text{and} \quad b = 0 \\ 1 & \text{for } x = 0 \quad \text{and} \quad b \neq 0 \\ 2 & \text{for } x \neq 0 \ \text{ and any } \ b. \end{cases}$$

Therefore the elements of the set

$$\{(a, b, 0, 0) \,|\, (a, b) \in R^2\}$$

are singular points of B, and

$$B \setminus \{(a, b, 0, 0) \,|\, (a, b) \in R^2\}$$

is a ruled hypersurface of R^4.

Fig.74 refers to some Runge-Kutta approximations of gradient lines obtained by a PC program of plotting (a=1, b=2, c=1,d=0; t=0; x∈{1;1.1;1.2;1.3}).

The catastrophe appears at passing through the bifurcation set D, since at this moment the number of equilibrium points is changed.

Let x_0 be an equilibrium point. If

$$\frac{d^2 f_{abcd}}{dx^2}(x_0) = 5x_0^4 + 3ax_0^2 + 2bx_0 + c < 0,$$

then the equilibrium point x_0 is asymptotically stable and therefore stable.

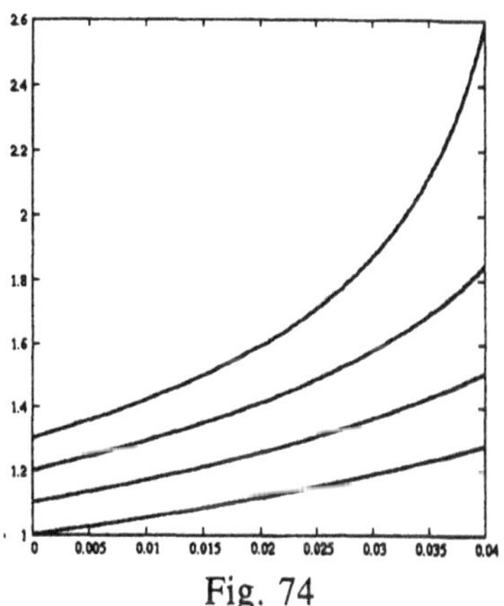

Fig. 74

5.7. EQUILIBRIUM POINTS OF GRADIENT OF ELLIPTIC UMBILIC

The standard *elliptic umbilic potential* is

$$(x, y) \to f_{abc}(x, y) = x^3 - 3xy^2 + a(x^2 + y^2) + bx + cy$$

where a, b, c are real parameters. Consequently, the general gradient lines of elliptic umbilic are solutions of the potential differential system

$$\frac{dx}{dt} = 3x^2 - 3y^2 + 2ax + b, \quad \frac{dy}{dt} = -6xy + 2ay + c. \tag{9}$$

The equilibrium set

$$M: 3x^2 - 3y^2 + 2ax + b = 0, \quad -6xy + 2ay + c = 0$$

is covered completely by the image of the Monge chart

$$r(x, y, a) = (x, y, a, 3(y^2 - x^2) - 2ax, 6xy - 2ay).$$

Thus M is a ruled submanifold of dimension 3 in R^5.

Denote by χ the catastrophe application. Then the function $\chi \circ r$ is defined by

$$\chi \circ r(x,y,a) = (a,\, 3(y^2 - x^2) - 2ax,\; 6xy - 2ay)$$

and it has the Jacobian

$$\begin{vmatrix} 0 & 0 & 1 \\ -6x-2a & 6y & -2x \\ 6y & 6x-2a & -2y \end{vmatrix} = 4[a^2 - 9(x^2+y^2)].$$

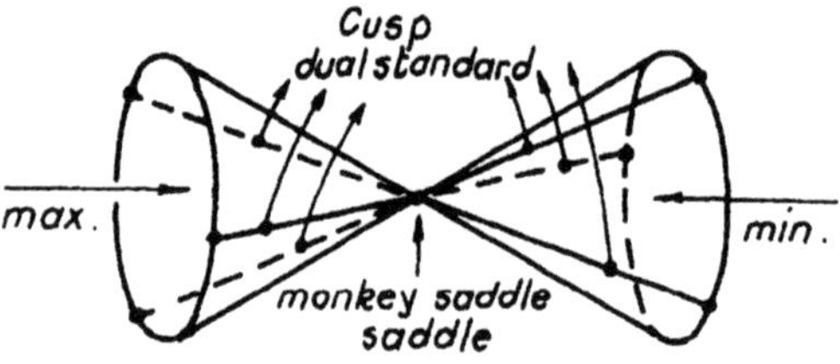

Fig. 75

Thus the points of the right circular cone (Fig.75)

$$\Sigma : x^2 + y^2 = \frac{a^2}{9}$$

are the singular points of $\chi \circ r$.

The set S of singularities of χ has the implicit Cartesian equations

$$3(x^2 - y^2) + 2ax + b = 0,\;\; -6xy + 2ay + c = 0,\;\; x^2 + y^2 = \frac{a^2}{9}.$$

Since the gradient vector fields

$$(6x+2a,\, -6y,\, 2x,\, 1,\, 0),\;\; (-6y,\, -6x+2a,\, 2y,\, 0,\, 1),\;\; \left(2x, 2y, \frac{-2a}{9}, 0, 0\right)$$

are linearly independent at every point of S excepting $(0,0,0,0,0)$, it follows that

$S \setminus \{(0,0,0,0,0)\}$ is a submanifold of dimension 2 in R^5.

The right circular cone Σ is the image of the application

$$(a,\theta) \to \left(\frac{a}{3}\cos\theta, \frac{a}{3}\sin\theta, a \right), \quad (a,\theta) \in R^2.$$

Therefore the bifurcation set B is characterized by the equations

$$b = -\frac{a^2}{3}(\cos 2\theta + 2\cos\theta), \quad c = \frac{a^2}{3}(\sin 2\theta - 2\sin\theta).$$

The intersection of B with the plane $a = 1$ is a *deltoid* or a *three-cusped hypocycloid*. The Jacobian of the map $(a,b) \to (b,c)$ has the expression

$$\frac{4a^3}{9}(1 - \cos 3\theta).$$

For that reason the points with $a = 0$ (the origin) or $\cos 3\theta = 1$, i.e., $\theta = 0, \frac{2\pi}{3}, \frac{4\pi}{3}$, are singular points of B. The remainder of the set B is a surface of R^3.

The equilibrium points of the differential system (9) are generated by the intersections of two families of hyperbolas

$$\left(x + \frac{a}{3} \right)^2 - y^2 - \frac{a^2 - 3b}{9} = 0, \quad -6xy + 2ay + c = 0.$$

If (x_0, y_0) is an equilibrium point, then the linear approximation of (9) around (x_0, y_0) is

$$\begin{cases} \dfrac{dx}{dt} = (6x_0 + 2a)(x - x_0) - 6y_0(y - y_0) \\[2ex] \dfrac{dy}{dt} = -6y_0(x - x_0) + (-6x_0 + 2a)(y - y_0). \end{cases} \tag{9'}$$

The symmetric matrix associated to this linear differential system has the characteristic equation

$$\lambda^2 - \beta\lambda + \gamma = 0, \quad \beta = 4a, \quad \gamma = 4a^2 - 36x_0^2 - 36y_0^2.$$

The roots (proper values)

$$\lambda_1 = 2a + 6\sqrt{x_0^2 + y_0^2}, \quad \lambda_2 = 2a - 6\sqrt{x_0^2 + y_0^2}$$

are real numbers, and the corresponding proper vectors are orthogonal.

The equilibrium point (x_0, y_0) of the linear differential system $(9')$ can be attractor, proper knot, improper knot or saddle point. Regarding the stability of this equilibrium point, the following propositions are true:

1) if $a > 0,\ a^2 - 9(x_0^2 + y_0^2) > 0$, then (x_0, y_0) is an unstable knot;

2) if $a < 0,\ a^2 - 9(x_0^2 + y_0^2) > 0$, then (x_0, y_0) is an asymptotically stable knot;

3) if $a^2 - 9(x_0^2 + y_0^2) < 0$, then (x_0, y_0) is a saddle point (unstable);

4) if $x_0 = y_0 = 0,\ a < 0$, then $(0,0)$ is a proper knot (asymptotically stable);

5) if $x_0 = y_0 = 0,\ a > 0$, then $(0,0)$ is an unstable proper knot.

Obviously the conditions 2) and 4) are equivalent to the fact that

$$\frac{1}{2} d^2 f_{abc}(x_0, y_0) = (a + 3x_0)dx^2 - 6y_0 dxdy + (a - 3x_0)dy^2$$

is negative definite. Also we recall that the asymptotic stability and the unstability from the linear differential system (9') transfer to the differential system (9).

The catastrophe takes place at passing through the bifurcation set.

Fig.76 presents some Runge-Kutta approximations of gradient lines obtained by a PC program of plotting with data: a=1/2, b=0, c=0; t=0; (1;1),(1.1;1),(1.2;1),(1.3;1).

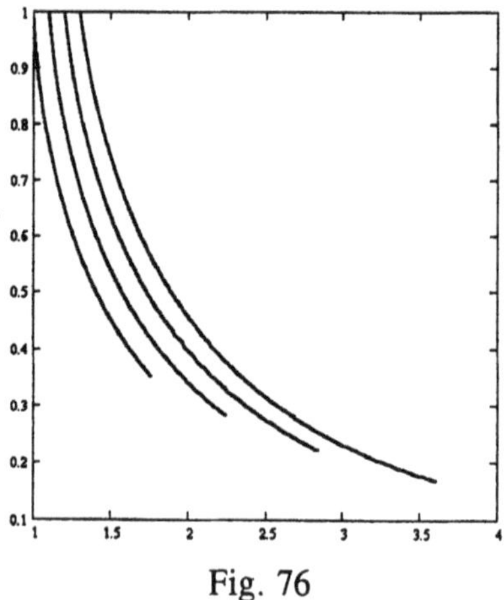

Fig. 76

Finally, we remark that $\Delta f_{abc} = 4a$. Thus the flow generated by $\text{grad} f_{abc}$ decreases the area if $a < 0$, increases the area if $a > 0$, or preserves the area if $a = 0$.

5.8. EQUILIBRIUM POINTS OF GRADIENT OF HYPERBOLIC UMBILIC

The standard *hyperbolic umbilic potential* is

$$(x,y) \to f_{abc}(x,y) = x^3 + y^3 + axy + bx + cy,$$

where a, b, c are real parameters. Its gradient lines are described by the potential differential system

$$\frac{dx}{dt} = 3x^2 + ay + b, \quad \frac{dy}{dt} = 3y^2 + ax + c. \tag{10}$$

The equilibrium set

$$M : 3x^2 + ay + b = 0, \; 3y^2 + ax + c = 0$$

is a ruled submanifold of dimension 3 in R^5. It can be realized as the image of the Monge chart

$$r(x,y,a) = (x,y,a, -3x^2 - ay, -3y^2 - ax).$$

If χ is the catastrophe map, then the Jacobian of $\chi \circ r$ is

$$\begin{vmatrix} 0 & 0 & 1 \\ -6x & -a & -y \\ -a & -6y & -x \end{vmatrix} = 36xy - a^2.$$

Thus the set of singularities of $\chi \circ r$ is the cone

$$\Sigma : 36xy = a^2.$$

The set of singularities of χ is

$$S : 3x^2 + ay + b = 0, \; 3y^2 + ax + c = 0, \; 36xy = a^2.$$

Since the gradient vector fields

$$(6x, a, y, 1, 0), \; (a, 6y, x, 0, 1), \; (36y, 36x, -2a, 0, 0)$$

are linearly independent at every point of S excepting $(0,0,0,0,0)$, it follows that $S \setminus \{(0,0,0,0,0)\}$ is a submanifold of dimension 2 in R^5. The bifurcation set is

$$B = \chi(S) = \{(a,b,c) \,|\, a = \pm 6\sqrt{xy}, \, b = -3x^2 \mp 6y\sqrt{xy}, \, c = -3y^2 \mp x\sqrt{xy}\}.$$

Excepting the singular points (the points at which the functions a, b, c are not differentiable, and the point at which the associated Jacobian matrix does not have the rank 2), the remainder of B is a surface in R^3.

The equilibrium points of the potential differential system (10) are generated by the intersections of families of parabolas

$$3x^2 + ay + b = 0 \quad \text{(with vertical axis)},$$
$$3y^2 + ax + c = 0 \quad \text{(with horizontal axis)}.$$

Denoting by (x_0, y_0) an equilibrium point, we find the linear differential approximation

$$\frac{dx}{dt} = 6x_0(x - x_0) + a(y - y_0), \quad \frac{dy}{dt} = a(x - x_0) + 6y_0(y - y_0). \tag{10'}$$

The matrix of the system $(10')$ is symmetric. Thus it admits real proper values, and it is diagonalizable. From the characteristic equation

$$\lambda^2 - \beta\lambda + \gamma = 0, \ \beta = 6(x_0 + y_0), \ \gamma = 36x_0 y_0 - a^2$$

we find the proper values

$$\lambda_1 = 3(x_0 + y_0) + \sqrt{9(x_0 - y_0)^2 + a^2}, \ \lambda_2 = 3(x_0 + y_0) - \sqrt{9(x_0 - y_0)^2 + a^2}.$$

The equilibrium point (x_0, y_0) of the linear differential system $(10')$ can be attractor, proper knot, improper knot or saddle point, having one of the following behaviors:

1) if $x_0 + y_0 > 0$, $36x_0 y_0 - a^2 > 0$, then (x_0, y_0) is an unstable knot;

2) if $x_0 + y_0 < 0$, $36x_0 y_0 - a^2 > 0$, then (x_0, y_0) is an asymptotically stable knot;

3) if $36x_0 y_0 - a^2 < 0$, then (x_0, y_0) is a saddle point (unstable);

4) if $x_0 = y_0 < 0$, $a = 0$, then (x_0, x_0) is an asymptotically stable proper knot;

5) if $x_0 = y_0 > 0$, $a = 0$, then (x_0, x_0) is an unstable proper knot.

The conditions of 2) and 4) are equivalent to the fact that

$$\frac{1}{2} d^2 f_{abc}(x_0, y_0) = 3x_0\, dx^2 + a\, dx\, dy + 3y_0\, dy^2$$

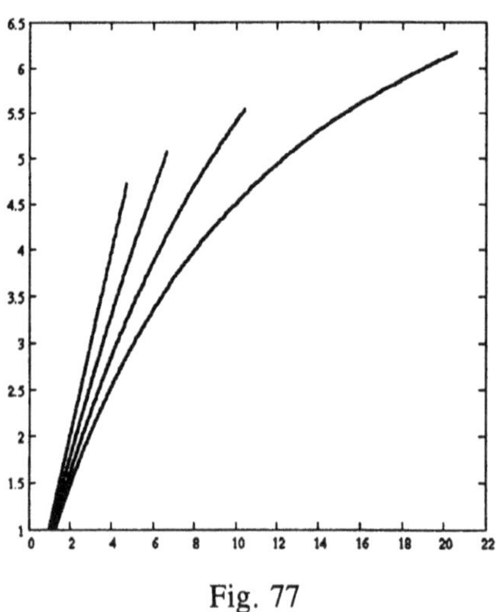

Fig. 77

is negative definite. They imply the asymptotic stability of the equilibrium position (x_0, y_0) of the differential system (10). The conditions 1), 3), 5) respectively implies the instability of the equilibrium position (x_0, y_0).

The catastrophe takes place at passing through the bifurcation set.

Fig.77 presents some Runge-Kutta approximations of gradient lines obtained by a PC program of plotting with data: a=1, b=0, c=0; t=0; (1;1),(1.1;1),(1.2;1),(1.3;1).

Since $\Delta f_{abc} = \operatorname{div} \operatorname{grad} f_{abc} = 6(x + y)$, the flow generated by $\operatorname{grad} f_{abc}$ decreases area in the semiplane $x + y < 0$ and increases area in the semiplane $x + y > 0$.

5.9. EQUILIBRIUM POINTS OF GRADIENT OF PARABOLIC UMBILIC

The standard *parabolic umbilic potential* is

$$(x,y) \to f_{abcd}(x,y) = x^2 y + y^4 + ax^2 + by^2 + ax + dy,$$

where a, b, c, d are real parameters. The gradient lines of this potential are solutions of the potential differential system

$$\frac{dx}{dt} = 2xy + 2ax + c, \quad \frac{dy}{dt} = 4y^3 + x^2 + 2by + d. \tag{11}$$

The equilibrium set

$$M : 2xy + 2ax + c = 0, \; 4y^3 + x^2 + 2by + d = 0$$

is a ruled manifold of dimension 4 in R^6. It is covered completely by the image of the Monge chart

$$r(x,y,a,b) = (x, y, a, b, -2xy - 2ax, -4y^3 - x^2 - 2by).$$

Let χ be the catastrophe map. The function

$$\chi \circ r(x,y,a,b) = (a, b, -2xy - 2ax, -4y^3 - x^2 - 2by)$$

has the Jacobian $6y^3 + 6ay^2 + by + ab - x^2$. It follows that the set of singular points of $\chi \circ r$ is

$$\Sigma : 6y^3 + 6ay^2 + by + ab - x^2 = 0,$$

and the singularities set of χ is $S = M \cap \Sigma$. It follows that $B = \chi(S)$.

Let (x_0, y_0) be an equilibrium point. The linear differential approximation around (x_0, y_0) is

$$\begin{cases} \dfrac{dx}{dt} = 2(y_0 + a)(x - x_0) + 2x_0(y - y_0) \\[2ex] \dfrac{dy}{dt} = 2x_0(x - x_0) + 2(6y_0^2 + b)(y - y_0). \end{cases} \tag{11'}$$

The characteristic equation of the symmetric matrix associated to this system is

$$\lambda^2 - \beta\lambda + \gamma = 0, \; \beta = 2(6y_0^2 + y_0 + a + b), \; \gamma = 4(6y_0^3 + 6ay_0^2 + by_0 - x_0^2 + ab).$$

The solutions

$$\lambda_{1,2} = 6y_0^2 + y_0 + a + b \pm \sqrt{4x_0^2 + (6y_0^2 - y_0 - a + b)^2}$$

are the proper values of the matrix.

The equilibrium point (x_0, y_0) of the linear differential system $(11')$ can be attractor, proper knot, improper knot, or saddle point:

1) if $\beta > 0$, $\gamma > 0$, then (x_0, y_0) is an unstable knot;

2) if $\beta < 0$, $\gamma > 0$, then (x_0, y_0) is asymptotically stable knot;

3) if $\gamma < 0$, then (x_0, y_0) is a saddle point (unstable);

4) if $x_0 = 0$, $6y_0^2 - y_0 - a + b = 0$, $6y_0^2 + y_0 + a + b < 0$, then $(0, y_0)$ is an asymptotically stable proper knot;

5) if $x_0 = 0$, $6y_0^2 - y_0 - a + b = 0$, $6y_0^2 + y_0 + a + b < 0$, then $(0, y_0)$ is an unstable proper knot.

Fig.78 refers to some Runge-Kutta approximations of gradient lines obtained by a PC program of plotting with data: a=1, b=1, c=0, d=0; t=0; (1;1),(1.1;1),(1.2;1),(1.3;1).

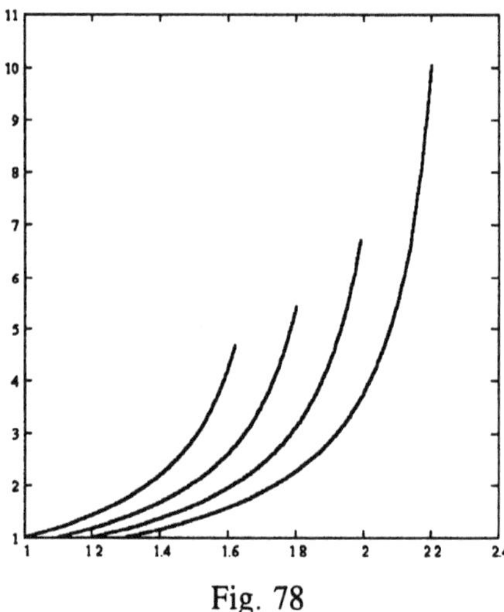

Fig. 78

The conditions for asymptotic stability are equivalent to the fact that

$$\frac{1}{2}d^2 f_{abcd}(x_0, y_0) = (y_0 + a)dx^2 + 2x_0 dx dy + (6y_0^2 + b)dy^2$$

is negative definite. The asymptotic stability (instability) for the linear differential system $(11')$ implies the asymptotic stability (instability) for the potential differential system (11).

The sign of the Laplacian

$$\Delta f_{abcd} = \text{div grad} f_{abc} = 2(6y^2 + y + a + b)$$

permits commentaries about the flow of $\text{grad} f_{abcd}$. Suppose $24(a+b) \leq 1$ and denote the roots of Δf_{abcd} by y_1, y_2; for $y \in (y_1, y_2)$, the flow decreases the area, and for $y \in (-\infty, y_1) \cup (y_2, \infty)$ the flow increases the area. If $24(a+b) > 1$, then the flow increases the area.

5.10. PROPOSED PROBLEMS

1. Which is the direction of the steepest increase for the function

$$f(x,y,z) = x \sin z - y \cos z$$

at the point $(0,0,0)$?

2. Find the points at which the gradient of the scalar field

$$f(x,y) = \ln\left(x + \frac{1}{y}\right)$$

is equal to

$$i - \frac{16}{9} j.$$

3. Consider the scalar fields

$$f(x,y) = 2x^3 + 3x^2y + 6y^2x + 5y^3, \; x > 0, \; y > 0,$$

$$f(x) = \sum_{i=1}^{n} \frac{x_i^2}{a_i^2}, \; x = (x_1, \dots, x_n) \in R^n.$$

Find the flow generated by $\text{grad} f$ and show that this flow increases the volume.

Hint. Convex scalar fields.

4. Determine the regions of R^n in which the flow generated by the gradient of the scalar field

$$f(x) = \left(\sum_{i=1}^{n} \frac{1}{x_i}\right)^{-1}$$

decreases or increases the volume.

Hint. It is enough to compute $d^2 f$; $x < 0$, dilation; $x > 0$, contraction.

5. One considers the potential differential systems associated to the following scalar fields:

$$f(x,y) = xy(a - x - y),\ f(x,y) = x^3 + y^3 - 3xy;$$
$$f(x,y) = (2ax - x^2)(2by - y^2),\ f(x,y) = \frac{a + bx + cy}{\sqrt{1 + x^2 + y^2}};$$
$$f(x,y) = \sin x + \sin y + \cos(x + y),\ 0 \le x \le \pi/4,\ 0 \le y \le \pi/4;$$
$$f(x,y) = x^3 y^2 (12 - x - y),\ x > 0,\ y > 0.$$

For each case, find the equilibrium points and study the stability of these points.

6. Let $f(x,y) = x^2 - xy + y^2 - x + y$ and $g(x,y) = x^4 + y^4 - x^2 - y^2$. Find the curves of steepest decrease, and then the minimum points.

7. Let us consider the scalar fields

$$f(x,y) = x^3 - 3xy^2,\ g(x,y) = x^3 + y^3,\ h(x,y) = x^2 y + y^4.$$

Determine the gradient lines. Draw the constant level curves and the gradient lines for each case.

8. Draw the constant level curves and the gradient lines for the elliptic umbilic, hyperbolic umbilic, and respectively parabolic umbilic.

Hint. Let (x_0, y_0) be an equilibrium point belonging to the constant level curve $f(x,y) = \alpha$. One uses the Taylor expansion of f around (x_0, y_0). Intersecting by the straight line $y - y_0 = t(x - x_0)$, we obtain the parametric equations of the constant level set.

9. Let us consider the Hamiltonian

$$H(p,q) = \frac{1}{2} \sum q_k^2 + V(p).$$

Study the completeness of the Hamiltonian vector field associated to H in the cases in which V is the fold, cusp, swallowtail, butterfly, elliptic umbilic, hyperbolic umbilic, and parabolic umbilic.

Hint. See theorems in 3.5, 3.6.

10. Let V be the electrostatic potential in a homogeneous dielectric of permitivity ε. Determine the intensity of the electric field and the distribution of the electric charge in the cases in which V is the fold, cusp, swallowtail, butterfly, elliptic umbilic, hyperbolic umbilic, and parabolic umbilic.

Hint. $E = -\operatorname{grad} V,\ k\rho_v = \varepsilon \operatorname{div} E$.

11. Show that the gradient lines of a function $f: R^n \to R$, with the property $\|\operatorname{grad} f\| = 1$, are straight lines.

6. FIELD HYPERSURFACES

The flow determined on a domain by a C^1 *vector field conserves the hypersurfaces generated by the field lines. These hypersurfaces are called field hypersurfaces (see 6.1).*

In thermodynamics, in the theory of Finsler spaces and in other applied or theoretical branches of science, some ideas are presented using homogeneous functions. The homogeneous functions of class C^1 *are solutions of Euler equations with partial derivatives of first order. The* C^∞ *homogeneous functions on* R^n *are homogeneous polynomials. The suprahomogeneous (subhomogeneous) functions of class* C^1 *are solutions of Euler inequalities with partial derivatives of first order (see 6.2).*

The flows generated on R^n *by torse forming vector fields preserve the ruled hypersurfaces; the flows generated on* R^n *by parallel vector fields preserve the cylindrical hypersurfaces; and the flows generated on* R^n *by concurrent vector fields preserve the conical hypersurfaces (see 6.3). The flows generated on* R^n *by Killing vector fields preserve the hypersurfaces of revolution (see 6.4).*

Any vector field X *can be viewed as a linear operator (see 1.5) and in this context we can speak about* $\mathrm{Ker}X$, $\mathrm{Im}X$, *proper values and proper vectors of* X, *etc. The properties of* X *connected to the fact that* X *is a linear operator are strongly related to the global properties of the flow generated by* X *(see 6.5).*

In cases in which the solutions of Cauchy problems attached to linear equations with partial derivatives of first order cannot be found by formulas, one can use a numerical method of calculus (the well-known grid method , see 6.6).

The chapter ends with proposed problems of 6.7, which make concrete some theoretical notions, asking for general solutions of some equations with partial derivatives of first order, solutions of Cauchy problems, the finding of field hypersurfaces, properties of homogeneous functions, proper values and proper vectors of some vector fields and approximate solutions for some Cauchy problems.

6.1. LINEAR EQUATIONS WITH PARTIAL DERIVATIVES OF FIRST ORDER

Let $X = (X_1, \ldots, X_n)$ be a C^1 vector field on an open and connected set $D \subset R^n$. Let $f : D \to R$ be a C^1 scalar field and $M : f(x) = c$ a level hypersurface attached to the function f. If the restriction of X to M is a vector field tangent to M (Fig.79), i.e., $(X, \mathrm{grad} f) = 0$ or $D_X f = 0$, then M is called a *field hypersurface* of X.

The field hypersurfaces associated to the vector field X are characterized by the *homogeneous linear equation with partial derivatives of first order*,

$$X_1(x)\frac{\partial f}{\partial x_1}(x)+\cdots+X_n(x)\frac{\partial f}{\partial x_n}(x)=0 \tag{1}$$

in the sense that these hypersurfaces are constant level sets attached to the solutions f of the equation (1).

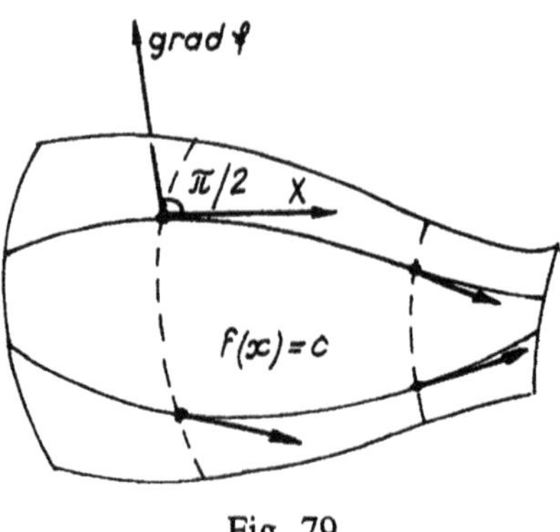

Fig. 79

Obviously, two collinear vector fields have the same field hypersurfaces, if we neglect the zero level set attached to the collinearity factor.

A field hypersurface is generated by field lines of $\boldsymbol{X}$. But it is known that the field lines of $\boldsymbol{X}$ are solutions of the symmetric differential system

$$\frac{dx_1}{X_1(x)}=\cdots=\frac{dx_n}{X_n(x)}, \tag{2}$$

called the *characteristic differential system* attached to the equation (1).

Paraphrasing the definition and the properties of the first integrals, it follows:

- Any first integral of the system (2) is a solution of the equation (1), and conversely.
- Let $f_1, \ldots, f_{n-1}$ be the $n-1$ functionally independent first integrals defined by the system (2) in a neighborhood of a point $x_0 \in D$ at which $\boldsymbol{X}(x_0) \neq 0$. A C^1 function f is a solution of the equation (1) on $U \subset D$ iff it is of the type $f=\phi(f_1,\ldots,f_{n-1})$. In other words the *general solution* f of the equation (1) is a C^1 arbitrary function ϕ of $n-1$ functionally independent first integrals $f_1, \ldots, f_{n-1}$ of the system (2).

If $f_1, \ldots, f_{n-1}$ are functionally independent first integrals of the system (2), then the general solution of the system (family of field lines) can be written in the form

$$f_1(x_1,\ldots,x_n)=c_1, \ldots, f_{n-1}(x_1,\ldots,x_n)=c_{n-1}.$$

Consequently the following conclusions are true:

- for finding the general solution of the equation (1) it is sufficient to determine the general solution of the system (2);
- for finding the general solution of the system (2) it is sufficient to find $n-1$

functionally independent solutions of the equation (1).

The first integrals are functions invariant with respect to the flow generated by the vector field X. Thus the field hypersurfaces of the vector field X are hypersurfaces invariant with respect to the flow generated by X.

Application. Let us find the general solution of the equation

$$yz\frac{\partial f}{\partial x}+zx\frac{\partial f}{\partial y}+xy\frac{\partial f}{\partial z}=0.$$

We attach the characteristic differential system

$$\frac{dx}{yz}=\frac{dy}{zx}=\frac{dz}{xy}.$$

First we remark that the axes of coordinates Ox, Oy, Oz are constituted only of zeros of the vector field $X(x,y,z)=(yz,zx,xy)$, and hence the equilibrium set is $Ox\cup Oy\cup Oz$. Then we find the integrable combinations $xdx-ydy=0$, $xdx-zdz=0$, and therefore the general solution of the characteristic system is $x^2-y^2=c_1$, $x^2-z^2=c_2$. There follows the general solution of the equation with partial derivatives, $f(x,y,z)=\phi(x^2-y^2,x^2-z^2)$, where ϕ is a C^1 arbitrary function. The field surfaces of X have the Cartesian implicit equations

$$\phi(x^2-y^2,x^2-z^2)=c.$$

Remarks. Let $M_c: f(x)=c$ be the family of field hypersurfaces of the field X. If X is a potential field, i.e., $X=\text{grad}\varphi$, then the field hypersurfaces M_c are orthogonal to the equipotential hypersurfaces $N_c:\varphi(x)=c$. More generally, if X is a biscalar vector field, i.e., $X=\psi\,grad\varphi$, then the field hypersurfaces M_c, that are not reduced to $M:\psi(x)=0$, are orthogonal to the hypersurfaces $N_c:\varphi(x)=c$. These statements are consequences of the implication

$$(X,\text{grad}f)=0\Rightarrow(\text{grad}\varphi,\text{grad}f)=0.$$

Let $f=\phi(f_1,\dots,f_{n-1})$ be the general solution of the equation (1) and

$$M_c:\phi(f_1(x),\dots,f_{n-1}(x))=c$$

the family of field hypersurfaces.

The *Cauchy problem* for the equation (1) consists in finding the field hypersurface M that contains a submanifold with $n-2$ dimensions $\Gamma: g(x_1,\dots,x_n)=0,\ h(x_1,\dots,x_n)=0.$ Under certain conditions, the Cauchy problem has a unique solution [39]. On the other hand, one observes that the hypersurface M, solution of the Cauchy problem, can be regarded as generated by the field lines

$$f_1(x)=c_1,\ \dots,f_{n-1}(x)=c_{n-1}$$

which meet the submanifold Γ. The equations

$$f_1(x) = c_1, \dots, f_{n-1}(x) = c_{n-1}, \; g(x) = 0, \; h(x) = 0$$

form an algebraic system of $n+1$ equations with n unknowns $x_1, \dots, x_n$. Eliminating $x_1, \dots, x_n$, we obtain the compatibility condition

$$\phi(c_1, \dots, c_{n-1}) = 0.$$

We reinterpret M as the geometrical locus of field lines satisfying this compatibility condition. By eliminating the parameters $c_1, \dots, c_{n-1}$ we find the field hypersurface

$$M : \phi(f_1(x), \dots, f_{n-1}(x)) = 0.$$

Application. Let there be given the equation

$$(x^2+y^2)\frac{\partial f}{\partial x} + 2xy\frac{\partial f}{\partial y} + xz\frac{\partial f}{\partial z} = 0.$$

Find the field surface passing through the circle

$$\Gamma : x = a, \; y^2 + z^2 = a^2.$$

Solution. We associate the characteristic symmetric system

$$\frac{dx}{x^2+y^2} = \frac{dy}{2xy} = \frac{dz}{xz},$$

and we remark that Oz consists of equilibrium points. Leaving aside the cases in which at most two denominators are zero, it follows that

$$\frac{dy}{2y} = \frac{dz}{z}, \quad \frac{d(x+y)}{(x+y)^2} = \frac{d(x-y)}{(x-y)^2},$$

from which we find the family of field lines

$$\frac{z^2}{y} = c_1, \quad \frac{1}{x-y} - \frac{1}{x+y} = \frac{2}{c_2}.$$

In this case the domains of definition of the first integrals

$$f_1 : R^3 \setminus xOz \to R, \; f_1(x,y,z) = \frac{z^2}{y};$$

$$f_2 : R^3 \setminus P \cup Q \to R, \; f_2(x,y,z) = \frac{1}{x-y} - \frac{1}{x+y}; \; P : x - y = 0, \; Q : x + y = 0$$

are not connected. The first integrals f_1, f_2 are functionally independent since the associated Jacobian matrix

$$J = \begin{bmatrix} 0 & -\dfrac{z^2}{y^2} & \dfrac{2z}{y} \\ -\dfrac{1}{(x-y)^2} + \dfrac{1}{(x+y)^2} & \dfrac{1}{(x-y)^2} + \dfrac{1}{(x+y)^2} & 0 \end{bmatrix}$$

has

$$\operatorname{rank} J = \begin{cases} 2 & \text{for } z \neq 0 \\ 1 & \text{for } z = 0. \end{cases}$$

The compatibility condition of the algebraic system

$$x = a,\ y^2 + z^2 = a^2,\ \frac{z^2}{y} = c_1,\ \frac{1}{x-y} - \frac{1}{x+y} = \frac{2}{c_2}$$

is $c_1 = c_2$. There follows the required field surface $M : y^2 + z^2 - x^2 = 0$ (a cone with the vertex at origin, Fig.80).

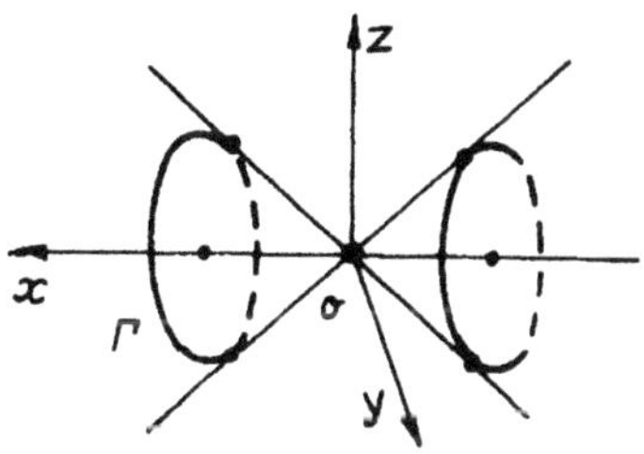

Fig. 80

Nonhomogeneous linear equations with partial derivatives of first order. By this terminology we mean equations of the form

$$X_1(x,f)\frac{\partial f}{\partial x_1} + \cdots + X_n(x,f)\frac{\partial f}{\partial x_n} = F(x,f), \tag{3}$$

where f is the unknown function. Here the solution f is required in implicit form

$$\phi(x, f(x)) = 0.$$

Taking partial derivatives we find

$$\frac{\partial \phi}{\partial x_i} + \frac{\partial \phi}{\partial f}\frac{\partial f}{\partial x_i} = 0,\ i = 1, \ldots, n$$

and so the equation (3) is transferred into an equation of type (1),

$$X_1(x,f)\frac{\partial \phi}{\partial x_1} + \cdots + X_n(x,f)\frac{\partial \phi}{\partial x_n} + F(x,f)\frac{\partial \phi}{\partial f} = 0 \tag{3'}$$

with the associated characteristic symmetric system

$$\frac{dx_1}{X_1(x,f)} = \cdots = \frac{dx_n}{X_n(x,f)} = \frac{df}{F(x,f)}. \tag{4}$$

One finds the general solution of the system (4), then the general solution ϕ of the equation $(3')$ and the algebraic equation $\phi(x, f(x)) = 0$ defines the general solution of the initial equation (3).

Remark. Let us consider the vector field $(X_1, \dots, X_n)$ and the diffeomorphism $x_{i'} = x_{i'}(x)$, $i = 1, \dots, n$. The new components $(X_{1'}, \dots, X_{n'})$ of the vector field are given by

$$X_{i'} = \sum_{i=1}^{n} \frac{\partial x_{i'}}{\partial x_i} X_i.$$

That is why the rectifying diffeomorphism is fixed by the linear equations with partial derivatives of the first order

$$\sum_{i=1}^{n} \frac{\partial x_{i'}}{\partial x_i} X_i = 0, \; i' = 1, \dots, n-1 \quad \text{(homogeneous)}$$

$$\sum_{i=1}^{n} \frac{\partial x_{n'}}{\partial x_i} X_i = 1 \quad \text{(nonhomogeneous)}.$$

The characteristic symmetric system attached to the nonhomogeneous equation,

$$\frac{dx_1}{X_1} = \dots = \frac{dx_n}{X_n} = \frac{dx_{n'}}{1}$$

shows that $x_{1'}, \dots, x_{n'-1'}$ must be first integrals of the differential system that determines the field lines, and $x_{n'}$ can be found as in 3.2.

Application. We consider the equation

$$\sum_{i,j=1}^{n} a_{ij} x_j \frac{\partial f}{\partial x_i}(x) = q(x), \tag{5}$$

where q is a positive (negative) quadratic form on R^n, and $A = [a_{ij}]$ is a real matrix whose proper values in the complex numbers C have strictly negative real parts. We shall show that this equation has a unique solution f in the class of negative (positive) quadratic forms defined on R^n.

One knows that the real vector space Q of quadratic forms on R^n is isomorphic to $R^{\frac{n(n+1)}{2}}$, and $D_{Ax} : Q \to Q$ is a linear operator. Under the specified conditions, it is sufficient to show that D_{Ax} is a bijection.

We denote by λ_i the proper values of the matrix A. Let us show that $\lambda_i + \lambda_j$ are proper values of D_{Ax}. For these we recall that the transpose matrix A^* has the same proper values as the matrix A. If

$$A^*u = \lambda u, \; A^*v = \mu v, \; f(x) = (u,x)(v,x),$$

then

$$\begin{aligned} D_{Ax} f(x) &= (u, Ax)(v,x) + (u,x)(v,Ax) \\ &= (A^*u, x)(v,x) + (u,x)(A^*v, x) = (\lambda + \mu) f(x) \end{aligned}$$

and hence $\lambda + \mu$ is the proper value of D_{Ax}. For simplicity suppose that $\lambda_i + \lambda_j$, $i \le j$ are different numbers. Then $\lambda_i + \lambda_j$ are all the proper values of the linear operator D_{Ax}. Since A has no opposite proper values, the linear operator D_{Ax} does not have the proper value zero, and therefore D_{Ax} is a bijection. In other words the equation (5) admits a unique quadratic form as solution.

Let us analyse the sign of the quadratic form f. For that we introduce the homogeneous linear differential system

$$\frac{dx}{dt} = Ax, \; A = [a_{ij}], \; x = {}^t[x_1, \dots, x_n]. \tag{6}$$

If $\alpha : R \to R^n$ is a solution of this system, then

$$\frac{d}{dt} f \circ \alpha = D_{Ax} f \circ \alpha = \left(\sum_{i,j=1}^{n} a_{ij} x_j \frac{\partial f}{\partial x_j} \right) \circ \alpha .$$

Suppose that q is not positive definite. If the quadratic form f is not negative definite, then there exists a nonvoid domain V^+ and by a theorem of 4.5 the equilibrium position $x = 0$ of the differential system (6) is unstable. But this result contradicts the hypothesis on the proper values of A; consequently the quadratic form f is negative definite.

Remarks. The preceding result can be reformulated in the following way. If $A = [a_{ij}]$ is a real matrix whose proper values in the complex numbers have strictly negative real parts, and $C = [c_{ij}]$ is a real symmetric positive (negative) definite matrix, then there exists a unique real symmetric negative (positive) definite matrix $B = [b_{ij}]$ satisfying $A^*B + BA = C$.

2) The characteristic symmetric system associated to the equation (5) is

$$\frac{dx_1}{\sum_j a_{1j} x_j} = \dots = \frac{dx_n}{\sum_j a_{nj} x_j} = \frac{df(x)(dx)}{q(x)} . \tag{7}$$

6.2. HOMOGENEOUS FUNCTIONS AND EULER'S EQUATION

A nonvoid set S of points in R^n is called a *cone with vertex at the origin* if simultaneously with the point x it contains also the point tx, for any $t > 0$. In other words, the nonvoid set S is a cone with vertex at the origin (Fig.81) if and only if simultaneously with x it contains the whole semi-straight line that joins the origin to the point x, excepting eventually the vertex (the origin).

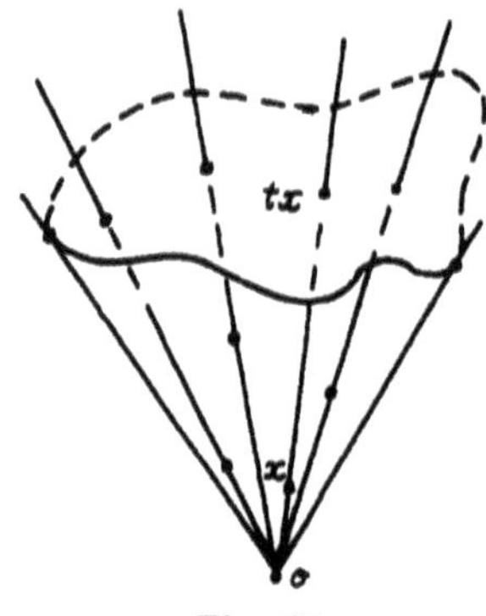

Fig. 81

Let S be a cone of R^n with vertex at the origin and $f: S \to R$ be a real function. If there exists a real number p such that

$$f(tx) = t^p f(x), \ \forall x \in S, \ \forall t > 0,$$

then f is called a *homogeneous function*, and p is called the *degree of homogeneity*.

Suppose that the origin belongs to the cone S and that the homogeneous function $f: S \to R$ is continuous at the origin. If $p < 0$, then

$$f(x) = \lim_{t \searrow 0} t^{-p} f(tx) = 0, \ \forall x \in S,$$

i.e., f is a constant on S; if $p > 0$, then

$$\lim_{t \searrow 0} f(tx) = \lim_{t \searrow 0} t^p f(x)$$

implies $f(0) = 0$.

Remarks. 1) If $p \in N$ ($p \in Z$, respectively $p \in (0, \infty)$), then the definition of the homogeneous function is extended to $t \in R$ ($t \in R \setminus \{0\}$, respectively $t \in [0, \infty)$). Obviously, the domain of definition must have the property that simultaneously with the point x it contains also the point tx.

2) If the cone S with vertex at the origin is an open set which does not contains all the points of a sphere with the centre at the origin, then the origin does not belong to S, but to the boundary ∂S of S.

Theorem. *Suppose that the cone S with vertex at the origin is an open set, and the function $f: S \to R$ is of class C^1. The function f is homogeneous of degree p if and only if* *it verifies the Euler equation*

$$\sum_{i=1}^{n} x_i \frac{\partial f}{\partial x_i}(x) = pf(x),\ x = (x_1, \ldots, x_n) \in S.$$

Proof. The case $p = 0$ is left for the reader. Suppose that the function f is homogeneous, $f(tx) = t^p f(x)$, $\forall t > 0$, with $p \neq 0$. Denote $u = tx$, i.e., $u_i = tx_i$, $i = 1, \ldots, n$, and differentiate both members of the preceding relation with respect to the parameter t, having in mind the chain formula for a composite function. We find

$$x_1 \frac{\partial f}{\partial u_1}(tx) + \cdots + x_n \frac{\partial f}{\partial u_n}(tx) = pt^{p-1} f(x).$$

For $t = 1$ we obtain the Euler equation.

Conversely, suppose that f satisfies the Euler equation,

$$\sum_{i=1}^{n} u_i \frac{\partial f}{\partial u_i}(u) = pf(u),\ u = (u_1, \ldots, u_n),\ p \neq 0.$$

We set $u_i = tx_i$ and we consider the function

$$\phi : (0, \infty) \to R,\ \phi(t) = \frac{1}{t^p} f(tx_1, \ldots, tx_n).$$

Differentiating with respect to t and using the Euler equation, we find

$$\phi'(t) = \frac{1}{t^{2p}}\left[t^p\left(x_1 \frac{\partial f}{\partial u_1} + \cdots + x_n \frac{\partial f}{\partial u_n}\right) - pt^{p-1} f(tx_1, \ldots, tx_n)\right]$$

$$= \frac{1}{t^{p+1}}\left[u_1 \frac{\partial f}{\partial u_1} + \cdots + u_n \frac{\partial f}{\partial u_n} - pf(u)\right] = 0,\ \forall t > 0.$$

It follows that $\phi(t) = c = \phi(1) = f(x_1, \ldots, x_n)$, $\forall t > 0$, or $f(tx) = t^p f(x)$, i.e., f is homogeneous of degree p.

Alternative. The Euler equation

$$\sum_{i=1}^{n} x_i \frac{\partial f}{\partial x_i}(x) = pf(x)$$

is a nonhomogeneous linear equation with partial derivatives of first order. The solution found with the method presented in 6.1 is proved to be a homogeneous function.

Theorem. *Any C^∞ homogeneous function on R^n is a homogeneous polynomial.*

Proof. Let $f: R^n \to R$ be a C^∞ homogeneous function with p as degree of homogeneity. By the preceding remarks, it is necessarily $p \geq 0$.

Let $n_0 > p$ be a natural number. Any partial derivative of order n_0 of the function f must vanish identically, as a homogeneous function on R^n with the degree of homogeneity $p - n_0 < 0$. Having in mind this result and using the Taylor formula, it follows that f is a polynomial, let us say of degree m, that can be written in the form

$$f = f_0 + f_1 + \cdots + f_m,$$

where f_i is a homogeneous polynomial of degree i and $f_m \neq 0$. The homogeneity condition together the hypothesis $f_m \neq 0$ imply $p = m$ and $f = f_m$ (i.e., $f_0 = f_1 = \cdots = f_{m-1} = 0$).

In the preceding conditions on S, the function $f: S \to R$ is called *suprahomogeneous of degree* p if

$$f(tx) \geq t^p f(x), \ \forall t > 0.$$

Analogously we can introduce the *subhomogeneous function of degree* p.

Theorem. *Suppose that the cone* S *with vertex at the origin is an open set, and the function* $f: S \to R$ *is of class* C^1. *The function* f *is suprahomogeneous of degree* p *if and only if it verifies the Euler inequality*

$$\sum_{i=1}^{n} x_i \frac{\partial f}{\partial x_i}(x) \leq p f(x), \ x = (x_1, \ldots, x_n) \in S.$$

Hint. Denoting $\varphi(t) = f(tx) - t^p f(x)$, the condition $\varphi(t) \geq \varphi(1) = 0$ implies $\varphi'(1) \leq 0$. Conversely $\phi(t) = \dfrac{1}{t^p} f(tx_1, \ldots, tx_n)$ and $\phi'(t) \leq 0$ imply $\phi(t) \geq \phi(1)$.

Generalization. Let S be a cone of R^n with vertex at the origin and $f: S^k \to R$ be a real function. If there exists a real number p such that

$$f(tx^1, \ldots, t^k x^k) = t^p f(x^1, \ldots, x^k), \quad \forall (x^1, \ldots, x^k) \in S^k, \ \forall t > 0,$$

then f is called a *k-homogeneous function*, and p is called the *degree of homogeneity*.

Suppose that the cone S with vertex at the origin is an open set, and the function $f: S^k \to R$ is of class C^1. The function f is k-homogeneous of degree p if and only if it verifies the generalized Euler equation

$$\sum_{j=1}^{k} \sum_{i=1}^{n} j x_i^j \frac{\partial f}{\partial x_i^j}(x^1, \ldots, x^k) = p f(x^1, \ldots, x^k),$$

where $x^j = (x_i^j)$, $j = 1, \ldots, k$.

Remark. The homogeneity is used in the theory of Finsler spaces, and the k-homogeneity is used in the theory of Finsler spaces of superior order [42].

6.3. RULED HYPERSURFACES

Ruled hypersurfaces. Let $m \in \{1, 2, \dots, n-2\}$. A hypersurface of R^n, $n \geq 3$, which can be generated by the motion of an m-plane G, which relies on a submanifold Γ with $n - m - 1$ dimensions, is called a *ruled hypersurface*; the m-plane G is called a *generator (ruling)*, and the submanifold Γ is called a *director submanifold*.

Theorem. *The field hypersurfaces of torse forming vector fields are ruled hypersurfaces.*

Proof. Suppose that X is a torse forming vector field, i.e.,

$$D_Z X = aZ + (Y, Z)X, \ \forall \, Z \in \mathcal{X}(R^n).$$

Particularly, $D_X X = bX$, where $b = a + (Y, X)$, and therefore the field lines of X are reparametrized straight lines. The field hypersurfaces $M : f(x) = c$ of the torse forming vector field X are ruled hypersurfaces, being generated by straight lines.

Open problem: Is the converse of the preceding theorem true or not?

Remark. The second fundamental form of a field hypersurface of a torse forming vector field cannot be definite. Indeed, starting with $D_X f = (X, \operatorname{grad} f) = 0$, and differentiating both members with respect to X, we find

$$(D_X X, \operatorname{grad} f) + (X, D_X \operatorname{grad} f) = 0$$

and hence $\operatorname{Hess} f(X, X) = 0$. As X is not identically zero, the last relation shows that $\operatorname{Hess} f$ cannot be (positive or negative) definite.

Cylindrical hypersurfaces. If the generator G moves preserving its director vector space, then the ruled hypersurface is called *cylindrical*.

Theorem. *A cylindrical hypersurface is a field hypersurface of a parallel vector field and conversely (Fig.82).*

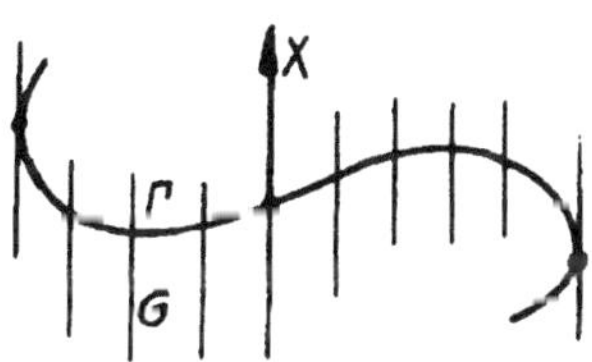

Fig. 82

Proof. Suppose that $b_1, \dots, b_m$ are orthogonal vectors generating the director vector space of G, and $b_{m+1}, \dots, b_n$ are orthogonal vectors generating the orthogonal complement of G in R^n. The set of m-planes parallel to G is represented analytically by the equations

$$(x, b_{m+1}) = c_{m+1}, \ldots, (x, b_n) = c_n, \ (c_{m+1}, \ldots, c_n) \in R^{n-m}. \tag{8}$$

The condition that the m-planes (8) rely on the $(n-m+1)$-dimensional submanifold

$$\Gamma : g_1(x) = 0, \ldots, g_{m+1}(x) = 0 \tag{9}$$

is obtained by eliminating $x = (x_1, \ldots, x_n)$ between the $n+1$ equations (8) and (9). One deduces

$$\phi(c_{m+1}, \ldots, c_n) = 0,$$

and therefore the cylindrical hypersurface is represented by the equation

$$\phi((x, b_{m+1}), \ldots, (x, b_n)) = 0. \tag{10}$$

Conversely, one can show that any hypersurface M of R^n characterized by an equation of type (10) is a cylindrical hypersurface.

Now we consider the function defined by $f(x) = \phi((x, b_{m+1}), \ldots, (x, b_n))$. Denoting $u_\alpha = (x, b_\alpha)$, $\alpha = m+1, \ldots, n$, we find

$$\frac{\partial f}{\partial x_j} = \sum_\alpha \frac{\partial \phi}{\partial u_\alpha} b_{\alpha j},$$

and hence

$$(b_1, \nabla f) = 0, \ldots, (b_m, \nabla f) = 0,$$

i.e., f is the solution of a system of homogeneous linear equations with partial derivatives of first order, equations attached to the parallel vector fields

$$X_1 = b_1, \ldots, X_m = b_m.$$

Conversely, if the parallel vector field $X = (a_1, \ldots, a_n)$ is given, then the field hypersurfaces are characterized by $M_c : f(x) = c$, where f is the general solution of the equation

$$a_1 \frac{\partial f}{\partial x_1} + \cdots + a_n \frac{\partial f}{\partial x_n} = 0.$$

Since the characteristic system

$$\frac{dx_1}{a_1} = \cdots = \frac{dx_n}{a_n}$$

has the general solution ($a_i \neq 0$, $i = 1, \ldots, n$, a hypothesis imposed by the procedure),

$$\frac{x_1}{a_1} - \frac{x_n}{a_n} = c_1, \ldots, \frac{x_{n-1}}{a_{n-1}} - \frac{x_n}{a_n} = c_{n-1},$$

it follows that

$$f(x) = \phi\left(\frac{x_1}{a_1} - \frac{x_n}{a_n}, \ldots, \frac{x_{n-1}}{a_{n-1}} - \frac{x_n}{a_n}\right)$$

and therefore M_c are cylindrical hypersurfaces, the generator G being a straight line, and Γ being an $(n-2)$-dimensional submanifold (Fig.82).

Corollary. *The field hypersurfaces of a vector field collinear to a parallel vector* *field are cylindrical hypersurfaces (we neglect the zero level set of the collinearity factor).*

Conical hypersurfaces. If the generator G passes through a fixed $(m-1)$-plane, then the ruled hypersurface is called *conical*, and the fixed $(m-1)$-plane is called the *vertex*.

Theorem. *A conical hypersurface with the vertex* $x_0 : x_1 = x_{10}, \dots, x_n = x_{n0}$ *is a field hypersurface of the concurrent vector field* $X = (x_1 - x_{10}, \dots, x_n - x_{n0})$ *and conversely (Fig.83).*

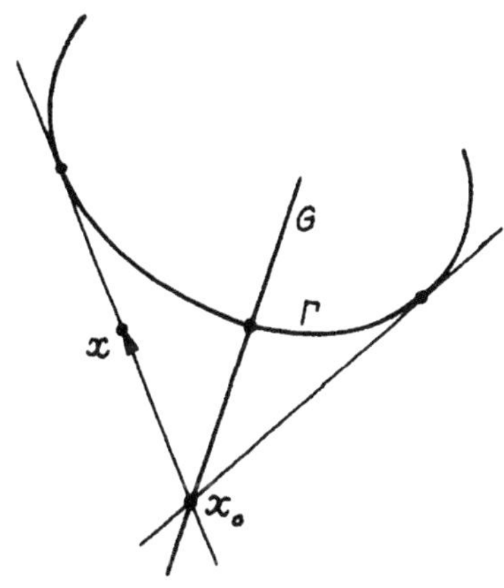

Fig. 83

Proof. The set of straight lines passing through the fixed point x_0 and not belonging to the hyperplane $x_n = x_{n0}$ is represented by the equations

$$x_1 - x_{10} = c_1(x_n - x_{n0}), \dots, x_{n-1} - x_{n-10} = c_{n-1}(x_n - x_{n0}), \ (c_1, \dots, c_{n-1}) \in R^{n-1}. \quad (11)$$

The condition that these straight lines rely on an $(n-2)$-dimensional manifold Γ of equations

$$g_1(x) = 0, \ g_2(x) = 0 \quad (12)$$

is obtained by eliminating $x = (x_1, \dots, x_n)$ between the $n+1$ equations (11) and (12). One deduces $\phi(c_1, \dots, c_{n-1}) = 0$, and hence the conical hypersurface is described by the equation

$$f(x_1, \dots, x_n) = \phi\left(\frac{x_1 - x_{10}}{x_n - x_{n0}}, \dots, \frac{x_{n-1} - x_{n-10}}{x_n - x_{n0}}\right) = 0. \quad (13)$$

Conversely, any hypersurface M of R^n characterized by an equation of type (13) is a conical hypersurface with the vertex x_0.

The function defined by $f(x_1, \dots, x_n)$ satisfies the equation

$$(x_1 - x_{10}) \frac{\partial f}{\partial x_1} + \dots + (x_n - x_{n0}) \frac{\partial f}{\partial x_n} = 0. \quad (14)$$

Obviously, the data (11), (12) and the equation (14) is a Cauchy problem.

We keep in mind that the field hypersurfaces of a concurrent vector field are conical hypersurfaces having as vertex a fixed point of R^n (Fig.83). The equation (14) is called the *homogeneous linear equation with partial derivatives of first order of the conical hypersurfaces with the vertex at the point* x_0.

Remarks. 1) Elimination of the straight lines belonging to the hyperplanes $x_n = x_{n0}$ is decided only by computation and therefore is not essential.

2) The general solution of the equation (14) is a homogeneous function with respect to $x_1 - x_{10}, \dots, x_n - x_{n0}$ having the degree of homogeneity equal to zero (see the Euler equation of 6.2).

3) Let V be a fixed $(m-1)$-plane. Without loss of generality we can suppose that V is given by the equations

$$x_1 = x_{10}, \dots, x_{n-m+1} = x_{n-m+10}.$$

The set of m-planes G passing through V is represented by

$$x_1 - x_{10} = c_1(x_{n-m+1} - x_{n-m+10}), \dots, x_{n-m} - x_{n-m0} = c_{n-m}(x_{n-m+1} - x_{n-m+10}), \qquad (15)$$

where $(c_1, \dots, c_{n-m}) \in R^{n-m}$. The condition that these m-planes rely on an $(n-m-1)$-dimensional submanifold Γ of equations

$$g_1(x) = 0, \dots, g_{m+1}(x) = 0 \qquad (16)$$

is obtained by eliminating $x = (x_1, \dots, x_n)$ between the $n+1$ equations (15), (16). One finds $\phi(c_1, \dots, c_{n-m}) = 0$ and therefore

$$f(x_1, \dots, x_n) = \phi\left(\frac{x_1 - x_{10}}{x_{n-m+1} - x_{n-m+10}}, \dots, \frac{x_{n-m} - x_{n-m0}}{x_{n-m+1} - x_{n-m+10}}\right) = 0$$

is the equation of a conical hypersurface with the vertex V. Also the function f generated by $f(x_1, \dots, x_n)$ satisfies

$$(x_1 - x_{10})\frac{\partial f}{\partial x_1} + \dots + (x_{n-m+1} - x_{n-m+10})\frac{\partial f}{\partial x_{n-m+1}} = 0.$$

Corollary. *The field hypersurfaces of a vector field which is collinear to a concurrent vector field are conical hypersurfaces (we neglect the zero level set of the collinearity factor).*

6.4. HYPERSURFACES OF REVOLUTION

A hypersurface of R^n, $n \geq 3$, which can be swept out by the rotation of a submanifold Γ, with the dimension $m \in \{1, 2, \dots, n-2\}$, around a fixed m-plane D is called a *hypersurface of revolution*; the m-plane D is called an *axis of revolution*, and the submanifold Γ is called a *generator* (Fig.84).

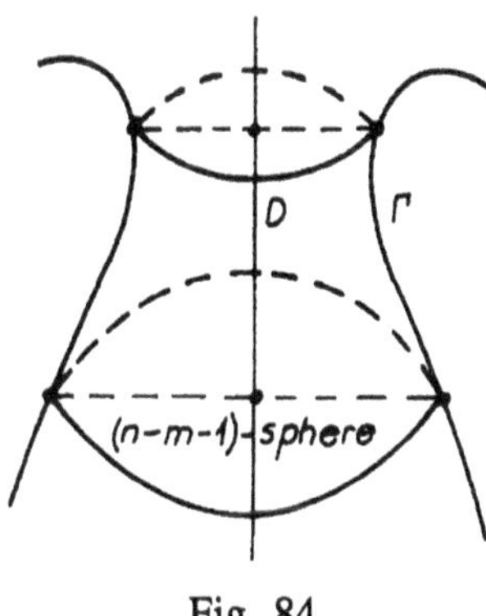

Fig. 84

Theorem. *A hypersurface of revolution is a field hypersurface of a Killing vector field of the form* Ax *and conversely.*

Proof. By hypothesis we disregard translations (parallel vector fields). Therefore we can suppose that the m-plane relying on the linearly independent vectors $b_1, \dots, b_m$ passes through the origin. Let

$$S : x_1^2 + \cdots + x_n^2 = r^2$$

be a hypersphere with centre at the origin (on the axis) and

$$P : (b_1, x) = 0, \dots, (b_m, x) = 0$$

the $(n-m)$-plane passing by the origin, orthogonal to D. The intersection $P \cap S$ is an $(n-m-1)$-sphere.

By the revolution around D, any point of

$$\Gamma : g_1(x) = 0, \dots, g_{n-m}(x) = 0$$

will move in an $(n-m)$-plane orthogonal to D and will describe an $(n-m-1)$-sphere with the centre on the revolution axis. Consequently the hypersurface of revolution can be viewed as the geometrical locus of the $(n-m-1)$-spheres with the centres on D, which pass through Γ, and whose $(n-m)$-planes are orthogonal to D. Thus the system

$$\sum_{j=1}^{n} x_j^2 = w_0, \ \sum_{j=1}^{n} b_{ij} x_j = w_i, \ i = 1, \dots, m, \ g_1(x) = 0, \dots, g_{n-m}(x) = 0$$

must be compatible. Eliminating $x = (x_1, \dots, x_n)$ between the $n+1$ equations, it follows that $\phi(w_0, w_1, \dots, w_m) = 0$ and therefore a hypersurface of revolution has a Cartesian equation of the form

$$f(x_1, \dots, x_n) = \phi\left(\sum_{j=1}^{n} x_j^2, \sum_{j=1}^{n} b_{1j} x_j, \dots, \sum_{j=1}^{n} b_{mj} x_j\right) = 0. \tag{17}$$

Conversely, it can be shown that a hypersurface M of R^n characterized by an equation of the type (17) is a hypersurface of revolution.

The function f defined by $f(x_1, \dots, x_n)$ has the partial derivatives

$$\frac{\partial f}{\partial x_j} = \frac{\partial \phi}{\partial w_0} 2x_j + \frac{\partial \phi}{\partial w_1} b_{1j} + \cdots + \frac{\partial \phi}{\partial w_m} b_{mj}, \; j = 1, \dots, n.$$

These equalities are n equations with $n+1$ unknowns $\frac{\partial \phi}{\partial w_0}, \frac{\partial \phi}{\partial w_1}, \dots, \frac{\partial \phi}{\partial w_m}$. Eliminating these unknowns between the n equations, we find the compatibility conditions that are in fact $n - m - 1$ homogeneous linear equations with partial derivatives of the first order, with the unknown function f. The coefficients of each such equation are the components of a Killing vector field, i.e., of the type Ax, where A is a skew-symmetric matrix.

Particularly, if $m = n - 2$, then the vector product of the $n - 1$ vectors $x, b_1, \dots, b_m$ can be written in the form Ax, where $A = [a_{ij}]$ is a skew-symmetric matrix of order n satisfying $Ab_1 = 0, \dots, Ab_m = 0$, and $x = {}^t[x_1, \dots, x_n]$. Using the matrix A we find a simple homogeneous linear equation with partial derivatives of the first order,

$$\sum_{i,j=1}^{n} a_{ij} x_j \frac{\partial f}{\partial x_i} = 0,$$

and, obviously, the vector field X of components $X_i(x) = \sum_{j=1}^{n} a_{ij} x_j$ is a Killing vector field.

For the converse theorem, let A be a skew-symmetric matrix, Ax be a Killing vector field, and $\nabla f(x) Ax = 0$ the equation with partial derivatives that characterizes the field hypersurfaces, written in the matrix language, where $\nabla f(x)$ is a line matrix and x is a column matrix. To show that the field hypersurfaces are hypersurfaces of revolution, it is enough to show that these are invariant with respect to the flow generated by the Killing vector field Ax, i.e., the equation $\nabla f(x) Ax = 0$ is invariant with respect to this flow. Indeed, the flow generated by the Killing vector field Ax is the diffeomorphism (rotation) $x = e^{At} y$, $t \in R$, with the inverse $y = e^{-At} x$. Since $\nabla f(x) = \nabla f(y) e^{-At}$, we find $\nabla f(y) e^{-At} A e^{At} y = 0$ and, considering that $e^{-At} A e^{At} = e^{-At} e^{At} A = A$, it remains that $\nabla f(y) Ay = 0$.

Variant for the converse theorem. If we have in mind that the family of orbits of a Killing vector field Ax is described by the Cartesian equations

$$\|x\|^2 = c_0, \; \|Ax\|^2 = c_1, \dots, \|A^{n-2} x\|^2 = c_{n-2},$$

it follows that

$$f(x) = \phi(\|x\|^2, \|Ax\|^2, \dots, \|A^{n-2} x\|^2),$$

with ϕ an arbitrary C^1 function, is the general solution of the equation $\nabla f(x) Ax = 0$. Consequently the field hypersurfaces are characterized by

$$\phi(\|x\|^2, \|Ax\|^2, \dots, \|A^{n-2} x\|^2) = c.$$

Corollary. *The field hypersurfaces of a vector field collinear to a Killing vector field Ax are hypersurfaces of revolution (one neglects the zero level set of the collinearity factor).*

6.5. PROPER VALUES AND PROPER VECTORS OF A VECTOR FIELD

Let $C^{\infty}(D)$ be the real vector space of real C^{∞} functions defined on the open connected set $D \subset R^n$. A vector field X of class C^{∞} on D can be viewed as a *linear operator on $C^{\infty}(D)$ via the formula*

$$X(f) = D_X f, \quad f \in C^{\infty}(D).$$

The properties of this linear operator are strongly related to the global properties of the flow generated by X.

A function $f \in C^{\infty}(D) \setminus \{0\}$ with the property $X(f) = \lambda f$, $\lambda \in R$, is called a *proper vector of X with respect to the proper value λ.*

Examples. 1) The proper vectors of the concurrent vector field $X = (x_1, \dots, x_n)$, $x \in D$ (a cone with vertex at the origin), are the homogeneous functions and the proper values are the corresponding degrees of homogeneity. If $x \in R^n$, then any proper value of X is a natural number m and the corresponding proper vector is a homogeneous polynomial of order m (see 6.2).

2) The nonzero functions that satisfy $X(f) = 0$, i.e., the nonzero elements of $\operatorname{Ker} X$, are proper vectors of X with respect to the proper value zero.

3) Let Ax be a linear vector field on R^n. The function $f: R^n \to R$, $f(x) = (x, y)$, y being a fixed vector of R^n, is a proper vector for Ax with respect to the proper value λ if and only if $Ay = \lambda y$, i.e., if and only if y is a proper vector of the matrix A with respect to the proper value λ.

Paraphrasing the results of 6.3 and 6.4, we arrive at the following conclusions:

- If $X = (a_1, \dots, a_n)$, $a_i \neq 0$, is a parallel vector field, then the function f defined by

$$f(x_1, \dots, x_n) = \phi\left(\frac{x_1}{a_1} - \frac{x_n}{a_n}, \dots, \frac{x_{n-1}}{a_{n-1}} - \frac{x_n}{a_n}\right),$$

with ϕ an arbitrary C^{ω} function, belongs to $\operatorname{Ker} X \setminus \{0\}$.

- If $X = (x_1 - x_{10}, \dots, x_n - x_{n0})$ is a concurrent vector field, then the function f defined by

$$f(x_1, \dots, x_n) = \phi\left(\frac{x_1 - x_{10}}{x_n - x_{n0}}, \dots, \frac{x_{n-1} - x_{n-10}}{x_n - x_{n0}}\right),$$

with ϕ an arbitrary C^{∞} function, belong to $\operatorname{Ker} X \setminus \{0\}$.

- Let $X(x) = Ax$ be a Killing vector field. The subset $\operatorname{Ker} X \setminus \{0\}$ consists of elements of the form

$$f(x) = \phi(\|x\|^2, \|Ax\|^2, \dots, \|A^{n-2}x\|^2),$$

where ϕ is a C^∞ arbitrary function.

Theorem. *1)* $f \in C^\infty(D) \setminus \{0\}$ *is a proper vector of* X *with respect to the proper value* λ *if and only if*

$$(f \circ \alpha)(t) = (f \circ \alpha)(0) e^{\lambda t}, \ t \in I$$

for any field line $\alpha : I \to D$ *of* X.

2) If every maximal field line of X *is periodic, then* X *admits only the proper value zero.*

Proof. If $\alpha : I \to D$ is a field line of X on D, and $f : D \to R$ is a C^∞ function, then

$$\frac{d}{dt}(f \circ \alpha) = X(f) \circ \alpha.$$

1) Let $X(f) = \lambda f$, λ being a given real number. It follows that

$$\frac{d}{dt}(f \circ \alpha) = \lambda (f \circ \alpha)$$

and therefore

$$(f \circ \alpha)(t) = A e^{\lambda t}, \ t \in I, \ A = (f \circ \alpha)(0).$$

Conversely, if the relation $(f \circ \alpha)(t) = A e^{\lambda t}$, $t \in I$, holds for a field line $\alpha : I \to D$ of X, then $X(f) = \lambda f$ on $\alpha(I)$. If the last equality holds for any field line of X, then $X(f) = \lambda f$ on D, and consequently λ is a proper value of X and f is a proper vector of X.

Remarks. 1) If $\alpha(0)$ is a zero of f, then $\alpha(I) \subset f^{-1}(0)$.

2) Let λ be a proper value and f be the corresponding proper vector of X. Since $f \neq 0$, there exists $x_0 \in D$ such that $f(x_0) \neq 0$. Let $\alpha : R \to D$ be a maximal field line of X starting from x_0 at the moment $t = 0$. If α is periodic of period $T > 0$, i.e., $\alpha(t) = \alpha(t + T)$, then it follows that $e^{\lambda t} = e^{\lambda(t+T)}$, $\forall\, t \in R$ and therefore $\lambda = 0$.

Counterexamples. 1) The function

$$f : R \times (0, \infty) \to R, \quad f(x,y) = \exp\left(\lambda \sin^{-1} \frac{x}{\sqrt{x^2 + y^2}}\right), \quad \lambda \neq 0,$$

is of class C^∞ and satisfies

$$y \frac{\partial f}{\partial x} - x \frac{\partial f}{\partial y} = \lambda f$$

on $R \times (0, \infty)$. It cannot be extended to a proper vector of the vector field $X(x,y) = (y, -x)$ on R^2. Indeed, the field lines of X are the periodic functions $\alpha(t) = (a \sin(t + b), a \cos(t + b))$, and therefore the only proper value of X on R^2 is zero.

2) The field lines of the vector field

$$X(x,y) = \left(\frac{y}{x^2+y^2}, \frac{-x}{x^2+y^2} \right), \quad (x,y) \in R^2 \setminus \{(0,0)\}$$

are the periodic curves $\alpha(t) = (a\sin(t+b), a\cos(t+b))$, $t \in R$, and hence the only proper value of X on $R^2 \setminus \{(0,0)\}$ is zero. This statement does not exclude the fact that the function

$$f: R \times (0,\infty) \to R, \quad f(x,y) = \exp\left(\lambda(x^2+y^2)\sin^{-1}\frac{x}{\sqrt{x^2+y^2}} \right), \quad \lambda \neq 0$$

is of class C^∞ and satisfies the equation

$$\frac{y}{x^2+y^2}\frac{\partial f}{\partial x} - \frac{x}{x^2+y^2}\frac{\partial f}{\partial y} = \lambda f$$

on $R^2 \times (0,\infty)$.

The relations between the properties of the linear operator X, and the global properties of the flow generated by X, are important in the case in which the flow preserves the volume. To describe these relations, one needs some knowledge of linear operator theory on Euclidean spaces (particularly on Hilbert spaces).

Suppose that D is an open convex bounded set of R^n with a piecewise C^∞ boundary ∂D. Then $\bar{D} = D \cup \partial D$ is a compact set of R^n. The set V of functions of class C^∞ on $\bar{D}$, which vanish on the boundary ∂D, is a real vector space. The scalar product on V is

$$(f,g) = \int_{\bar{D}} f(x)g(x)dx$$

and therefore V is a Euclidean space.

Theorem. *A C^∞ vector field on $\bar{D}$ whose flow conserves the volume is a skew-symmetric linear operator on the Euclidean vector space V.*

Proof. We take into account the hypotheses $f|_{\partial D} = 0$, $\operatorname{div}X = 0$ (a solenoidal vector field) and the Gauss-Ostrogradski formula [12, p.308],

$$\int_{\bar{D}} (\operatorname{div}X)dx = \int_{\partial D} (X,N)d\sigma,$$

where N is the (exterior) unit normal vector field on ∂D. It follows that

$$(X(f),g) = \int_{\bar{D}} X(f)(x)g(x)dx = \int_{\bar{D}} X(fg)(x)dx - \int_{\bar{D}} f(x)X(g)(x)dx$$

$$= \int_{\bar{D}} div(fgX)(x)dx - \int_{\bar{D}} f(x)g(x)(\operatorname{div}X)(x)dx - \int_{\bar{D}} f(x)X(g)(x)dx$$

$$= \int_{\partial \bar{D}} (fgX,N)d\sigma - \int_{\bar{D}} f(x)g(x)(\operatorname{div}X)(x)dx - \int_{\bar{D}} f(x)X(g)(x)dx$$

$$= -\int_{\bar{D}} f(x)X(g)(x)dx = -(f,X(g)), \ \forall f, g \in V.$$

Corollary. *The single (real) proper value of the* C^∞ *vector field* $X : V \to V$, *whose flow preserves the volume, is zero.*

Proof. This is a property of skew-symmetric linear operators; in our case the relations $X(f) = \lambda f$, $f \neq 0$, $(X(f), f) = 0$ imply $\lambda = 0$.

For examples of vector fields whose flows conserve the volume, see 3.7 - 3.13.

Remark. Let us consider the equation $X(f) = Ff$, alternatively written $X(\ln|f|) = f$, where $F : D \to R$ is a fixed function. For any field line $\alpha : I \to D$ of the vector field X one satisfies

$$\frac{d}{dt} \ln|f(\alpha(t))| = F(\alpha(t))$$

or

$$f(\alpha(t)) = f(\alpha(t_0)) \exp \int_{t_0}^{t} F(\alpha(t))\, dt.$$

If we know the functions F and f, then from their properties and the preceding relation it devolves properties of the field lines α and of the vector field X.

6.6. GRID METHOD

In the case in which the solution f of a Cauchy problem attached to a linear equation with partial derivatives of first order is not obtained by formulas, one appeals to the *grid numerical method*, by means of which is obtained a table of values of the function f.

To simplify the exposition, let us consider the Cauchy problem

$$a \frac{\partial f}{\partial x} + \frac{\partial f}{\partial y} = F(x,y), \quad f(x,0) = g(x),$$

where F, g, f are C^1 real functions on $[c,d] \times [0,T]$. This problem has the exact solution

$$f(x,y) = g(x - ay) + \int_0^y F(at - ay + x, t)\, dt.$$

The numerical method for finding a table of values of the function f consists of the following: one replaces the domain $[c,d] \times [0,T]$ by a rectangular grid of double step h, k ($h > 0, k > 0$ suitably selected, Fig.85), i.e., by a discrete set of points M_{pq} having the coordinates $x_p = ph$, $y_q = qk$, $p, q \in Z$, $q \geq 0$; one determines the values of the function f at the grid point M_{pq} replacing the Cauchy problem by a system with finite differences.

Algorithm. One fixes the numbers h and k, and one denotes $F_{pq} = F(ph, qk)$, $g_p = g(ph)$, $f_{pq} = f(ph, qk)$. Then the Cauchy problem is replaced by the system with finite differences,

$$\frac{f_{pq+1} - f_{pq}}{k} + a \frac{f_{p+1q} - f_{pq}}{h} = F_{pq}, \quad f_{p0} = g_p,$$

where a, F_{pq}, g_p are known real numbers, and the sequence $\{f_{pq}\}$, $p, q \in Z$, $q \geq 0$, is a double sequence of real numbers that is determined term by term (Fig. 86).

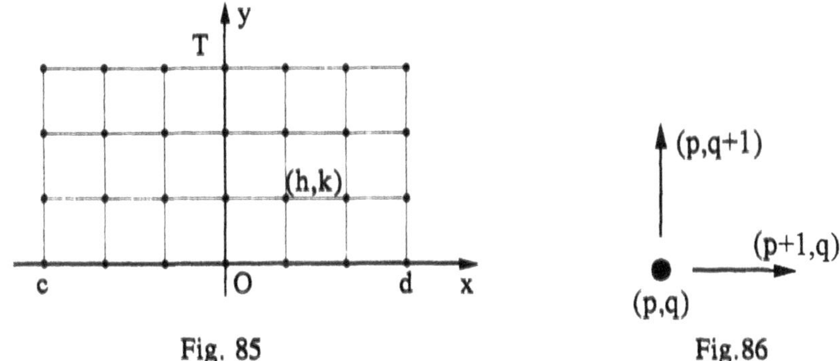

Fig. 85 Fig. 86

Theorem. *If the steps* h, k *of the grid satisfy the condition* $0 \leq -\dfrac{ak}{h} \leq 1$, *then*

$$\sup_{p,q \in Z} |f_{p,q} - f(ph, qk)| \leq nk|\eta(h,k)|,$$

where

$$\lim_{(h,k) \to (0,0)} \eta(h,k) = 0,$$

and n *is a fixed natural number.*

The inequality in the theorem gives an estimate of the error in the approximation $f(ph, qk) \approx f_{pq}$. In conclusion, the theorem says that if $(h,k) \to (0,0)$ and n is sufficiently large, constrained by the condition nk = constant, then

$$\lim_{(h,k) \to (0,0)} \sup |f_{pq} - f(ph, qk)| = 0$$

and therefore the grid method is convergent.

6.7. PROPOSED PROBLEMS

1. Show that the functions defined respectively by

$$f(x) = x_i + x_j + x_k, \quad g(x) = x_i x_j x_k, \quad x = (x_1, \dots, x_n) \in R^n,$$

i, j, k being fixed, are solutions of the equation

$$x_i(x_j - x_k)\frac{\partial f}{\partial x_i} + x_j(x_k - x_i)\frac{\partial f}{\partial x_j} + x_k(x_i - x_j)\frac{\partial f}{\partial x_k} = 0.$$

2. Verify that the function defined by

$$f(x) = \frac{x_1 - x_3}{x_1 - x_4}\,\frac{x_2 - x_4}{x_2 - x_3}$$

is a solution of the equations

$$\sum_{i=1}^{4} \frac{\partial f}{\partial x_i} = 0, \ \sum_{i=1}^{4} x_i \frac{\partial f}{\partial x_4} = 0, \ \sum_{i=1}^{4} x_i^2 \frac{\partial f}{\partial x_i} = 0.$$

3. Let

$$\boldsymbol{X}_1 = (1,0,0),\ \boldsymbol{X}_2 = (0,1,0),\ \boldsymbol{X}_3 = (0,0,1),\ \boldsymbol{X}_4 = (-x_2, x_1, 0),$$
$$\boldsymbol{X}_5 = (0, -x_3, x_2),\ \boldsymbol{X}_6 = (x_3, 0, -x_1),\ (x_1, x_2, x_3) \in \boldsymbol{R}^3,$$

be Killing vector fields linearly independent in $\mathcal{X}(\boldsymbol{R}^3)$. Determine the field surfaces.

4. For each vector field, find the family of field surfaces:

1) $\boldsymbol{V} = 2(x^2 - y^2)\boldsymbol{i} + 2xy\boldsymbol{j} + xyz\boldsymbol{k}$,
2) $\boldsymbol{V} = x(x+z)\boldsymbol{i} + y(y+z)\boldsymbol{j} + (x^2 - xy)\boldsymbol{k}$,
3) $\boldsymbol{V} = (z + e^x)\boldsymbol{i} + (z + e^y)\boldsymbol{j} + (z^2 - e^{x+y})\boldsymbol{k}$,
4) $\boldsymbol{V} = (xy^3 - 2x^4)\boldsymbol{i} + (2y^4 - x^3y)\boldsymbol{j} + 9z(x^3 - y^3)\boldsymbol{k}$,
5) $\boldsymbol{V} = xy\boldsymbol{i} - y\sqrt{1-y^2}\,\boldsymbol{j} + (z\sqrt{1-y^2} - 2ax)\boldsymbol{k}$,
6) $\boldsymbol{V} = (x^2 + y^2)\boldsymbol{i} + 2xy\boldsymbol{j} + xz\boldsymbol{k}$.

Hint. 1) $z^2 = e^y \varphi\left(y^2 e^{\frac{x^2}{y^2}}\right)$, 2) $\ln x + \dfrac{z}{y} = \varphi\left(\ln y + \dfrac{z}{x}\right)$, 3) $y + ze^{-x} = \varphi(x + ze^{-y})$,

4) $x^3y^3z = \varphi(xy^{-2} + yx^{-2})$, 5) $yz + ax(y + \sqrt{1-y^2}) = \varphi(xe^{\arcsin y})$, 6) $z^2 = y\varphi\left(\dfrac{x^2 - y^2}{y}\right)$.

5. Find the solution of the Cauchy problem

$$z(x+z)\frac{\partial z}{\partial x} - y(y+z)\frac{\partial z}{\partial y} = 0,\ z(1,y) = \sqrt{y}.$$

6. Being given the vector field

$$\boldsymbol{V} = x^2(y+z)\boldsymbol{i} - y^2(z+x)\boldsymbol{j} + z^2(y-x)\boldsymbol{k},$$

determine the field surface passing through the curve

$$xy = a,\ x + y = b.$$

7. Solve the following Cauchy problems:

1) $x\dfrac{\partial z}{\partial y} - y\dfrac{\partial z}{\partial x} = 0, \quad z(x,0) = \varphi(x)$,

2) $\dfrac{\partial z}{\partial x} + \dfrac{\partial z}{\partial y} = z^2, \quad z(x,0) = \varphi(x)$,

3) $\dfrac{\partial z}{\partial y} = xz\dfrac{\partial z}{\partial x}, \quad z(x,0) = x$,

4) $x\frac{\partial f}{\partial x}+y\frac{\partial f}{\partial y}+\frac{\partial f}{\partial z}=f,\ f(x,y,0)=\varphi(x,y).$

Hint. 1) $z=\varphi(\sqrt{x^2+y^2})$, 2) $z=\dfrac{\varphi(x-y)}{1-y\varphi(x-y)}$, 3) $x=ze^{-yz}$, 4) $f=\varphi(xe^{-z},ye^{-z})e^{z}$.

8. Show that the harmonic polynomials in two variables are homogeneous polynomials.

Hint. $(x+iy)^n=P_n(x,y)+iQ_n(x,y)$ implies $\frac{\partial P_n}{\partial x}=nP_{n-1}$, $\frac{\partial P_n}{\partial y}=-nQ_{n-1}$,

$$\frac{\partial Q_n}{\partial x}=nQ_{n-1},\ \frac{\partial Q_n}{\partial y}=nP_{n-1},\ P_{n+1}=xP_n-yQ_n,\ Q_{n+1}=yP_n+xQ_n.$$

Therefore

$$x\frac{\partial P_n}{\partial x}+y\frac{\partial P_n}{\partial y}=n(xP_{n-1}-yQ_{n-1})=nP_n,\ x\frac{\partial Q_n}{\partial x}+y\frac{\partial Q_n}{\partial y}=nQ_n.$$

9. Let $f:R^{2n}\to R$ be a C^∞ function on $R^{2n}\setminus R^n$, where $R^n=\{(x,y)\in R^{2n}\mid y=0\}$. If $f(x,0)=0$ and if the partial function $y\to f(x,y)$ is homogeneous of degree $p>0$, then f is continuous on R^n.

10. Let us consider the vector fields

$$(y,-x,0),\ (x,y,z),\ (x^2,yx,xz),\ (xy,y^2,yz),\ (xz,yz,z^2).$$

Show that the family of cones $x^2+y^2=c^2z^2$, where c is a real parameter, is invariant with respect to the flow generated by each of the given vector fields.

The same problem for the vector fields

$$(1,0,y),\ (x,0,z),\ (x^2,xy-z,xz),\ (0,1,x),\ (0,y,z),\ (xy-z,y^2,yz)$$

and the hyperbolic paraboloid $z=xy$.

11. Show that the flows generated by vector fields $(1,x)$, $(x,2y)$, (x^2-y,xy) conserve the parabola $x^2-2y=0$.

12. The vector fields $\boldsymbol{X}=(1,2x,3y)$, $\boldsymbol{Y}=(x,2y,3z)$, $\boldsymbol{Z}=(0,1,3x)$ and the real function $f(x,y,z)=3xy-z-2x^3$ are given. Verify that:

1) the function f is an invariant with respect to a one parameter group generated by $\boldsymbol{X}$ and respectively $\boldsymbol{Z}$;

2) the function f is a proper vector of $\boldsymbol{Y}$ with respect to the proper value 3.

13. Analyse the existence of proper values and proper vectors for the vector fields $\boldsymbol{X}=(X_1,\dots,X_n)$ in the cases

$$1)\ X_i(x)=\sum_{j\neq i}x_j,\quad i,j=1,\dots,n;\ 2)\ X_i(x)=\prod_{j\neq i}x_j,\quad i,j=1,\dots,n.$$

Hint. $\operatorname{div} X = 0$.

The same problem for homothetic, affine and projective vector fields.

14. Using the grid method, approximate the solutions of the following Cauchy problems

1) $\dfrac{\partial f}{\partial x} = \dfrac{\partial f}{\partial y}$, $f(x,0) = \sin \pi x$, $(x,y) \in [0,1] \times [0,1]$, $h = k = 0{,}2$;

2) $\dfrac{\partial f}{\partial x} + \dfrac{\partial f}{\partial y} = y \sin x$, $f(x,0) = \cos x$, $(x,y) \in \left[0, \dfrac{\pi}{2}\right] \times [0, 1]$, $h = 0{,}1$; $k = 0{,}05$.

15. Find the Gauss curvature and the mean curvature of a field surface in R^3.

16. Let $f: R^n \to R$ be a function with the property $\|\operatorname{grad} f\| = 1$. Show that the field surfaces of $\operatorname{grad} f$ are ruled surfaces.

7. BIFURCATION THEORY

Bifurcation theory deals with the study of the influence of parameter variation upon equilibrium points and nonconstant field lines, having applications in biology, chemistry, physics, engineering, etc (or in detail in the domains mentioned in the introduction to Chapter 5). From these we shall present only the basic ideas and examples, noting however that the general theory requires supplementary knowledge of functional analysis, topology and dynamical systems.

In 7.1 we describe the bifurcation in the equilibrium set, underlining the role of the implicit function theorem in this problem. Simultaneously we recall the classification of points of a plane curve given by an implicit Cartesian equation, and give examples of bifurcation in cases that the equilibrium set is a quartic, bicylindric quartic, hypoped quartic and spherical rodonee of index 2, respectively.

The notion of centre manifold, which derives from the notion of invariant set, is presented in 7.2. Then bifurcation of the local flow is commented on (see 7.3) in the sense of passing from open field lines to closed field lines, taking as models a linear differential system and a nonlinear differential system (a model from biology), both with two unknown functions.

In 7.2 we present the Hopf theorem of bifurcation in a simplified version, but sufficient in generality to be applied to essential concrete cases such as the Van der Pol equation from the theory of electrical circuits, the Lorenz differential system which describes the dynamical turbulance of a fluid and the Goodwin differential system which models a biochemical process.

The problems of 7.5 refer to the equilibrium set, bifurcation in the equilibrium set, the existence of centre manifolds, stability of equilibrium points, and flow bifurcation (with applications in chemistry and the theory of reactors).

7.1. BIFURCATION IN THE EQUILIBRIUM SET

Bifurcation means a division in two, a splitting apart, a change. In dynamical systems, the object of bifurcation theory is to study the changes that occur when the parameters change.

Let $X(x, c) = (X_1(x, c), \dots, X_n(x, c))$, $x = (x_1, \dots, x_n) \in R^n$, be a C^∞ vector field on R^n which depends on the vector parameter $c = (c_1, \dots, c_m) \in R^m$. The space R^n is called the *state space*, and R^m is called the *control space* for the differential system

$$\frac{dx_1}{dt} = X_1(x_1, \dots, x_n; c_1, \dots, c_m), \dots, \frac{dx_n}{dt} = X_n(x_1, \dots, x_n; c_1, \dots, c_m). \tag{1}$$

The subset E of $R^n \times R^m$ characterized by the Cartesian implicit equations

$$X_1(x,c) = 0, \ldots, X_n(x,c) = 0, \ x \in R^n, \ c \in R^m \tag{2}$$

is called the *equilibrium set*, since its projection on R^n consists only of equilibrium points of the differential system (1). The set E is a submanifold of dimension m of $R^n \times R^m$ only if the vector field X has certain properties (for example, to satisfy the hypotheses in the implicit function theorem, $\det\left[\frac{\partial X_i}{\partial x_j}(x,c)\right] \neq 0$). Generally, the equilibrium set consists of isolated points or graphs of implicit functions defined by the algebraic system (2). These graphs are called *branches* of the equilibrium set.

Let χ be the restriction of the projection $\pi : R^n \times R^m \to R^m$, $\pi(x,c) = c$ to the equilibrium set E. The subset S of E containing the singular points of the function $\chi : E \to R^m$, i.e., the points at which the rank of the Jacobian matrix $J(\chi)$ is smaller than m, is called the *set of singularities*. Taking into account the explicit expression of the Jacobian of χ, it comes out that S is characterized by the equations

$$X_i(x,c) = 0, \ \det\left[\frac{\partial X_i}{\partial x_j}(x,c)\right] = 0, \ i,j = 1, \ldots, n.$$

Suppose that (x_0, c_0) is not an isolated point of equilibrium set E. If (x_0, c_0) is a singular point of E with the property that there exist at least two branches $E_1 : x = \varphi(c)$ and $E_2 : x = \psi(c)$ of E such that $\varphi(c_0) = \psi(c_0) = x_0$ and $E_1 \cap E_2 = \{(x_0, c_0)\}$, then the point c_0 is called the *bifurcation point* of the branches.

The image $B = \chi(S) \subset R^m$ is called the *bifurcation set* of the equilibrium points. The bifurcation set B is observable, and the number and the nature of critical points are changed on B.

The isolated equilibrium points and the disjoint branches of E have no direct connection to bifurcations.

Classification of points of a plane curve defined by a Cartesian implicit equation

Let us consider the curve $\Gamma : F(u,v) = 0$, where $F : R^2 \to R$ is a C^∞ function.

1) A point of Γ at which $\frac{\partial F}{\partial u} \neq 0$ or $\frac{\partial F}{\partial v} \neq 0$ is called a *regular point*. At such a point, the implicit function theorem works, i.e., there exists a unique function $u = u(v)$ or $v = v(u)$ whose graph passes through the considered point and is included in Γ.

2) A point $M_0(u_0, v_0)$ of Γ at which $\frac{\partial F}{\partial v}(M_0) \neq 0$ and $\frac{du}{dv}$ changes sign on passing of v through v_0 (or $\frac{\partial F}{\partial u}(M_0) \neq 0$ and $\frac{dv}{du}$ changes sign on passing of u through u_0) is called

a *regular point of crossing*.

3) A point of Γ at which $\frac{\partial F}{\partial u} = 0$, $\frac{\partial F}{\partial v} = 0$ is called a *singular point*.

4) A singular point of the curve Γ, in which at least one derivative of order two of F is not zero, and through which pass two and only two branches of the curve Γ having distinct tangents, is called a *double point* (Fig.87.a).

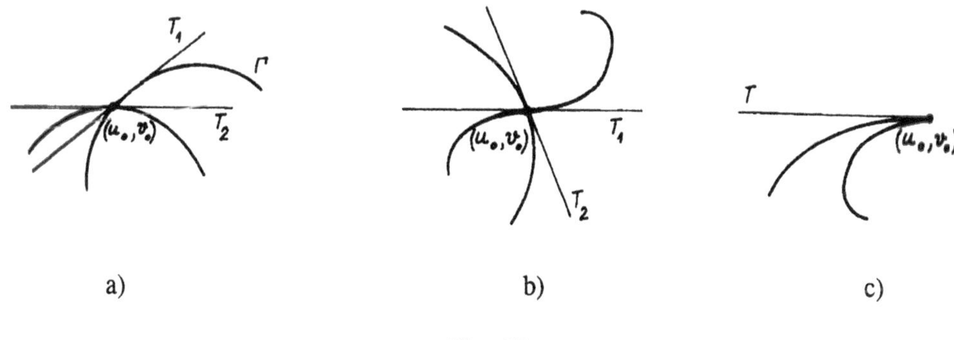

Fig. 87

5) A double point $M_0(u_0, v_0)$ of Γ, for which $\frac{du}{dv}$ $\left(\text{or } \frac{dv}{du}\right)$ changes sign on one branch, at passing of v through v_0 (of u by u_0), is called *a double singular point of crossing* (Fig. 87.b).

6) A singular point of Γ at which two branches of Γ have a contact of order two is called a *cusp point*. At such a point the two branches have the same tangent (Fig.87.c).

7) An isolated point of Γ is called a *conjugate point*.

8) A singular point of Γ at which all the second derivatives of the function F vanish is called a *singular point of higher order*.

Let $(u_0, v_0) \in \Gamma$ be a singular point for which the Hessian $d^2F(u_0, v_0)$ is not identically zero. If $\det d^2F(u_0, v_0) > 0$, then (u_0, v_0) is an isolated (conjugate) point of Γ; if $\det d^2F(u_0, v_0) < 0$, then (u_0, v_0) is a double point of Γ; if $\det d^2F(u_0, v_0) = 0$, then (u_0, v_0) is a cusp point of Γ. At a double or cusp point, the directions (l, m) of the tangents to Γ are given by

$$l^2 \frac{\partial^2 F}{\partial u^2}(u_0, v_0) + 2lm \frac{\partial^2 F}{\partial u \partial v}(u_0, v_0) + m^2 \frac{\partial^2 F}{\partial v^2}(u_0, v_0) = 0.$$

The conjugate point and the double point of the curve Γ are isolated critical points of the function F.

Applications. 1) Let us consider the differential equation (with separable variables)

$$\frac{dx}{dt} = c^4 - c^2 + \frac{x^2}{4},$$

where c is a real parameter. The equilibrium points set E is described by the algebraic equation $c^4 - c^2 + \frac{x^2}{4} = 0$ or equivalently $x = \pm 2|c|\sqrt{1-c^2}$, $c \in [-1,1]$. Note that $(0,0)$ is a unique singular point of E (quartic [68]). This is a cusp point (Fig.88).

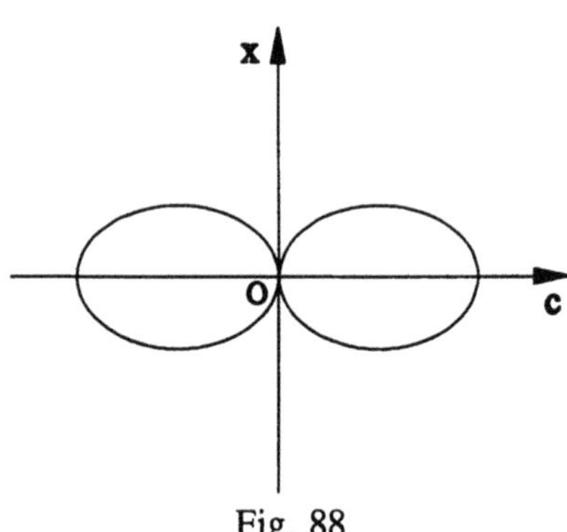

Fig. 88

The branches

$$x = -2|c|\sqrt{1-c^2},\ x = 2|c|\sqrt{1-c^2},\ c \in [-1,1]$$

of E bifurcate one from another at $c = 0$.

2) Let us now consider the autonomous differential system

$$\frac{dx}{dt} = x^2 + c^2 - 1,\ \frac{dy}{dt} = y^2 + c^2 - 1,$$

where c is a real parameter. The set of equilibrium points

$$E: x^2 + c^2 - 1 = 0,\ y^2 + c^2 - 1 = 0,\ c \in [-1,1]$$

is a bicylindric quartic [96], i.e., the intersection of two cylinders whose axes are orthogonal, with respect to the Cartesian frame $Oxyc$ (Fig.89). The curve E has two singular points, namely $(0,0,\pm 1)$.

The branches of the curve E,

$$x = \pm\sqrt{1-c^2},\ y = \pm\sqrt{1-c^2},\ c \in [-1,1],$$

bifurcate one from another at $c = -1$ and at $c = 1$.

3) We will illustrate the bifurcation in the equilibrium set by means of the autonomous differential system

$$\frac{dx}{dt} = x^2 + y^2 + c^2 - 4,\ \frac{dy}{dt} = (x-1)^2 + y^2 - 1,$$

where c is a real parameter. The set of equilibrium points is

$$E: x^2 + y^2 + c^2 - 4 = 0,\ (x-1)^2 + y^2 - 1 = 0.$$

Obviously, $c \in [-2,2]$ and E is a hypoped quartic (spherical lemniscate [96]), i.e., the intersection between a sphere and a cylinder of rotation tangent interior to the sphere, with respect to the Cartesian frame $Oxyc$ (Fig.90).

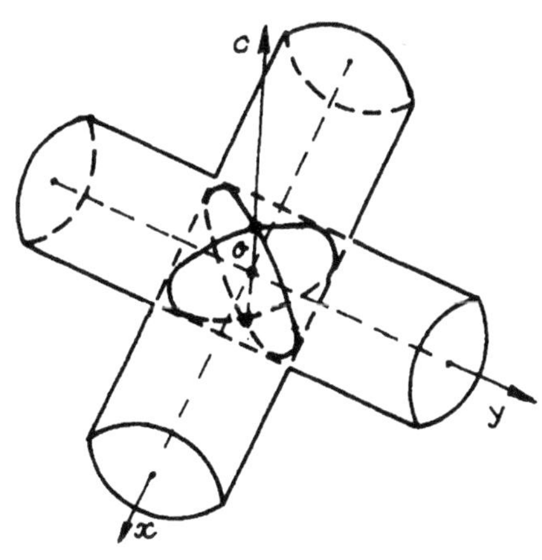

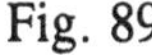
Fig. 89

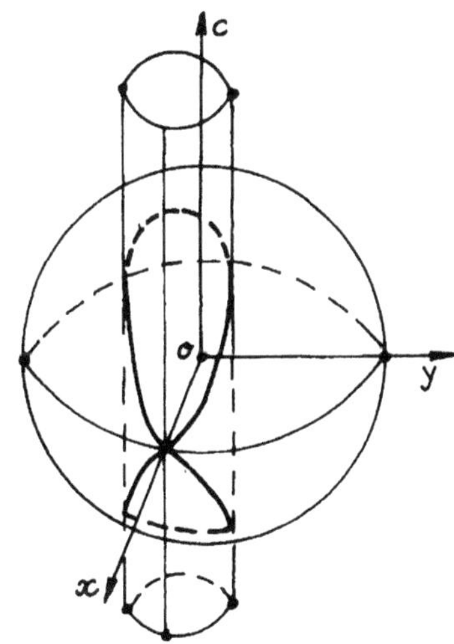

Fig. 90

The branches of E,

$$x = \frac{4 - c^2}{2}, \; y = \pm \frac{|c|}{2}\sqrt{4 - c^2}, \; c \in [-2,2],$$

bifurcate one from another at $c = 0$. The unique singular point of the curve E has the coordinates $x = 2$, $y = 0$, $c = 0$.

4) We consider the autonomous differential system

$$\frac{dx}{dt} = x^2 + y^2 + c^2 - 1, \; \frac{dy}{dt} = y^2 - x^2 + c(x^2 + y^2),$$

where c is a real parameter. Here the set of equilibrium points,

$$E : x^2 + y^2 + c^2 - 1 = 0, \; y^2 - x^2 + c(x^2 + y^2) = 0, \; c \in [-1,1]$$

is a spherical rodonee of index 2 [96]. Indeed, the curve E admits the periodic parametric representation

$$x = \sin 2u \cos u, \; y = \sin 2u \sin u, \; c = \cos 2u, \; u \in R$$

and therefore E is the curve $v = 2u$ situated on the sphere

$$x = \sin v \cos u, \; y = \sin v \sin u, \; c = \cos v, \; u, v \in R,$$

of unit radius. The singular points of the curve E are characterized by

$$x^2 + y^2 + c^2 - 1 = 0,\ y^2 - x^2 + c(x^2 + y^2) = 0,\ \begin{vmatrix} 2x & 2y \\ 2x(c-1) & 2y(c+1) \end{vmatrix} = 0$$

and therefore they are $(0, 0, \pm 1)$. The branches of E,

$$x = \pm (1 + c)\sqrt{\frac{1 - c}{2}},\quad y = \pm (1 - c)\sqrt{\frac{1 + c}{2}},\quad c \in [-1, 1],$$

bifurcate one from another at $c = -1$ and at $c = 1$ (Fig.91).

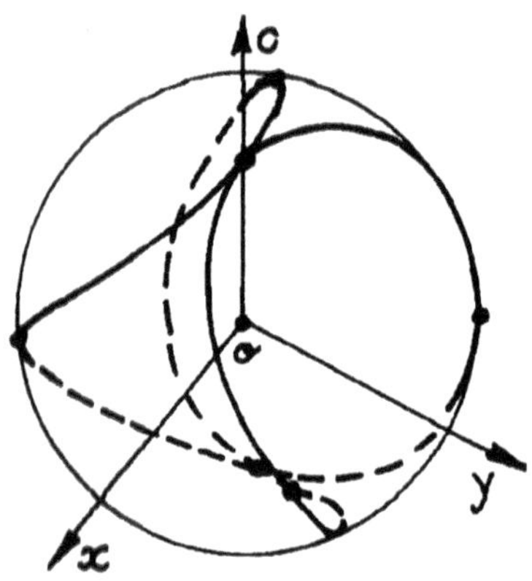

Fig. 91

7.2. CENTRE MANIFOLD

Let $X = (X_1, \ldots, X_n)$ be a C^∞ vector field on R^n and

$$\frac{dx_i}{dt} = X_i(x),\ i = 1, \ldots, n \tag{3}$$

the autonomous differential system that describes the field lines of X.

A subset $S \subset R^n$ is called a *locally invariant set* for the differential system (3) if, for every $x_0 \in S$, the field line $x(t)$ of X determined by the initial conditions $x(0) = x_0$ lies in S for $t \in (-\varepsilon, \varepsilon)$. If $\varepsilon = \infty$, then S is called an *invariant set*.

The void set and R^n are locally invariant. The orbits of the vector field X are locally invariant nonvoid sets (of minimal dimension) and any nonvoid locally invariant set is a union of orbits. Consequently, the field hypersurfaces are locally invariant sets.

The orbits that are equilibrium points are invariant and hence the equilibrium set is invariant.

The union and the intersection of two locally invariant sets are locally invariant sets.

Now we consider a special autonomous differential system

$$\frac{dx}{dt} = Bx + f(x,y), \quad \frac{dy}{dt} = Cy + g(x,y), \tag{4}$$

where $x \in R^n$, $y \in R^m$, and B , C are real matrices. Suppose that the proper values of B are purely imaginary, the proper values of C have strictly negative real parts, and the functions f and g are C^∞ and satisfy the conditions

$$f(0,0) = 0,\ f'(0,0) = 0,\ g(0,0) = 0,\ g'(0,0) = 0$$

(by f' we understand the Jacobian matrix of f).

Since the proper values in complex numbers of a real matrix exist in pairs (a complex number and its conjugate), the trace of the matrix B (the sum of the proper values) is equal to zero, and the trace of the matrix C is strictly negative. Therefore, at $(0,0)$ the divergence of the vector field $(Bx+f(x,y), Cy+g(x,y))$ is strictly negative. By continuity, the divergence remains strictly negative on a neighborhood of $(0,0)$, and hence the flow generated by the vector field on this neighborhood decreases the volumes.

Let $S : y = h(x)$ be a locally invariant set of the differential system (4). If h is of class C^1 and $h(0) = 0$, $h'(0) = 0$, then S is called a *centre manifold.*

The centre manifold is often used in bifurcation theory. As a submanifold of $R^n \times R^m$, the centre manifold is tangent to R^n at the origin.

Theorem [10]. *If the matrices* B, C *and the functions* f, g *satisfy the preceding conditions, then the differential system (4) admits a centre manifold* $S : y = h(x)$, $\|x\| < \delta$.

We shall illustrate the technique of proof on the example

$$\frac{dx_1}{dt} = x_2, \quad \frac{dx_2}{dt} = 0, \quad \frac{dy}{dt} = -y + g(x_1, x_2), \tag{4'}$$

where g is a C^∞ function with $g(x_1, x_2) = O(x_1^2 + x_2^2)$ when $(x_1, x_2) \to (0,0)$.

Let $\psi : R^2 \to R$ be a C^∞ function with $\psi(x) = 1$ for $\|x\| \le 1$, and $\psi(x) = 0$ for $\|x\| \ge 2$. Define $G(x_1, x_2) = \psi(x_1, x_2)\, g(x_1, x_2)$ and show that

$$\frac{dx_1}{dt} = x_2, \quad \frac{dx_2}{dt} = 0, \quad \frac{dy}{dt} = -y + G(x_1, x_2) \tag{4''}$$

admits a centre manifold $y = h(x_1, x_2)$, $(x_1, x_2) \in R^2$. Since the restriction of G to the disc of radius 1 with centre at the origin is g, it follows that there exists $\delta > 0$ such that $y = h(x_1, x_2)$, $x_1^2 + x_2^2 < \delta$ is a local centre manifold for the differential system $(4')$.

The first two equations of $(4'')$ admit the solution $x_1(t) = c_1 + c_2 t$, $x_2(t) = c_2$, $t \in R$, where $x_i(0) = c_i$, $i = 1, 2$. If $y(t) = h(x_1(t), x_2(t))$ is a solution of the third equation of $(4'')$, then

$$\frac{d}{dt} h(c_1 + c_2 t, c_2) = - h(c_1 + c_2 t, c_2) + G(c_1 + c_2 t, c_2).$$

This first order nonhomogeneous linear differential equation admits the solution

$$h(c_1 + c_2 t, c_2) = e^{-t}\left(h(c_1, c_2) + \int_0^t e^s G(c_1 + c_2 s, c_2)\, ds \right).$$

The condition

$$\lim_{t \to -\infty} h(c_1 + c_2 t, c_2) e^t = 0$$

implies

$$h(c_1, c_2) = \int_{-\infty}^0 e^s G(c_1 + c_2 s, c_2)\, ds,$$

facts which determine properly the function h, since G has compact support. By construction, $y = h(c_1, c_2)$, $(c_1, c_2) \in R^2$ is a centre manifold for the differential system $(4'')$ and the restriction to $c_1^2 + c_2^2 < \delta$ is a centre manifold of the differential system $(4')$.

From these examples it follows that [10]:

- the centre manifold is not necessarily unique, and the intersection of centre manifolds is not void;

- if the functions f and g are analytical, it is not necessary that h be of class C^∞ or analytical.

Application. The differential system

$$\frac{dx}{dt} = -x^3, \quad \frac{dy}{dt} = -y$$

admits a family with two parameters of centre manifolds

$$y = h(x, c_1, c_2) = \begin{cases} c_1 \exp \dfrac{-x^2}{2} & \text{for } x < 0 \\ 0 & \text{for } x = 0 \\ c_2 \exp \dfrac{-x^2}{2} & \text{for } x > 0. \end{cases}$$

Indeed, $(0,0)$ is an equilibrium point, the equation $\dfrac{1}{2x^2} = t + k_1$, where k_1 is an arbitrary constant, defines the general solution of the differential equation $\dfrac{dx}{dt} = -x^3$, and $y = k_2 e^{-t}$, k_2 being an arbitrary constant, is the general solution of the differential equation $\dfrac{dy}{dt} = -y$. Thus we obtain the orbits $(0,0)$ and

$$y = \begin{cases} c_1 \exp \dfrac{-x^2}{2} & \text{for } x < 0 \\ c_2 \exp \dfrac{-x^2}{2} & \text{for } x > 0, \end{cases}$$

c_1, c_2 being arbitrary constants. These orbits are pictured in Fig.92 $(c_1 < c_2)$ having as basis the following table of variation, worked out for $c_1 > c_2 > 0$:

x	$-\infty$		0		∞
y'	0	−	0 | 0	+	0
y	c_1	↘	0 | 0	↗	c_2

The centre manifold (the union of the preceding two families of orbits) is drawn in Fig.93 $(c_1 < c_2)$, adding to the preceding remarks that $x \to h(x, c_1, c_2)$ is a C^∞ function.

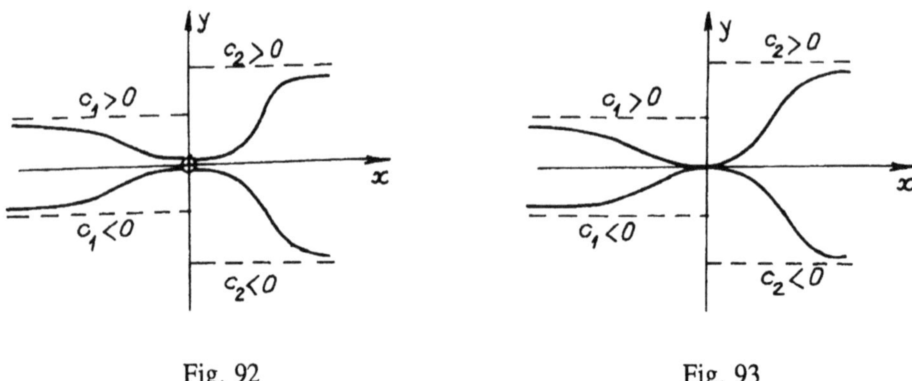

Fig. 92 Fig. 93

7.3. FLOW BIFURCATION

Let us consider the C^{∞} vector field $X(x,c)$, $x \in R^n$, $c \in R^m$ and the associated autonomous differential system

$$\frac{dx}{dt} = X(x,c). \tag{5}$$

Let V be an open set of R^m which contains the point c_0 and $x = x(c)$, $c \in V$, an isolated equilibrium point of the differential system (5). We say that $c = c_0$ is a *bifurcation point* for the differential system (5), if at $c = c_0$ there appears a changing of the qualitative properties of the local flow in the sense that in any neighborhood of c_0 there exist the points a and b such that the local phase portraits for $c = a$ and $c = b$ are not topologically equivalent.

Suppose that the linear approximation of (5) about the point $x(c)$ is

$$\frac{dx}{dt} = A(c)x. \tag{6}$$

The points c_0 that are candidates for producing the bifurcation are those in which the matrix $A(c_0)$ has also proper values with zero real part. Indeed, if all the proper values of the matrix $A(c_0)$ have nonzero real parts, then for $\| c - c_0 \|$ sufficiently small, the solutions of the differential system (5) behave locally like those of the linear differential system (6) and hence $c = c_0$ is not a bifurcation point. Furthermore, since we are interested especially in the bifurcation of stable phenomena, it is necessary to add the hypothesis that the matrix $A(c_0)$ has no proper values with strictly positive real part.

Applications. 1) Linear differential system. The most simple example of flow bifurcation is encountered for the homogeneous linear differential system

$$\frac{dx}{dt} = cx - y, \ \frac{dy}{dt} = x + cy, \ c \in R,$$

attached to the Killing vector field $(cx - y, x + cy)$ on R^2. With the notations of 4.3, we have

$$\beta = 2c, \ \gamma = 1 + c^2 > 0, \ \beta^2 - 4\gamma = -4 < 0.$$

Since $\gamma = 1 + c^2 > 0, \ \gamma > \frac{\beta^2}{4}, \ \forall c \in R$, the isolated equilibrium point $(0,0)$ is (1) an asymptotically stable focus, (2) a centre for $c = 0$, (3) an unstable focus for $c > 0$ (Fig.54). Thus, $c_0 = 0$ is the value of c at which one produces flow bifurcation: from spiral orbits coming toward $(0,0)$ we pass to closed orbits (concentric ellipses, around $(0,0)$ and then to spiral orbits starting near $(0,0)$. This bifurcation takes place since the passing of c from negative values, through zero, to positive values causes the point (β, γ) to traverse the axis $O\gamma$ at a point for which $\gamma > 0$.

Naturally, we must ask if the linear homogeneous differential system

$$\frac{dx}{dt} = a_{11}x + a_{12}y, \ \frac{dy}{dt} = a_{21}x + a_{22}y$$

can produce also another type of bifurcation different from those previously described. The theory of 4.3 and Fig.52 give the answer to this question. Indeed, if a_{ij}, $i,j = 1,2$, are differentiable functions of c, it is possible to obtain closed field lines only if $\beta = 0$ and $\gamma > 0$. Hence, either we have a proper bifurcation of the preceding type, or we have a pathological bifurcation which appears at passing through $(0,0)$ of the point $(0,\gamma)$ which moves on the positive semiaxis $O\gamma$. The pathology is connected to the fact that for $\gamma = 0$ we have a straight line of equilibrium points and not an isolated equilibrium point.

2) Nonlinear differential system. Certain aspects of the interactions between two populations, one being predatory and one prey, are modeled by the nonlinear autonomous differential system [59]

$$\frac{dx}{dt} = x(x(1-x) - y), \ \frac{dy}{dt} = \alpha\left(x - \frac{1}{c}\right)y \tag{7}$$

on $x \geq 0$, $y \geq 0$, where α is a fixed strictly positive number, and c is a strictly positive parameter.

The equilibrium points of the system (7) are $(0,0)$, $(1,0)$ and $(c^{-1}, c^{-1}(1 - c^{-1}))$, $c > 1$. With respect to the Cartesian frame $Oxyc$, the equilibrium set E is composed from the open semiaxis Oc, open semistraight $D: x = 1, \ y = 0, \ c > 0$ and the curve $\Gamma: x = \frac{1}{c}, \ y = \frac{1}{c}\left(1 - \frac{1}{c}\right)$, $c > 1$, that appear as intersection of two cylindrical surfaces, $\Sigma_1: x = \frac{1}{c}$, $c \geq 1$ with generators parallel to Oy, and $\Sigma_2: y = \frac{1}{c}\left(1 - \frac{1}{c}\right)$, $c \geq 0$ with generators parallel to Ox. The surface Σ_1 is a part of a hyperbolic cylinder. The shape of

Σ_2 is determined by the shape of the graph of the real function $y = \frac{1}{c}\left(1 - \frac{1}{c}\right)$, $c > 1$ (Fig.95) which follows from the table

c	1		2		3		∞
y′	| 1	+	0	-		-	0
y″	|	-		-	0	+	
y	| 0	↗	1/4	↘	2/9	↘	0

Fig.95 contains Σ_1, Σ_2, $E = Oc \cup D \cup \Gamma$ and the projection of E on the plane xOy, which is the parabolic arc $\gamma_1 : y = x(1 - x)$, $0 < x \leq 1$, $c = 0$. One observes that at the point $c = 1$ is produced a bifurcation of equilibrium points.

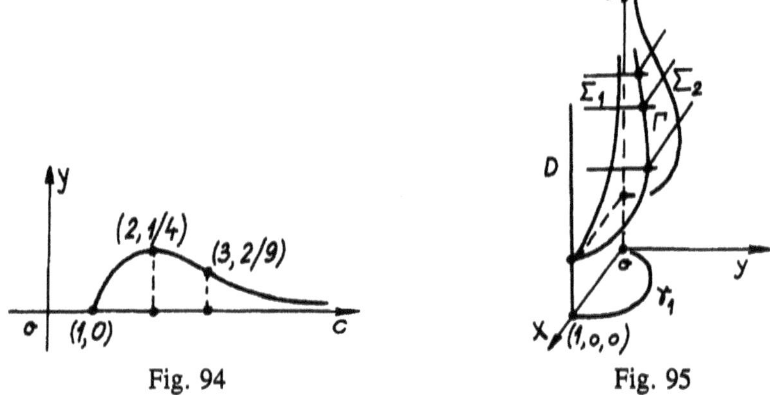

Fig. 94 Fig. 95

In the sequel we shall consider the linear approximation of (7), the theory of 4.3 and Fig.52.

The linear approximation of the differential system (7) in the neighborhood of the equilibrium point $(0,0)$ is $\frac{dx}{dt} = 0$, $\frac{dy}{dt} = -\frac{\alpha}{c}y$. Thus, with the notations of 4.3 we have $\beta = -\frac{\alpha}{c} < 0$, $\gamma = 0$ and therefore in Fig.52 the point (β, γ) lies on the negative semiaxis $O\gamma'$. The family of field lines $x = k_1$, $y = k_2 \exp\left(-\frac{\alpha}{c}t\right)$, $t \in R$, shows the behavior of the flow around $(0,0)$.

Now we consider the equilibrium point $(1,0)$. The matrix of the linear approximation of the differential system (7) in a neighborhood of $(1,0)$ is $\begin{bmatrix} -1 & -1 \\ 0 & \alpha(1-c^{-1}) \end{bmatrix}$.

Thus $\beta = -1 + \alpha(1-c^{-1})$, $\gamma = -\alpha(1-c^{-1})$. For $0 < c < 1$ we have $\frac{dx}{dt} < 0$, $\frac{dy}{dt} < 0$, which helps to show that for any initial condition $x(0) \geq 0$, $y(0) \geq 0$ we have $\lim_{t\to\infty} x(t) = 1$, $\lim_{t\to\infty} y(t) = 0$. For $c > 1$ we have $\gamma < 0$ and Fig.52 shows that $(1,0)$ is a saddle point.

Let us consider the equilibrium point $(c^{-1}, c^{-1}(1-c^{-1}))$, $c > 1$. The linear approximation of the differential system (7) in a neighborhood of this point has the matrix

$$\begin{bmatrix} c^{-1}(1-2c^{-1}) & -c^{-1} \\ \alpha c^{-1}(1-c^{-1}) & 0 \end{bmatrix}$$

and so $\beta = c^{-1}(1-2c^{-1})$, $\gamma = \alpha c^{-2}(1-c^{-1}) > 0$.

If $c = 2$, then $\beta = 0$, $\gamma = \frac{\alpha}{8} > 0$ and the equilibrium point $\left(\frac{1}{2}, \frac{1}{4}\right)$ is a centre (Fig.52).

If $c < 2$, then $\beta < 0$ and therefore the equilibrium point is either a focus $\left(\text{for } \gamma > \frac{\beta^2}{4}\right)$, or an asymptotically stable knot $\left(\text{for } \gamma < \frac{\beta^2}{4}\right)$. If $c > 2$, then $\beta > 0$ and hence the equilibrium point is either a focus $\left(\text{for } \gamma > \frac{\beta^2}{4}\right)$, or an unstable knot $\left(\text{for } \gamma < \frac{\beta^2}{4}\right)$. We specify that for c sufficiently close to 2 we have two foci, and the inequality $\gamma > \frac{\beta^2}{4}$ is equivalent to $\alpha > \frac{(1-2c^{-1})^2}{4(1-c^{-1})}$. The next table contains all the possibilities and shows that for a certain value of α, the bifurcation takes place at passing through $c = 2$. Denoting $a = \frac{(1-2c^{-1})^2}{4(1-c^{-1})}$, we can draw up the table

$\alpha > a$	$\alpha < a$
$c < 2$ asymptotically stable focus	asymptotically stable knot
$c = 2$ centre	impossibility since $\alpha > 0$
$c > 2$ unstable focus	unstable knot

7.4. HOPF THEOREM OF BIFURCATION

Now we shall analyse the fashion in which the periodic solutions of some autonomous differential systems appear from the variation of equilibrium points with respect to some parameters. Necessarily the corresponding vector fields X are neither potential, nor biscalar, nor vector fields for which $(D_X X, X)$ is not zero at any point, since these do not admit closed nonconstant field lines (see 5.1, 8.4, 9.1). Also, the bifurcation of periodic flow cannot appear for vector fields defined on R, but only for vector fields defined on R^n, $n \geq 2$.

Let $X(x,c) = (X_1(x,c), \dots, X_n(x,c))$ be a C^∞ vector field on R^n, $n \geq 2$, which depends on the real parameter c and

$$\frac{dx_1}{dt} = X_1(x,c), \dots, \frac{dx_n}{dt} = X_n(x,c) \tag{8}$$

be the differential system that determines the field lines of X. Suppose that the algebraic system

$$X_1(x,c) = 0, \dots, X_n(x,c) = 0$$

admits an isolated solution $x_1 = x_1(c), \dots, x_n = x_n(c)$, $c \in I$. This is an isolated equilibrium point of the differential system (8).

Let

$$\frac{dx}{dt} = A(c)x, \; A(c) = \left[\frac{\partial X_i}{\partial x_j}(x(c), c)\right]$$

be the linear differential system that approximates (8) in a neighborhood of the equilibrium point $x = x(c)$. Denote by $\lambda_1(c), \dots, \lambda_n(c)$ the proper values (in the set of complex numbers) of the matrix $A(c)$ and suppose

$$\lambda_1(c) = \alpha(c) + i\beta(c), \; \lambda_2(c) = \alpha(c) - i\beta(c) = \overline{\lambda_1}(c).$$

If $n > 2$, one adds the hypothesis

$$\text{Re}\,\lambda_3(c) < 0, \dots, \text{Re}\,\lambda_n(c) < 0, \; c \in I.$$

Suppose that there exists an isolated value $c_0 \in I$ such that $\alpha(c_0) = 0$, $\beta(c_0) \neq 0$, $\frac{d\alpha}{dc}(c_0) > 0$ (this means that at passing of c by c_0, the function $c \to \alpha(c)$ passes from negative values to positive values; obviously one can consider also the opposite inequality). The value c_0 is called the *critical value* of the parameter c.

In the preceding hypotheses, E.Hopf has shown that one and only one of the following three situations can occur.

Situation 1. *The equilibrium point is a centre, i.e., there exist an infinite set of concentric closed orbits around* $x_0 = x(c_0)$. *In this case, for* $c \neq c_0$, *but neighbor with* c_0, *there exist no periodic orbits around* $x(c)$.

Situation 2. *There exists a number* $b > c_0$ *such that for every* $c \in (c_0, b)$ *there exists one and only one closed orbit around the equilibrium point* $x(c)$ *in a neighborhood of this point. This family with one parameter of closed orbits bifurcates at the equilibrium point* $x(c)$ *in the sense that, if* $c \to c_0$, *then the diameter of the closed orbits varies with* $|c - c_0|^{\frac{1}{2}}$. *In this case, for* $c \leq c_0$, $c \in I$, *there do not exist closed orbits neighbor to* $x(c)$.

Situation 3. *There exists a number* $a < c_0$ *such that for every* $c \in (a, c_0)$ *there exists a closed orbit and only one around the equilibrium point* $x(c)$ *in a neighborhood of this point. This family with one parameter of closed orbits bifurcates in the fashion explained before. For* $c \geq c_0$ *there do not exist closed orbits neighbor to* $x(c)$.

Instead of the proof we shall comment on the geometry of the Hopf theorem. The hypotheses

$$\mathrm{Re}\,\lambda_3(c) < 0, \dots, \mathrm{Re}\,\lambda_n(c) < 0, \ c \in I, \ \alpha(c_0) = 0, \ \beta(c_0) \neq 0$$

guarantee that the contribution of the proper functions associated to $\lambda_3, \dots, \lambda_n$ to the solution of the linear approximation tends to zero for $t \to \infty$, while the contribution of proper functions associated to λ_1 and λ_2 survives.

We recall that: 1) to every real proper value one associates a 1-dimensional real proper space (straight line in R^n) which contains the equilibrium point $x_j = x_j(c_0)$, $j = 1, \dots, n$; 2) to every pair of complex conjugate proper values one associates a 2-dimensional real proper space (plane in R^n) which contains the equilibrium point (in the phase space). Having this in mind, it follows that, being given a point $x^* = (x_1^*, \dots, x_n^*)$ neighbor to the equilibrium point $x_j = x_j(c_0)$, $j = 1, \dots, n$, the field line through x^* tends in time either to the equilibrium point, or to the plane of the equilibrium point generated by the proper functions (*sine, cosine*) associated to λ_1 and λ_2. Thus we concentrate the Hopf theorem on the remark that in case we stop at the linear approximation, then the interesting evolution (the part of the solution which does not disappear) occurs in a plane containing the equilibrium point.

Recent proofs [29, 32, 38] of the Hopf theorem exploit the fact that for a nonlinear differential system there exists (in the phase space) a 2-dimensional submanifold (surface) which contains the equilibrium point and which plays the role of the plane from the linear differential system associated to λ_1 and λ_2. This surface is called a *centre manifold*. Thus, for any $n \geq 2$, the only topological possibilities of appearance of closed orbits, except for the equilibrium points, are exactly the possibilities in the case $n = 2$. The hypotheses "X of class

C^{∞}, $\beta(c_0) = 0$, $\frac{d\alpha}{dc}(c_0) > 0$" limit the possible cases to those already presented.

Remarks. 1) Because of the centre manifold existence, the Hopf bifurcations are 2-dimensional phenomena.

2) The inequality $\frac{d\alpha}{dc}(c_0) < 0$ can be transformed in the opposite inequality, replacing c with $c_0 - c$, $\frac{1}{c}$, etc respectively.

3) If the differential system depends on many parameters, then from the context it is necessary to discover the parameter whose variation produces Hopf bifurcation.

4) In the hypotheses of Hopf bifurcation, it turns out that $\operatorname{div} A(c)x|_{c=c_0} = \operatorname{trace} A(c_0) < 0$. By continuity, $\operatorname{div} A(c)x$ remains strictly negative in a neighborhood of c_0, and therefore the family of flows generated by $A(c)x$, $c \in (c_0 - \varepsilon, c_0 + \varepsilon)$, decreases the volume.

Applications. 1) **Van der Pol equation.** The differential equations of the electric circuit RLC sketches in Fig.20 are

$$i_C = \frac{dv_C}{dt}, \; v_L = L\frac{di_L}{dt}, \; v_R = \phi(i_R), \; i_R = i_L = -i_C, \; v_R + v_L = v_C,$$

where $i's$ are currents on the branches indicated by indices and $v_R = \phi(i_R)$ is the generalized Ohm's law (characteristic of the resistor R). Denoting $i_L = x$, $v_C = -\left(\frac{L}{C}\right)^{\frac{1}{2}} y$, $t = (LC)^{\frac{1}{2}}\tau$, the preceding differential equations are written

$$\frac{dx}{d\tau} = -y - f(x), \; \frac{dy}{d\tau} = x,$$

where $f(x) = \left(\frac{L}{C}\right)^{\frac{1}{2}} \phi(x)$. If the resistance is described by the function $f(x) = -\mu x + x^3$, then the preceding differential system is a representation of the Van der Pol differential equation of order two. The parameter μ controls the magnitude of "negative resistance."

For any μ, the point $x = 0$, $y = 0$ is an equilibrium point. The matrix of the linear approximation has the proper values

$$\lambda_{1,2} = \frac{\mu \pm \sqrt{\mu^2 - 4}}{2}.$$

These are: (1) real negative, for $\mu \le -2$, (2) complex conjugate with negative real part, for $-2 < \mu < 0$, (3) complex conjugate with positive real part, for $0 < \mu < 2$, (4) real positive, for $\mu \ge 2$.

If $\mu < 0$, then the equilibrium point $(0,0)$ is asymptotically stable. If μ increases passing by zero, the equilibrium point $(0,0)$ loses stability due to the proper values $\lambda_{1,2} = \alpha(\mu) \pm i\beta(\mu)$, where $\alpha(\mu) = \frac{\mu}{2}$, $\beta(\mu) = \sqrt{1 - \alpha^2(\mu)}$. Since $\alpha'(0) = \frac{1}{2} > 0$, one applies the Hopf theorem: there exists a family of periodic orbits that bifurcates at $(0,0)$.

2) **Lorenz system.** The autonomous differential system

$$\frac{dx}{dt} = -\sigma x + \sigma y, \quad \frac{dy}{dt} = -xz + rx - y, \quad \frac{dz}{dt} = xy - bz,$$

where σ, r, b are real parameters, was the mathematical model accepted by Lorenz for the dynamical turbulence of a fluid [37]. The solutions of this system are defined on the whole real line (see 3.6).

Assuming σ and b have fixed values, and r remains as parameter, we shall look for bifurcation with respect to r.

If $\sigma \neq 0$ and $b(r-1) > 0$, then the equilibrium points of the Lorenz system are

$$x = 0,\ y = 0,\ z = 0;$$
$$x = \pm\sqrt{b(r-1)},\ y = \pm\sqrt{b(r-1)},\ z = r-1.$$

We stop at the equilibrium point

$$x_0 = \sqrt{b(r-1)},\ y_0 = \sqrt{b(r-1)},\ z_0 = r-1,$$

which leads to more interesting results. The Jacobian matrix, i.e., the matrix of the linear approximation in a neighborhood of the point (x_0, y_0, z_0) is

$$\begin{bmatrix} -\sigma & \sigma & 0 \\ 1 & -1 & -x_0 \\ x_0 & x_0 & -b \end{bmatrix}.$$

This matrix has the characteristic polynomial

$$\lambda^3 + (\sigma + b + 1)\lambda^2 + b(r+\sigma)\lambda + 2b\sigma(r-1).$$

Taking into account that the polynomial of order three, having the real root α and purely imaginary roots $\pm i\beta$, is $\lambda^3 - \alpha\lambda^2 + \beta^2\lambda - \alpha\beta^2$, we arrive at the conclusion that the critical value r_0 of the parameter r must satisfy the relations

$$\alpha = -(\sigma + b + 1),\ \pm i\beta = \pm i\sqrt{b(r_0 + \sigma)},\ 2b\sigma(r_0 - 1) = b(r_0 + \sigma)(\sigma + b + 1).$$

From the last relation it follows that

$$r_0 = \frac{\sigma(\sigma + b + 3)}{\sigma - b - 1},$$

and

$$b(r_0 + \sigma) = \frac{2b\sigma(\sigma + 1)}{\sigma - b - 1}$$

is positive if $\sigma > b + 1$.

Suppose $\sigma > 0$, $b > 0$ and hence $r > 1$. Taking into account that the solution λ of the characteristic equation

$$\lambda^3 + (\sigma + b + 1)\lambda^2 + b(r + \sigma)\lambda + 2b\sigma(r - 1) = 0$$

is a function of r, by taking the derivative of both members, we find

$$\lambda'(r) = \frac{-b(\lambda + 2\sigma)}{3\lambda^2 + 2(\sigma + b + 1)\lambda + b(r + \sigma)}.$$

It follows that

$$\alpha'(r_0) = \operatorname{Re}\lambda'(r_0) = \frac{b(\sigma - b - 1)}{2[\beta^2(r_0) + (\sigma + b + 1)^2]} > 0.$$

With these we have proved that we are in the conditions of the Hopf theorem and hence the loss of stability at $r = r_0$ leads to a bifurcation of Hopf type.

3) **Goodwin system**. The differential system

$$\frac{dx}{dt} = \frac{1}{1 + z^n} - ax, \quad \frac{dy}{dt} = x - by, \quad \frac{dz}{dt} = y - cz,$$

where a, b, c are real strictly positive parameters, and n is a fixed natural number, models biochemical processes with negative feedback (see 4.4).

We fix a and b, and allow c as parameter. We study the presence of Hopf bifurcation with respect to the parameter c.

The equilibrium point of the differential system is (x_0, y_0, z_0) with $x_0 = bcz_0$, $y_0 = cz_0$, where z_0 is the strictly positive solution of the algebraic equation

$$\frac{1}{1 + z^n} = abcz$$

(see 4.4). The linear approximation of the differential system around (x_0, y_0, z_0) has the matrix

$$\begin{bmatrix} -a & 0 & \dfrac{-nz_0^{n-1}}{1 + z_0^n} \\ 1 & -b & 0 \\ 0 & 1 & -c \end{bmatrix},$$

and the characteristic polynomial of this matrix has the expression

$$\lambda^3 + (a+b+c)\lambda^2 + (ba+ac+bc)\lambda + abc + \frac{n z_0^{n-1}}{1 + z_0^n}.$$

Indentifying this polynomial with the polynomial of degree three that admits the real root α and the purely imaginary roots $\pm i\beta$ (see the preceding example), we deduce that the critical values c_0 (if they exist) of c must satisfy

$$\alpha = -(a+b+c_0),\ \beta^2 = ab + (a+b)c_0,$$

$$abc_0 + \frac{n z_0^{n-1}}{1 + z_0^n} = (a+b+c_0)[ab + (a+b)c_0].$$

Denoting

$$a + b = A,\ ab = B,\ \frac{n z_0^{n-1}}{1 + z_0^n} = D,$$

the last equation can be written

$$A c_0^2 + A^2 c_0 + AB - D = 0.$$

For $A^3 - 4AB + 4D \geq 0$, this last equation has real roots and, if we add the condition $D > AB$, the root

$$c_0 = \frac{-A^2 + \sqrt{A^4 - 4A^2B + 4AD}}{2A}$$

is strictly positive.

The implicit equation

$$\lambda^3 + (a+b+c)\lambda^2 + (ab+ac+bc)\lambda + abc + \frac{n z_0^{n-1}}{1 + z_0^n} = 0$$

defines λ as a function of c, and the derivative of this function is obtained by differentiating both members of the preceding equation with respect to c. It follows that

$$3\lambda^2\lambda' + \lambda^2 + 2(A+c)\lambda\lambda' + A\lambda + (B+Ac)\lambda' + B = 0$$

and hence

$$\lambda'(c) = \frac{-\lambda^2 - A\lambda - B}{3\lambda^2 + 2(A+c)\lambda + B + Ac}.$$

From this we find

$$\alpha'(c_0) = \text{Re}\,\lambda'(c_0) = \frac{-(A+c_0)^2 + A(A+c_0) - B}{3(A+c_0)^2 - 2(A+c_0)^2 + B + Ac_0} = \frac{-c_0^2 - Ac_0 - B}{-\beta^2(c_0) + (A+c_0)^2} < 0.$$

Consequently, at passing of c by c_0, the stability of the equilibrium point is lost and the Hopf bifurcation appears. The symmetry of the characteristic polynomial with respect to a, b, c allows any one parameter a, b, c to fulfil the role described before.

4) The biochemical processes with positive feedback described by the differential system

$$\frac{dx}{dt} = \frac{1+z^n}{k+z^n} - ax, \quad \frac{dy}{dt} = x - by, \quad \frac{dz}{dt} = y - cz,$$

where $a, b, c \in (0,\infty)$, $k > 1$ are parameters, and $n \in N$ is fixed, do not profit by Hopf bifurcation with respect to the parameter c (and hence not with respect to a or b) for the equilibrium point (x_0, y_0, z_0) with $x_0 = bcz_0$, $y_0 = cz_0$, where z_0 is one positive solution of the equation

$$\frac{1+z^n}{k+z^n} = abcz$$

(see 4.4). Indeed, the characteristic polynomial of the matrix of the linear approximation in the neighborhood of (x_0, y_0, z_0) is

$$\lambda^3 + (a+b+c)\lambda^2 + (ab+ac+bc)\lambda + abc - \varphi'(z_0) = 0,$$

where

$$\varphi(z) = \frac{1+z^n}{k+z^n}$$

and therefore

$$\varphi'(z_0) > 0,$$

and its identification with the polynomial

$$\lambda^3 - \alpha\lambda^2 + \beta^2\lambda - \alpha\beta^2,$$

which has the real root α and the purely imaginary roots $\pm i\beta$, gives the system

$$\alpha = -(a+b+c_0),\ \beta^2 = ab + (a+b)c_0,\ abc_0 - \varphi'(z_0) = (a+b+c_0)[ab + (a+b)c_0].$$

But the last equation of this algebraic system, of degree 2 with respect to c_0, does not admit a strictly positive solution, as required by the hypothesis on c in this problem.

7.5. PROPOSED PROBLEMS

1. Verify that the equilibrium set attached to the differential system

$$\frac{dx}{dt} = cy + x(x^2+y^2),\ \frac{dy}{dt} = -cx + y(x^2+y^2)$$

admits no bifurcation.

2. Let us consider the differential systems

$$\begin{cases} \dfrac{dx}{dt} = cx - cy - x^2 + y^2 \\ \dfrac{dy}{dt} = cy + xy, \end{cases} \quad \begin{cases} \dfrac{dx}{dt} = 3cx - 5cy - x^2 + y^2 \\ \dfrac{dy}{dt} = 2cx - xy, \end{cases} \quad \begin{cases} \dfrac{dx}{dt} = 3cx - 3cy - x^2 + y^2 \\ \dfrac{dy}{dt} = cx - xy, \end{cases}$$

$$\begin{cases} \dfrac{dx}{dt} = cx - x^2 - xy \\ \dfrac{dy}{dt} = -2cx + 2cy + xy - y^2, \end{cases} \quad \begin{cases} \dfrac{dx}{dt} = cy + xy \\ \dfrac{dy}{dt} = -cx + cy + x^2 + y^2, \end{cases}$$

where c is a real parameter. For each case, find the equilibrium set, the bifurcation set, specifying the values of c at which is produced the bifurcation of equilibrium points. Discuss the stability of equilibrium points with respect to the parameter c.

3. Verify that for any real number α the set

$$M_\alpha - \{(x,y) | y = \alpha e^{1/x}, x < 0\} \cup \{(x,y) | x \geq 0, y = 0\}$$

is the centre manifold of the differential system

$$\frac{dx}{dt} = x^2,\ \frac{dy}{dt} = -y.$$

4. Show that the analytic differential system

$$\frac{dx}{dt} = -x^2, \quad \frac{dy}{dt} = -y + x^2$$

has no analytic centre manifold.

Hint. It results the divergent series $y = \sum_{n=2}^{\infty} (n-1)!\, x^n$.

5. Let the vector field

$$X(x,y,z,c) = ((c-1)x - y + xz,\ x + (c-1)y + yz,\ cz - (x^2 + y^2 + z^2)),$$

where c is a real parameter. Show that if $c \in \left(\frac{1}{2}, 1\right)$, then X has a periodic field line in a plane. Determine the zeros of the field and study their stability.

Hint. $\alpha(t) = (R(c)\cos t,\ R(c)\sin t,\ 1 - c)$.

6. We consider the change of variables

$$x = r\cos\theta, \quad y = r\sin\theta, \quad z = z.$$

What becomes the differential system attached to the vector field X in the preceding problem?

7. Let

$$X(x,y,z,c) = (cx - y,\ x + cy,\ -z + xy),$$

where c is a real parameter. Study the stability of the equilibrium point $(0,0,0)$. For $c = 0$, described the initial conditions that produce periodic solutions.

8. Some autocatalytic chemical reactions with diffusion are described by the differential system

$$\frac{dx}{dt} = -(b+1)x + x^2 y + a, \quad \frac{dy}{dt} = bx - x^2 y,$$

where a and b are strictly positive parameters. Determine the equilibrium point and analyse its stability. Study if the variation of b generates bifurcation.

9. We consider two containers separated by a common membrane of diffusion. Let x_1, x_2, x_3 be the concentrations of three chemical substances situated in one container and y_1, y_2, y_3, respectively, the concentrations of the same substances in the other container. Suppose that the diffusion takes place and that the functions $x = (x_1, x_2, x_3)$, $y = (y_1, y_2, y_3)$ are

connected by the differential system

$$\frac{dx}{dt} = Ax + B(y-x) + \varphi(x), \quad \frac{dy}{dt} = Ay + B(x-y) + \varphi(y),$$

where

$$A = \begin{bmatrix} -0.1 & -1 & 0.8 \\ 1 & -0.1 & 0 \\ 0.8 & 0 & -0.1 \end{bmatrix}, \quad B = \begin{bmatrix} 0.01 & 0 & 0 \\ 0 & 0.01 & 0 \\ 0 & 0 & \frac{c}{2} \end{bmatrix}, \quad \varphi(x) = \begin{bmatrix} -x_1 x_2 \\ 0 \\ 0 \end{bmatrix} \quad c \in R.$$

Study the Hopf bifurcation.

Hint. The values of bifurcation for c are $c_1 = 0.2314$ and $c_2 = 1.9953$. Three of the proper values, -0.1 and $-0.1 \pm 0.6i$ are also proper values of $2A$. The other three are proper values of $A - 2B$.

10. The dynamical behaviour of two reactors with mobile reservoirs, with reaction of thc first order and recycling, is described by the Kubicek differential system [35]:

$$\frac{dx_1}{dt} = 0.2\,x_3 - x_1 + \alpha\,(1 - x_1)\exp_\gamma x_2$$

$$\frac{dx_2}{dt} = 0.2\,x_4 - x_2 + 12\,\alpha\,(1 - x_1)\exp_\gamma x_2 - 2\,x_2$$

$$\frac{dx_3}{dt} = 5\,\alpha\,[x_1 - x_3 + 0.2\,(1 - x_3)\exp_\gamma x_4]$$

$$\frac{dx_4}{dt} = 5\,\alpha\,[x_2 - x_4 + 2.4\,(1 - x_3)\exp_\gamma x_4 - 2\,x_4],$$

where $\exp_\gamma x = \exp\left(\dfrac{x}{1 + \dfrac{x}{\gamma}}\right)$, $\gamma = 1000$, and α is a real parameter. Show that, at the points $\alpha_1 = 0.09556;\ \alpha_2 = 0.1574;\ \alpha_3 = 0.2730$, the Hopf bifurcation is produced.

8. SUBMANIFOLDS ORTHOGONAL TO FIELD LINES

The theory exposed in this chapter has as basis the concept of transversality: the Euclidean space R^n *is the direct sum of orthogonal subspaces* R *and* R^{n-1}.

The submanifolds orthogonal to field lines are solutions of Pfaff equations attached to vector fields. Like sections orthogonal to orbits, they give the best information about evolution of the physical system described locally by the vector field. Their definition and the standard examples are given in 8.1.

The complete integrability of a Pfaff equation, on an open and connected set D, *is equivalent to the fact that through every point of the set* D *passes a hypersurface orthogonal to field lines (see 8.2). This is a good theoretical result, but with small chances of applicability. A compensating factor is the Frobenius theorem, which one reduces the problem of complete integrability to performing some simple computations (see 8.3).*

The complete integrability of a Pfaff equation is established by the notions of local potential or local biscalar vector fields. The most suitable examples for such cases are the Newtonian vector fields, the electrostatic vector fields, the torse forming vector fields and the vector fields which describe thermodynamical systems. In the case of space with three dimensions, the condition of (local) biscalarity is reduced to orthogonality between the given vector field and its rotor (see 8.4).

A vector field defines an (n-1)-dimensional transversal distribution, which may or may not be integrable. If this distribution is integrable, then its integral hypersurfaces determine a stratification of the open and connected set on which one works; if this distribution is not integrable, then the set of all its integral manifolds is a nonholonomic space (see 8.5). The general theory of nonholonomic spaces is applicable to Analytical Mechanics, Thermodynamics, etc [136].

The orbits of a vector field can be expressed (locally) in three fashions: as intersections of families of hypersurfaces, as intersections between families of hypersurfaces and nonholonomic spaces or as intersection of nonholonomic spaces (see 8.6).

In 8.7 we analyse facts that lead to the definition of nonholonomic hyperquadrics, proving an original theorem (with respect to the references). In 8.8 we mention open problems regarding dependence on parameters of submanifolds orthogonal to field lines.

Section 8.9 develops the theory of extrema constrained by a Pfaff system, proves the existence of C^1 *curves containing a given sequence of points and applies the result to free extrema, analyses the relations between constrained extrema and uniformly constrained extrema, and gives a result regarding extrema on star-shaped sets with respect to integral curves of a Pfaff system.*

Section 8.10 recalls that integral submanifolds of the Gibbs-Pfaff equation are curves or surfaces, defines 10 simple thermodynamic systems, refers to the minima of the energy of a thermodynamic system, and describes simple interactions between thermodynamic systems.

The problems proposed in 8.11 refer to complete integrable Pfaff equations, biscalar vector fields, distributions, nonholonomic quadrics, intersections of surfaces and nonholonomic surfaces, extrema with nonholonomic constraints, etc.

The field lines and their orthogonal submanifolds are correlate intuitively. However, there exists an ontological difference between the notion of field lines and those of submanifolds orthogonal to field lines. For example, in the mathematical representation of mechanical phenomena, the field line shows the trajectory described by a particle in motion in the field domain, as soon as one can find a particle which is sensitive to the given field (the field line reflects the corpuscular intuitions), while a submanifold orthogonal to field lines shows the equal possibility of moving of an infinity of particles (i.e., a submanifold orthogonal to field lines reflects the undulatory intuitions).

8.1. SUBMANIFOLDS ORTHOGONAL TO FIELD LINES

Let $X = (X_1, \dots, X_n)$ be a C^1 vector field on an open connected set $D \subset R^n$, $n \geq 2$, without zeros on D. To the vector field X one attaches a family of hyperplanes Ω_x, $x \in D$, every hyperplane Ω_x being determined by a point x and the normal vector $X(x)$. Obviously, the hyperplane Ω_x is orthogonal to the field line passing through the point x.

The submanifolds M of D, with the property that the restriction of X to M is a vector field normal to M, are called *submanifolds orthogonal to the field lines of* X.

Let M be a submanifold of D and T_xM be the tangent space to M at $x \in M$. The submanifold M is orthogonal to the field lines of X if and only if $T_xM \subset \Omega_x \subset T_xD = T_xR^n$, $\forall x \in D$ (the submanifold M is tangent at every point $x \in M$ to the hyperplane Ω_x). The dimension of a submanifold orthogonal to the field lines of X can be at most $n - 1$.

Since $(dx_1, \dots, dx_n)$ is a vector from the hyperplane Ω_x, it follows that the submanifold orthogonal to the field lines of X are characterized by the equation

$$X_1(x)dx_1 + \cdots + X_n(x)dx_n = 0, \ n \geq 2 \tag{1}$$

which is called a *Pfaff equation* on D.

The submanifolds of D orthogonal to field lines of X are called *integral manifolds* (or *solutions*) of the Pfaff equation (1).

Locally, any integral manifold M of dimension $p \in \{1, \dots, n-1\}$ of the Pfaff equation (1) is characterized

(I) either by an immersion $f = (f_1, \dots, f_n) : V \subset R^p \to M$,

$$u = (u_1, \dots, u_p) \to f(u) = (f_1(u), \dots, f_n(u))$$

which satisfies the orthogonality conditions

$$\sum_{i=1}^{n} X_i(f(u)) \frac{\partial f_i}{\partial u_j} = 0, \ j = 1, \dots, p;$$

(II) or by a system of implicit Cartesian equations $F_1(x) = 0, \ldots, F_{n-p}(x) = 0$ attached to the submersion $F = (F_1, \ldots, F_{n-p}) : U \subset D \to R^{n-p}$, with the property that the Pfaff equation (1) is a consequence of the equations

$$F_1(x) = 0, \ldots, F_{n-p}(x) = 0, \; dF_1(x) = 0, \ldots, dF_{n-p}(x) = 0.$$

The notion of 1-dimensional integral manifold can be extended in the following fashion: any immersion $\alpha : I \to D$, $\alpha(t) = (x_1(t), \ldots, x_n(t))$ is called an *integral curve* of the Pfaff equation (1) if

$$X_1(\alpha(t)) \frac{dx_1}{dt} + \cdots + X_n(\alpha(t)) \frac{dx_n}{dt} = 0. \qquad (1')$$

The existence of integral curves is obvious, being conditioned by a single differential equation $(1')$ with n unknown functions. As a result, one observes that by every point x of D passes an infinity of integral curves of the Pfaff equation (1) (Fig.96). The existence of integral manifolds of dimension $p \in \{2, \ldots, n-2\}$ depends on the rank of the matrix

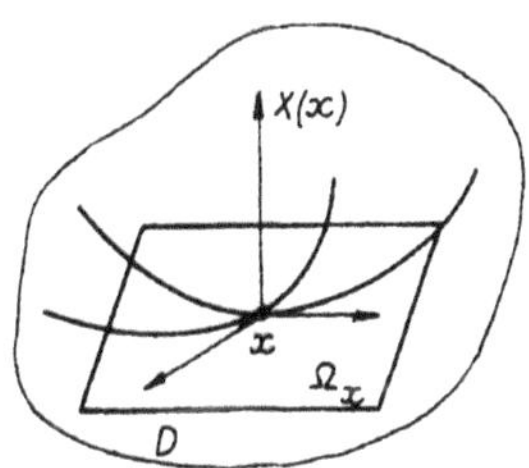

Fig. 96

$$\operatorname{rot} X = \left[\frac{\partial X_i}{\partial x_j} - \frac{\partial X_j}{\partial x_i} \right]$$

and the dimension n. For example:

Theorem. *If* $n = 2m+1$ *and* $\operatorname{rank} \operatorname{rot} X = 2m$, *then the highest dimension of the integral manifolds of the Pfaff equation (1) is equal to* m.

Proof. By a theorem of Darboux, changing the system of coordinates, the Pfaff equation (1) can be reduced to the canonical form

$$dz - \sum_{\alpha=1}^{m} y_\alpha \, dx_\alpha = 0. \qquad (1'')$$

In these adapted coordinates, the m-plane M described by the equations $x_\alpha = \overset{0}{x}_\alpha$, $z = z_0$, $\alpha = 1, \ldots, m$ is an m-dimensional integral manifold, and the general maximal integral manifold of dimension m is given by

$$z = f(x_1, \ldots, x_n), \quad y_1 = \frac{\partial f}{\partial x_1}, \ldots, \quad y_m = \frac{\partial f}{\partial x_m},$$

where f is an arbitrary C^2 function.

Let us show that there exists no integral manifold of the Pfaff equation (1") whose dimension is higher than m. For that we shall use the almost contact metric structure ϕ, ξ, η, g associated to the contact form

$$\eta = dz - \sum y_\alpha \, dx_\alpha ,$$

i.e., the tensor fields

$$\phi = \begin{bmatrix} 0 & \delta_{\alpha\beta} & 0 \\ -\delta_{\alpha\beta} & 0 & 0 \\ 0 & y_\beta & 0 \end{bmatrix}, \ \xi = \begin{bmatrix} 0 \\ 0 \\ 1 \end{bmatrix}, \ \eta = [-y_\alpha, 0, 1]$$

$$g = \begin{bmatrix} \delta_{\alpha\beta} + y_\alpha y_\beta & 0 & -y_\alpha \\ 0 & \delta_{\alpha\beta} & 0 \\ -y_\beta & 0 & 1 \end{bmatrix}, \ \mathrm{rot}\,\eta = -2g\phi$$

which verify

$$\phi^2 = -I + \xi\eta, \ \eta\xi = 1, \ \phi\xi = 0, \ \eta\phi = 0,$$

$${}^t\eta = g\xi, \ {}^t\phi g \phi = g - {}^t\eta\eta .$$

Suppose Σ is an integral manifold of dimension p given as an immersion of class C^2,

$$\begin{cases} x_\alpha = x_\alpha(u) \\ y_\alpha = y_\alpha(u) \ , u = (u_1, \dots, u_p) \\ z = z(u), \end{cases}$$

which satisfies

$$\frac{\partial z}{\partial u_l} - \sum y_\alpha(u) \frac{\partial x_\alpha}{\partial u_l} = 0, \ l = 1, \dots, p.$$

(an orthogonality condition between ξ and $v_l^h = \left(\frac{\partial x_\alpha}{\partial u_l}, \frac{\partial y_\alpha}{\partial u_l}, \frac{\partial z}{\partial u_l} \right)$, with respect to the Riemannian metric g). Differentiating with respect to u_k and subtracting the equations obtained by interchanging l and k, we obtain

$$g_{ih}(\phi_j^h v_l^j) v_k^i = 0,$$

and consequently the vectors v_k^h and $\phi_j^h v_l^j$ are orthogonal. On the other hand the vector ξ

is orthogonal to $\phi_j^h v_l^j$. Hence $2p+1$ vectors ξ, v_k^h, $\phi_j^h v_l^j$ are linearly independent. Therefore $p \le m$.

Remark. The integral manifold of dimension $p \le n-2$ passing through the point x_0, and tangent to the linearly independent vectors $(a_l^\alpha, b_l^\alpha, c_l)$, $l = 1, \dots, p$, is not unique, since for $p \le n-2$ the condition of being an integral manifold is too weak.

The problem of existence and uniqueness of the integral hypersurfaces (n-1)-dimensional submanifolds of $D \subset R^n$) by every point x of D is the most difficult, but also the most important. In the next sections we shall show that this problem is reduced to the existence of a local scalar field whose constant level sets are integral hypersurfaces of the Pfaff equation.

Paraphrasing the known results in the theory of irrotational vector fields (see 2.1), we reach the following

Theorem. *Let* $X = (X_1, \dots, X_n)$ *be an irrotational vector field on* D, *without zeros, and* $x_0 = (x_{10}, \dots, x_{n0})$ *a point in* D.

1) If D *is an n-dimensional interval, then the constant level hypersurfaces of the function*

$$f: D \to R,\ f(x) = \sum_{i=1}^{n} \int_{x_{i0}}^{x_i} X_i(x_{10}, x_{20}, \dots, x_{i-10}, x_i, \dots, x_n)\, dx_i$$

are orthogonal to the field lines of X.

2) If D *is a convex set, then the constant level hypersurfaces of the function*

$$f: D \to R,\ f(x) = \int_0^1 (X(x_0 + t(x - x_0)), x - x_0)\, dt$$

are orthogonal to the field lines of X.

Hint. It turns out that $X = \operatorname{grad} f$.

Remark. The circulation of the vector field X along a curve orthogonal to field lines of X is zero.

8.2. COMPLETELY INTEGRABLE PFAFF EQUATIONS

Let $X = (X_1, \dots, X_n)$ be a C^1 vector field on an open connected set $D \subset R^n$, $n \ge 2$, without zeros on D, and

$$X_1(x)dx_1 + \dots + X_n(x)dx_n = 0 \tag{2}$$

be the Pfaff equation associated to this field. The Pfaff equation (2) is called *exact* if the vector field X is potential, i.e., if there exists $f: D \to R$ of class C^2 such that

$$\frac{\partial f}{\partial x_i}(x) = X_i(x), \; i = 1, \ldots, n,$$

or, equivalently,

$$df(x) = \sum_{i=1}^{n} X_i(x) dx_i .$$

Consequently (see 2.1), on an open, connected and simply connected set $D \subset R^n$, the equation (2) is exact if and only if the vector field X is irrotational.

Suppose that the Pfaff equation (2) is not exact. Sometimes there exists a nonconstant function $\mu : D \to R \setminus \{0\}$ of class C^1 such that

$$\mu(x) X_1(x) dx_1 + \cdots + \mu(x) X_n(x) dx_n = 0$$

is an exact equation, i.e., there exists $F: D \to R$ of class C^2 such that

$$\frac{\partial F}{\partial x_i}(x) = \mu(x) X_i(x), \; i = 1, \ldots, n,$$

or, equivalently,

$$dF(x) = \mu(x) \sum_{i=1}^{n} X_i(x) dx_i .$$

The function μ is called an *integrant factor* and satisfies the system of equations with partial derivatives (a consequence of Schwartz's theorem for F)

$$\frac{\partial (\mu X_i)}{\partial x_j}(x) = \frac{\partial (\mu X_j)}{\partial x_i}(x), \; i \neq j.$$

The locally exact Pfaff equations and the Pfaff equations that admit locally integrant factors are called *completely integrable Pfaff equations*.

Theorem. *The Pfaff equation (2) is completely integrable if and only if by every point $x_0 \in D$ there passes an integral hypersurface of the equation.*

Proof. Suppose that the Pfaff equation (2) is locally exact, i.e., for every $x_0 \in D$ there exists an open set $U \subset D$ that contains x_0, and a C^2 scalar field $f: U \to R$ such that $df(x) = \sum_{i=1}^{n} X_i(x) dx_i = 0$ on U. Then through $x_0 \in D$ passes the integral hypersurface $f(x) = f(x_0)$.

Suppose that the Pfaff equation (2) admits the local integrant factor μ, i.e., for every $x_0 \in D$ there exists an open set $U \subset D$ that contains x_0, and $\mu : U \to R \setminus \{0\}$ of class C^1, and $F : U \to R$ of class C^2 such that

$$dF(x) = \sum_{i=1}^{n} \mu(x) X_i(x) dx_i = 0.$$

Then through $x_0 \in D$ passes the integral hypersurface $F(x) = F(x_0)$.

Assume that through every point of D passes an integral hypersurface of the Pfaff equation (2), the family of hypersurfaces being locally described by $G(x) = c$. It follows that

$$dG(x) = \sum_{i=1}^{n} \frac{\partial G}{\partial x_i}(x) dx_i = 0.$$

Since the Pfaff equation (2) must be a consequence of these relations, we have either $\frac{\partial G}{\partial x_i}(x) = X_i(x)$ or $\frac{\partial G}{\partial x_i}(x) = \mu(x) X_i(x)$, i.e., the Pfaff equation (2) is either locally exact or admits a local integrant factor.

The set of all integral hypersurfaces of a completely integrable Pfaff equation is called the *general solution* of the equation.

Finally, we remark that the Pfaff equation (2) is completely integrable if and only if there exist the local scalar fields λ and f such that $X = \lambda \operatorname{grad} f$ (Fig.97). Here the constant level hypersurfaces of f (a family with one parameter of hypersurfaces) are orthogonal to the field lines of X. To fix one of these hypersurfaces it is sufficient to give a point through which it passes.

Complements. Let σ be a bounded region from a hypersurface in $D \subset R^n$ described by the completely integrable Pfaff equation $\sum_{i=1}^{n} X_i(x) dx_i = 0$ and by a point which is contained in the hypersurface. The hypersurface σ is orientable since the normal vector field X does not vanish on σ.

Let $Y = (Y_1, \ldots, Y_n)$ be a C^1 vector field on D and $N = \frac{X}{\|X\|}$ the unit normal vector field on σ.

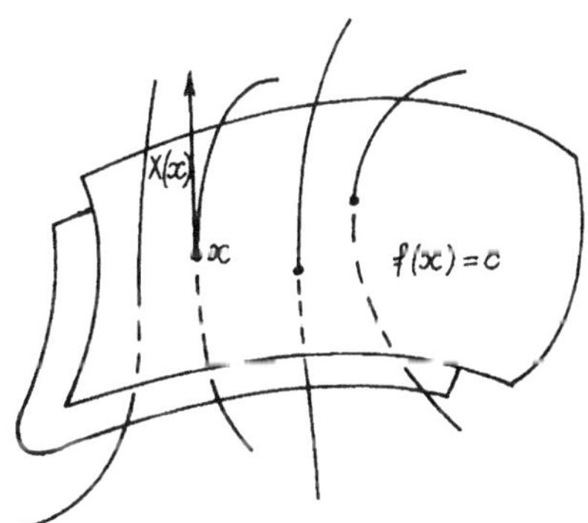

Fig. 97

The number

$$\int_\sigma (Y, N)\, d\sigma$$

is called the *flux of* Y *at traversing* σ.

We remark that the flux of $X = (X_1, \dots, X_n)$ at traversing σ (a hypersurface orthogonal to field lines of X) is strictly positive, and the extrema of the real function

$$Y \to \int_\sigma (Y, N)\, d\sigma, \ \|Y\| = 1$$

are attained on the versors fields

$$-\frac{X}{\|X\|}, \ \frac{X}{\|X\|}.$$

Application. Find the general solutions of the following Pfaff equations:

1) $x_1(x_1^2 + x_2^2 - a^2)\, dx_1 + x_2(x_1^2 + x_2^2 + a^2)\, dx_2 = 0$, $(x_1, x_2) \in R^2$,

2) $(1 + \sin x_1)\, dx_1 + (2 + \sin x_2)\, dx_2 + \cdots + (n + \sin x_n)\, dx_n = 0$,

$$(x_1, \dots, x_n) \in R^n,$$

3) $x_1(x_2 - 1)(x_3 - 1)\, dx_1 + x_2(x_3 - 1)(x_1 - 1)\, dx_2 + x_3(x_1 - 1)(x_2 - 1)\, dx_3 = 0$,

$$x_i > 1.$$

Answer. 1) Denote

$$X_1(x_1, x_2) = x_1(x_1^2 + x_2^2 - a^2), \ X_2(x_1, x_2) = x_2(x_1^2 + x_2^2 + a^2).$$

Since

$$\frac{\partial X_1}{\partial x_2}(x) = \frac{\partial X_2}{\partial x_1}(x) = 2x_1 x_2, \ \forall\, x = (x_1, x_2) \in R^2,$$

the Pfaff equation is exact. We find

$$f(x) = \int_0^{x_1} t(t^2 + x_2^2 - a^2)\, dt + \int_0^{x_2} t(0^2 + t^2 + a^2)\, dt = \frac{x_1^4}{4} + \frac{x_2^4}{4} + \frac{x_1^2 x_2^2}{2} + \frac{a^2 x_2^2}{2} - \frac{a x_1^2}{2}.$$

The general solution of the Pfaff equation is defined by $f(x) = c$.

2) Let $X_i(x) = i + \sin x_i$, $i = 1, \dots, n$, $x = (x_1, \dots, x_n) \in R^n$. The vector field $X = (X_1, \dots, X_n)$ is irrotational, and R^n is a convex set. We compute

$$f(x) = \int_0^1 (X(tx), x)\, dt = \int_0^1 \sum_{i=1}^n (i + \sin t x_i) x_i\, dt = \sum_{i=1}^n (i x_i - \cos x_i).$$

The general solution is defined by $f(x) = c$, where c is an arbitrary constant.

3) The set $D = \{(x_1, x_2, x_3) \in R^3 \mid x_1 > 1, x_2 > 1, x_3 > 1\}$ is open, connected and simply connected. Denoting

$$X_1(x) = x_1(x_2 - 1)(x_3 - 1), \; X_2(x) = x_2(x_3 - 1)(x_1 - 1),$$
$$X_3(x) = x_3(x_1 - 1)(x_2 - 1), \; x = (x_1, x_2, x_3),$$

one establishes that

$$\mu(x) = (x_1 - 1)^{-1}(x_2 - 1)^{-1}(x_3 - 1)^{-1}$$

is a solution of the system of partial differential equations

$$\frac{\partial(\mu X_i)}{\partial x_j} = \frac{\partial(\mu X_j)}{\partial x_i}, \quad i, j = 1, 2, 3.$$

Therefore μ is an integrant factor. By multiplication with μ, the Pfaff equation can be written in the equivalent form

$$\left(1 + \frac{1}{x_1 - 1}\right) dx_1 + \left(1 + \frac{1}{x_2 - 1}\right) dx_2 + \left(1 + \frac{1}{x_3 - 1}\right) dx_3 = 0$$

or

$$d[x_1 + x_2 + x_3 + \ln(x_1 - 1)(x_2 - 1)(x_3 - 1)] = 0.$$

There follows the general solution

$$x_1 + x_2 + x_3 + \ln(x_1 - 1)(x_2 - 1)(x_3 - 1) = c.$$

8.3. FROBENIUS THEOREM

Let $D \subset R^n$, $n \geq 2$, be an open connected set, and $X = (X_1, \dots, X_n)$ be a C^1 vector field on D, which vanishes nowhere. The search for complete integrability of the Pfaff equation

$$X_1(x)dx_1 + \cdots + X_n(x)dx_n = 0, \tag{2'}$$

using the definitions in the preceding paragraph, is difficult. That is why we present an alternative due to Frobenius that, in concrete situations, is reduced to doing simple computations.

Theorem. *1) For $n = 2$, the Pfaff equation (2′) is completely integrable.*

2) For $n \geq 3$, the Pfaff equation (2′) is completely integrable if and only if

$$X_i\left(\frac{\partial X_k}{\partial x_j} - \frac{\partial X_j}{\partial x_k}\right) + X_j\left(\frac{\partial X_i}{\partial x_k} - \frac{\partial X_k}{\partial x_i}\right) + X_k\left(\frac{\partial X_j}{\partial x_i} - \frac{\partial X_i}{\partial x_j}\right) = 0, \; i, j, k = 1, \dots, n.$$

Proof. 1) For $n = 2$, the Pfaff equation (2′) is reduced to an ordinary differential equation whose general solution (family of curves) is assured by the (local) existence and uniqueness theorem.

2) Let $n \geq 3$. If the Pfaff equation $(2')$ is locally exact, then

$$\operatorname{rot} \boldsymbol{X} = \left[\frac{\partial X_i}{\partial x_j} - \frac{\partial X_j}{\partial x_i}\right] = 0$$

and the conditions in the theorem are satisfied. If the Pfaff equation is not exact, but admits locally an integrant factor μ, i.e., there exist the C^1 local scalar field μ, and the C^2 local scalar field F such that

$$\frac{\partial F}{\partial x_i}(x) = \mu(x) X_i(x),$$

then the functions

$$X_i = \frac{1}{\mu}\frac{\partial F}{\partial x_i}, \; i = 1, \ldots, n$$

satisfy the conditions in the theorem.

Suppose that the relations in the theorem hold true. If $\operatorname{rot}\boldsymbol{X} = 0$, then the Pfaff equation $(2')$ is called *exact*. If there exists $x_0 \in D$ such that $\operatorname{rot}\boldsymbol{X}(x_0) \neq 0$, then we accept $X_i(x_0) \neq 0$, i being fixed, and by continuity there exists an open set $U \subset D$ that contains x_0, and on which these relations are maintained. Replacing $x_1, \ldots, x_{i-1}, x_{i+1}, \ldots, x_n$ with $u_1, \ldots, u_{i-1}, u_{i+1}, \ldots, u_n$ respectively and x_i with z, the conditions in the theorem imply

$$\frac{\partial f_\beta}{\partial u_\alpha} + \frac{\partial f_\beta}{\partial z} f_\alpha = \frac{\partial f_\alpha}{\partial u_\beta} + \frac{\partial f_\alpha}{\partial z} f_\beta, \tag{*}$$

where $f_\alpha = -\dfrac{X_\alpha}{X_i}$, $\alpha, \beta \in J = \{1, \ldots, i-1, i+1, \ldots, n\}$, and the Pfaff equation is written in the form

$$dz = \sum_{\alpha \in J} f_\alpha(u_1, \ldots, u_{i-1}, z, u_{i+1}, \ldots, u_n) du_\alpha . \tag{**}$$

The relations (*) are equivalent to

$$\frac{\partial^2 z}{\partial u_\alpha \partial u_\beta} = \frac{\partial^2 z}{\partial u_\beta \partial u_\alpha},$$

which are nothing else but the conditions of complete integrability of the system of equations with partial derivatives

$$\frac{\partial z}{\partial u_\alpha} = f_\alpha(u_1, \dots, u_{i-1}, z, u_{i+1}, \dots, u_n), \ \alpha \in J,$$

equivalent to the equation with total differentials (**) and hence with the Pfaff equation $(2')$ on the set U. Therefore, by the point x_0 of U passes the integral hypersurface $x_i = x_i(x_1, \dots, x_{i-1}, x_{i+1}, \dots, x_n)$, i being fixed.

Commentary. According to the preceding theorem, to the Pfaff equation $(2')$ one can attach n^3 functions $f_{ijk} : D \to R$,

$$f_{ijk} = X_i\left(\frac{\partial X_k}{\partial x_j} - \frac{\partial X_j}{\partial x_k}\right) + X_j\left(\frac{\partial X_i}{\partial x_k} - \frac{\partial X_k}{\partial x_i}\right) + X_k\left(\frac{\partial X_j}{\partial x_i} - \frac{\partial X_i}{\partial x_j}\right), \ i, j, k = 1, \dots, n.$$

Since $f_{ijk} = f_{jki} = f_{kij}$, $f_{ijk} = -f_{ikj}$, $f_{ijk} = -f_{kji}$, $f_{ijk} = -f_{jik}$, only C_n^3 of the functions f_{ijk} can be linearly independent (namely those for which $i < j < k$). For example: if $n = 3$, there remains only one function f_{123}; if $n = 4$, there remain four functions $f_{123}, f_{124}, f_{134}, f_{234}$; if $n = 5$, there are ten functions, etc.

If one function f_{ijk}, $i < j < k$, is not the function zero, then the Pfaff equation is not completely integrable. This is equivalent to the fact that there exists a point $x_0 \in D$ such that each integral manifold passing through x_0 (and one integral manifold passes anyhow!) is of dimension at most $n - 2$.

Even if the Pfaff equation $(2')$ is not completely integrable, it can admit as solutions some hypersurfaces. In this case both the Pfaff equation $(2')$ and the algebraic equations $f_{ijk}(x) = 0$, $i < j < k$ must be conditioned identities with respect to the Cartesian or parametric equations of these hypersurfaces. For example, the Pfaff equation $xz\,dx + z(2x - y)\,dy - x^2 dz = 0$ is not completely integrable since $f_{123}(x, y, z) = 2xz(x - y)$, but admits the solution $z = 0$ (xOy plane).

Remarks. 1) For $n = 3$, the condition of complete integrability is $(\boldsymbol{X}, \mathrm{rot}\boldsymbol{X}) = 0$.

2) On the Riemannian manifold (R^n, δ_{ij}) the vector fields can be identified with 1-forms without altering the mathematical contents and the possibilities of representation of concrete problems. Thus, instead of the vector field $\boldsymbol{X} = (X_1, \dots, X_n)$, it is often preferable to use the attached differential 1-form $\omega(x) = X_1(x)dx_1 + \cdots + X_n(x)dx_n$, and the Pfaff equation is written simply $\omega = 0$. Denoting by $d\omega$ the exterior differential of the 1-form ω, one proves that the equation $\omega = 0$ is completely integrable if and only if $\omega \wedge d\omega = 0$, in fact equivalent to the Frobenius conditions of integrability. The highest dimension of the integral manifolds of the Pfaff equation $\omega = 0$ is imposed by the dimension n and by $\mathrm{rank}(d\omega)$.

8.4. BISCALAR VECTOR FIELDS

Let $X = (X_1, \dots, X_n)$ be a C^1 vector field on an open connected set D of R^n. Suppose there exist two scalar fields, λ of class C^1 and f of class C^2 on D such that $X = \lambda\,\mathrm{grad} f$. If λ and f are functionally independent, then the vector field X is called *biscalar*. If λ and f are functionally dependent, then one proves that X is a potential vector field.

The field lines of a biscalar vector field are reparametrizations of gradient lines (hence they cannot be closed curves).

The results in preceding sections show that a C^1 vector field, on an open and connected set, which vanishes nowhere, is locally potential or biscalar if and only if it admits a family of hypersurfaces orthogonal to its field lines. Consequently, the C^1 vector fields on R^2, which vanish nowhere, are either locally potential or locally biscalar, and the following theorem of characterization of local biscalar vector fields hold true for the cases $n \geq 3$.

Theorem. *Let $D \subset R^n$, $n \geq 3$, be an open connected set and $X = (X_1, \dots, X_n)$ be a C^1 rotational vector field on D, without zeros on D. The vector field X is locally biscalar if and only if*

$$X_i\left(\frac{\partial X_k}{\partial x_j} - \frac{\partial X_j}{\partial x_k}\right) + X_j\left(\frac{\partial X_i}{\partial x_k} - \frac{\partial X_k}{\partial x_i}\right) + X_k\left(\frac{\partial X_j}{\partial x_i} - \frac{\partial X_i}{\partial x_j}\right) = 0, \quad i, j, k = 1, \dots, n.$$

Applications. 1) Let D be an open and connected set of R^n. A vector field $X = (X_1, \dots, X_n)$ on D is called *torse forming* if there exists a scalar field a on D and a vector field $Y = (Y_1, \dots, Y_n)$ on D (all of suitable class) such that

$$\frac{\partial X_i}{\partial x_j} = a\delta_{ij} + X_i Y_j, \quad i, j = 1, \dots, n,$$

where δ_{ij} is the Kronecker symbol. Any torse forming vector field X is locally either a potential or a biscalar vector field, since it satisfies the condition of complete integrability of the Frobenius theorem.

2) Let $x_1, \dots, x_n$ be the *state parameters* of a thermodynamical system. We assimilate $x = (x_1, \dots, x_n)$ with a point in R^n called *state,* and suppose that the set of all states is an open cone D with vertex at the origin, which does not contain the origin in its interior (reason imposed by the theory of homogeneous functions, see 6.2). One postulates that the local evolution of the thermodynamical system is described by a vector field $X = (1, X_2, \dots, X_n)$, where $X_2, \dots, X_n$ are C^1 homogeneous functions having degree of homogeneity equal to zero on D. A curve that is orthogonal to field lines is called an

adiabatic path. By an *evolution* we understand either a field line of X or an adiabatic path of X. The second principle of thermodynamics is equivalent to the fact that X is a certain biscalar field, namely $X = T\,\mathrm{grad}\,S$, where T is the thermodynamic temperature, and S is the entropy of the system. Obviously, the entropy is constant along adiabatic paths.

The condition that X is locally a biscalar vector field has a simple expression in the case $n = 3$, namely $(X, \mathrm{rot}X) = 0$. This relation shows that the surfaces orthogonal to field lines of X are found between the field surfaces of $\mathrm{rot}\,X$ (eddy surfaces). Starting from this remark and leaving aside the irrotational vector fields, J.Bertrand gave the following algorithm for obtaining the local functionally independent scalar fields λ and f for which $X = \lambda\,\mathrm{grad}f$.

Bertrand's algorithm. Suppose $(X, \mathrm{rot}\,X) = 0$. Let $\varphi_1(x,y,z) = c_1$, $\varphi_2(x,y,z) = c_2$ be the field lines of $\mathrm{rot}X$ (eddy lines) expressed by the first integrals φ_1 and φ_2. Since

$$(\mathrm{grad}\,\varphi_1, \mathrm{rot}X) = 0,\ (\mathrm{grad}\varphi_2, \mathrm{rot}X) = 0,$$

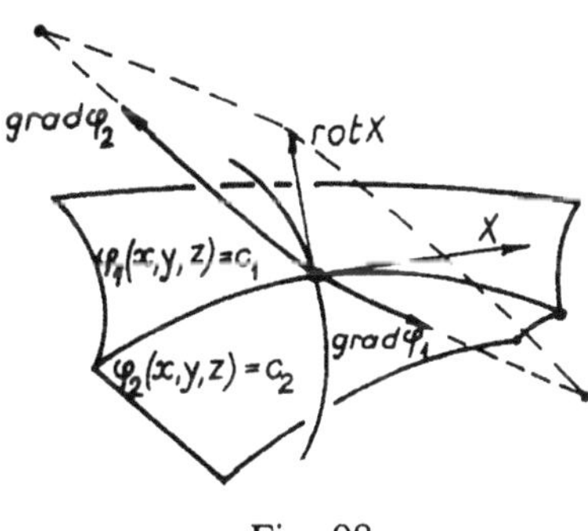

Fig. 98

There follows the coplanarity of the vector fields $X, grad\,\varphi_1$, $grad\,\varphi_2$, i.e., (Fig. 98)

$$X = \alpha\,\mathrm{grad}f_1 + \beta\,\mathrm{grad}\,f_2,\ \alpha^2 + \beta^2 \neq 0.$$

This new expression of X permits writing of the Pfaff equation in the form

$$\alpha\,d\varphi_1 + \beta\,d\varphi_2 = 0.$$

Let us prove that $\frac{\alpha}{\beta}$, for $\beta \neq 0$, depends only on the first integrals φ_1 and φ_2. Indeed, the relations

$$X = \alpha\,\mathrm{grad}f_1 + \beta\,\mathrm{grad}\,f_2,\ (X, \mathrm{rot}X) = 0$$

imply

$$\left(\mathrm{grad}\,\frac{\alpha}{\beta}, \mathrm{grad}\,\varphi_1 \times \mathrm{grad}\,\varphi_2\right) = 0,$$

and the mixed product is the Jacobian of the functions $\frac{\alpha}{\beta}$, φ_1, φ_2. It follows that

$$\frac{\alpha}{\beta} = E(\varphi_1, \varphi_2), \quad \frac{d\varphi_2}{d\varphi_1} + E(\varphi_1, \varphi_2) = 0.$$

The general solution $f(\varphi_1, \varphi_2) = c$ of this differential equation represents the family of surfaces orthogonal to the field lines of X. When this is the case, from the identity $X = \lambda \operatorname{grad} f$ one finds λ.

Applications. 1) $X = (x,y,z) = (yz, x(z-x), -xy)$ is locally a biscalar field. Indeed, $\operatorname{rot} X = (-2x, 2y, -2x)$ and therefore $(X, \operatorname{rot} X) = 0$.

Zeros of X are the points of the straight lines Oy, Oz and $D : y = 0,\ x = z$. Since the preceding theory eliminates these points, one considers that the domain of definition of X is $R^3 \setminus (Oy \cup Oz \cup D)$.

The family of eddy lines of X is the general solution of the symmetric differential system

$$\frac{dx}{-x} = \frac{dy}{y} = \frac{dz}{-x},$$

i.e., $xy = c_1$, $x - z = c_2$. It follows that

$$X(x,y,z) = \alpha \operatorname{grad}(xy) + \beta \operatorname{grad}(x-z) = \alpha\,(y,x,O) + \beta\,(1,0,-1)$$

and by identification we find $\alpha = z - x$, $\beta = xy$, i.e.,

$$X(x,y,z) = (z-x) \operatorname{grad}(xy) + xy \operatorname{grad}(x-z).$$

The equation $yzdx + x(z-x)dy - xydz = 0$ is written $(z-x)d(xy) + xyd(x-z) = 0$ and hence $xy = c(x-z)$ represents the family of surfaces orthogonal to the field lines of X.

From the identity $X = \lambda \operatorname{grad} \frac{xy}{x-z}$ we find $\lambda = -(x-z)^2$.

2) Let $X = (X_1, X_2, X_3)$ be the Killing vector field of components

$$X_1(x) = 2x_2 - 3x_3, \quad X_2(x) = x_3 - 2x_1, \quad X_3(x) = 3x_1 - x_2$$

which verify the biscalarity relation $(X, \operatorname{rot} X) = 0$. This means that X is locally biscalar or that the Pfaff equation $(2x_2 - 3x_3)dx_1 + (x_3 - 2x_1)dx_2 + (3x_1 - x_2)dx_3 = 0$ is completely integrable.

Zeros of X are characterized by

$$2x_2 - 3x_3 = 0, \quad x_3 - 2x_1 = 0, \quad 3x_1 - x_2 = 0,$$

i.e., they are the points of the straight lines of equations $3x_1 - x_2 = 0,\ 2x_1 - x_3 = 0$. These zeros are eliminated from the domain of definition by the preceding theory.

We determine the first integrals of eddy lines characterized by the differential system

$$\frac{dx_1}{-2} = \frac{dx_2}{-6} = \frac{dx_3}{-4}.$$

It follows that

$$\varphi_1(x) = 3x_1 - x_2,\quad \varphi_2(x) = 2x_1 - x_3,$$

which are functionally independent.

We write $X = \alpha\,\mathrm{grad}\,\varphi_1 + \beta\,\mathrm{grad}\,\varphi_2$ and by identification we obtain

$$\alpha(x) = 2x_2 - x_3,\quad \beta(x) = x_2 - 3x_1.$$

With these, the Pfaff equation is written as

$$(2x_2 - x_3)\,d(3x_1 - x_2) + (x_2 - 3x_1)\,d(2x_2 - x_3) = 0,\quad d\left(\frac{3x_1 - x_2}{2x_2 - x_3}\right) = 0.$$

The general solution of this Pfaff equation is defined by

$$\frac{3x_1 - x_2}{2x_2 - x_3} = c,$$

i.e., it is a part of a pencil of planes, less the axis of the pencil that contains zeros of X. From the identity

$$X = \lambda\,\mathrm{grad}\frac{3x_1 - x_2}{2x_2 - x_3}$$

follows

$$\lambda = \frac{1}{(2x_2 - x_3)^2}.$$

The symmetric differential system

$$\frac{dx_1}{2x_2 - 3x_3} = \frac{dx_2}{x_3 - 2x_1} = \frac{dx_3}{3x_1 - x_2}$$

shows that the orbits of X have the implicit Cartesian equations

$$x_1 + 3x_2 + 2x_3 = c_1,\quad x_1^2 + x_2^2 + x_3^2 = c_2$$

and therefore they are circles. The axis of the preceding pencil of direction $(-1, -3, -2)$ is nothing else than the oriented normal, passing through the origin, common to the planes $x_1 + 3x_2 + 2x_3 = c$ (Fig. 99).

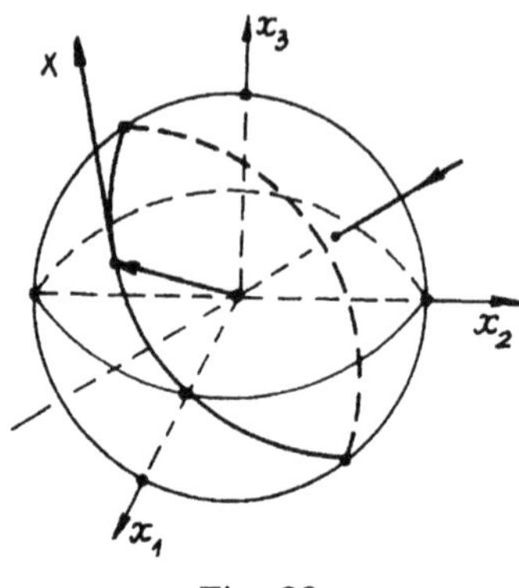

Fig. 99

8.5. DISTRIBUTION ORTHOGONAL TO A VECTOR FIELD

Let D be an open connected set of R^n, $n \geq 2$. Let $X = (X_1, \ldots, X_n)$ be a C^1 vector field without zeros on D, and

$$X_1(x)\,dx_1 + \cdots + X_n(x)\,dx_n = 0 \qquad (2'')$$

the Pfaff equation associated to X on D. If the Pfaff equation $(2'')$ is completely integrable and has the general solution $M_c : f(x) = c$, then D can be regarded as the union of the constant level hypersurfaces M_c (which are disjoint sets). In other words, a completely integrable Pfaff equation produces a stratification (foliation) of D by hypersurfaces.

Suppose that the Pfaff equation $(2'')$ is not completely integrable (it follows that $n \geq 3$), i.e., the vector field X does not possess a family of hypersurfaces orthogonal to the field lines. Even in this case the Pfaff equation determines a stratification of D by integral manifolds of maximum dimensions, but this stratification is essentially different from those in the completely integrable case, since every stratum has a dimension between 1 and $n-2$ depending on $\operatorname{rank} \operatorname{rot} X$ (accidentally, the dimension can be $n-1$), and by a point can pass different integral manifolds with the same dimension.

The two situations described previously can be included in a more general theory in the following fashion. We denote by $T_x D$ the tangent space to D at the point x. For a fixed point $x \in D$, the equation $(2'')$ represents the hyperplane Ω_x determined by the point x and by the normal vector $X(x)$. The correspondence $x \to \Omega_x \subset T_x D$ defines a function Ω on D which is an (n-1)-dimensional distribution, called the *distribution orthogonal to the vector field* X. A vector field Y belongs to the distribution Ω if $Y(x) \in \Omega_x$, $\forall x \in D$, or equivalent $(X, Y) = 0$ on D. Obviously, for every $x \in D$ there exists a neighborhood U of x and $n-1$

vector fields $Y_1, \dots, Y_{n-1}$ of class C^1 on U such that $\{Y_1(x), \dots, Y_{n-1}(x)\}$ generates Ω_x, $x \in U$ (see also 3.2 from which it follows that $Y_1, \dots, Y_{n-1}$ can be gradient fields). The set $\{Y_1, \dots, Y_{n-1}\}$ is called a *local basis* of the distribution Ω.

The distribution Ω is called *involutive* if the allegiance $Y, Z \in \Omega$ and Y, Z of class C^1 imply $[Y, Z] \in \Omega$. The integral manifolds of the Pfaff equation $(2'')$ are called *integral manifolds of the distribution* Ω. The distribution Ω is called *integrable* if the Pfaff equation $(2'')$ is completely integrable.

Now, let us give a variant of the Frobenius theorem for the distribution Ω.

Theorem. *The distribution Ω is integrable if and only if it is involutive.*

Proof. Suppose that Ω is integrable, i.e., the Pfaff equation $(2'')$ is completely integrable or locally $X = \operatorname{grad} f$. Then the allegiance $Y, Z \in \Omega$ means $(\operatorname{grad} f, Y) = 0$, $(\operatorname{grad} f, Z) = 0$. Computing the derivatives with respect to Z and Y respectively, we find

$$\operatorname{Hess} f(Y, Z) + (\operatorname{grad} f, D_Z Y) = 0, \ \operatorname{Hess} f(Z, Y) + (\operatorname{grad} f, D_Y Z) = 0,$$

and by subtraction we obtain $(\operatorname{grad} f, [Y, Z]) = 0$, i.e., $[Y, Z] \in \Omega$. Thus Ω is involutive.

Suppose that Ω is involutive and $\{Y_1, \dots, Y_{n-1}\}$ is a local basis of Ω. Then

$$(X, Y_\alpha) = 0, \ [X, [Y_\beta, Y_\gamma]) = 0, \ \alpha, \beta, \gamma = 1, \dots, n-1.$$

Since

$$(D_{Y_\beta} X, Y_\gamma) + (X, D_{Y_\beta} Y_\gamma) = 0, \ (D_{Y_\gamma} X, Y_\beta) + (X, D_{Y_\gamma} Y_\beta) = 0,$$

we have

$$0 = (X, [Y_\beta, Y_\gamma]) = (X, D_{Y_\beta} Y_\gamma - D_{Y_\gamma} Y_\beta) = (D_{Y_\beta} X, Y_\gamma) - (D_{Y_\gamma} X, Y_\beta) = (\operatorname{rot} X)(Y_\beta, Y_\gamma).$$

We fix the local frame field $\{Z_1 = Y_1, \dots, Z_{n-1} = Y_{n-1}, Z_n = X\}$ and we remark that the functions (see 8.3)

$$f_{ijk} = X_i (\operatorname{rot} X)_{jk} + X_j (\operatorname{rot} X)_{ki} + X_k (\operatorname{rot} X)_{ij}$$

constitute the components of a tensor field of order three. The components of this tensor field with respect to the fixed frame are

$$f_{ABC} = \sum_{i,j,k} f_{ijk} Z^i_A Z^j_B Z^k_C = X_A (\operatorname{rot} X)_{BC} + X_B (\operatorname{rot} X)_{CA} + X_C (\operatorname{rot} X)_{AB},$$

$$A = \alpha, n; \ B = \beta, n; \ C = \gamma, n,$$

where

$$X_A = \sum_i X_i Z^i_A, \ (\operatorname{rot} X)_{AB} = \sum_{i,j} (\operatorname{rot} X)_{ij} Z^i_A Z^j_B$$

are respectively the components of X and $\operatorname{rot} X$. The relations

$$X_\alpha = 0, \ (\operatorname{rot} X)_{\beta\gamma} = 0$$

and the properties referring to the indices of the functions f_{ABC} show that $f_{ABC} = 0$. These last relations and the fact that Z^i_A is a nonsingular matrix imply $f_{ijk} = 0$. Thus the Pfaff equation is completely integrable, and hence Ω is integrable.

Assume that the Pfaff equation ($2''$) is not completely integrable. As we have shown in 8.1, through every point x of D pass surely an infinity of integral curves of the Pfaff equation (Fig.96), even when we fix a tangent vector to D at x. Also there exists a subset U of D with the property that any two points of U are joined by an integral curve of the Pfaff equation ($2''$), a property which can be interpreted in the sense that a noncompletely integrable Pfaff equation on U is not a "constraint for positions (points)."

This old conjecture, appearing in the work of Caratheodory [9] and Vrănceanu [136], [137], is translates into the next theorem.

Chow's Theorem. *If there exists a local basis $\{Y_1, \dots, Y_{n-1}\}$ of the distribution Ω on D such that the vector fields $Y_1, \dots, Y_{n-1}$ and all their repeated Lie brackets generate $T_x D$ at every point $x \in D$, then any two points $x_1, x_2 \in D$ can be joined by a finite concatenation of field lines of $Y_1, \dots, Y_{n-1}$ (concatenation of integral curves of the Pfaff equation, Fig.100).*

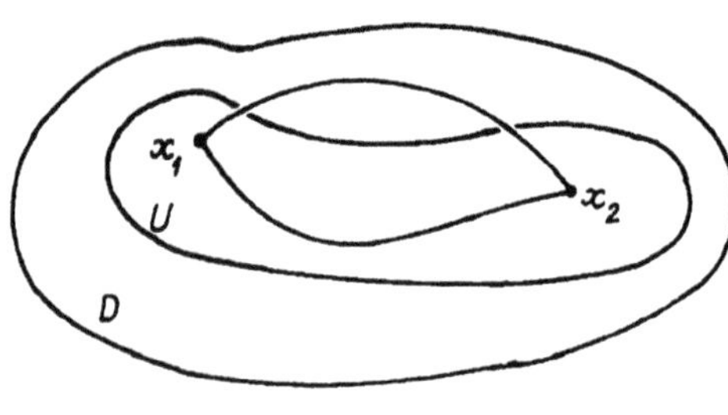

Fig. 100

Let X be a vector field on $D \subset R^n$ which is not locally potential or locally biscalar (it follows that $n \geq 3$) and Ω be its orthogonal distribution (which is not integrable). The set of all integral manifolds of the distribution Ω is called a *nonholonomic manifold defined by the set D and the vector field X on D*. A nonholonomic manifold has a structure which is completely different from those defined on D by a family of hypersurfaces orthogonal to the field lines, though locally these are similar by the existence of tangent hyperplanes (see also 8.7).

Remark. The differential geometry of the nonholonomic manifolds [136],[137] is a creation of the Romanian geometer Gh. Vrănceanu (1900 - 1979).

Let $X = (X_1, \dots, X_n)$ be a C^1 vector field on the open and connected set D and

$$X_1(x)dx_1 + \cdots + X_n(x)dx_n = 0 \tag{3}$$

the Pfaff equation associated to X on D. The preceding theory refers to the Pfaff equation on the open set $D_* = \{x \in D \mid X(x) \neq 0\}$. In the case that X has zeros on D, we extend this theory. Thus, by a solution of the Pfaff equation (3) we understand either an integral manifold fixed by a point $x_0 \in D$ and a given tangent space or the set of zeros of X on D denoted by $Z(X)$. Obviously $Z(X)$ is not a submanifold of D except in particular cases.

Zeros of the vector field X are called *singular points* of the *nonholonomic manifold* defined by the Pfaff equation (3).

Applications. 1) The most simple and maybe the most famous nonholonomic space in R^3 can be obtained extending the equality $y' = \frac{dy}{dx}$. For this is enough to denote $y' = z$ and to interpret the triple (x,y,z) as a point in R^3, since $dy - zdx = 0$ is a not a completely integrable Pfaff equation.

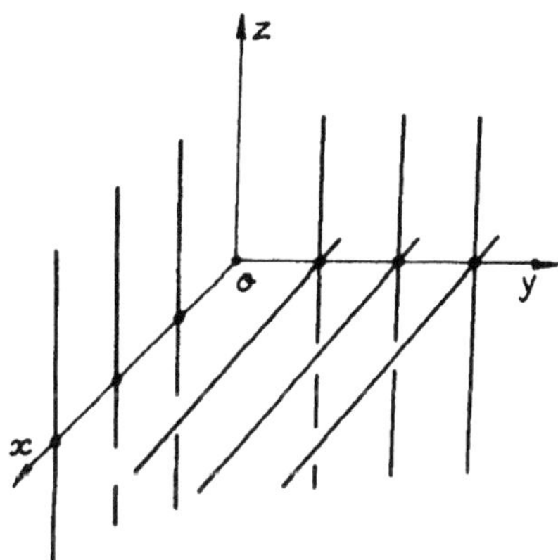

Fig. 101

The nonholonomic space Σ : $dy - zdx = 0$ has no singular point. It consists in integral curves containing all the straight lines that are parallel to Oz, i.e., the straight lines of equations $x = x_0$, $y = y_0$. Particularly, the intersection of Σ with the plane yOz is the family of straight lines $x = 0$, $y = c_1$, and the intersection to the plane xOz is the Ox- axis and the family of straight lines $y = 0$, $x = c_2$ (Fig.101).

The vector fields $Y_1 = (1, z, 0)$, $Y_2 = (0, 0, 1)$ determine a global basis of the distribution described by the Pfaff equation $dy - zdx = 0$. Since Y_1, Y_2, $[Y_1, Y_2] = (0, -1, 0)$ are linearly independent at each point of R^3, any two points of R^3 are joined by a concatenation of field lines of Y_1, Y_2. The orbits of Y_1 are the straight lines $y = c_1 x + c_2$, $z = c_1$ and the orbits of Y_2 are the straight lines $x = c_1$, $y = c_2$.

2) The Goodwin vector field $X = (x, y, z) = \left(\frac{1}{1 + z^n} - ax,\ x - by,\ y - cz \right)$ admits only curves that are orthogonal to the field lines, since $(X, \mathrm{rot}\, X) \neq 0$ and the surface of Cartesian equation $(X, \mathrm{rot}\, X) = 0$ is not orthogonal to the field lines.

3) Let us consider the Pfaff equation $dz - xdy + ydx = 0$ on R^3. We remark that the vector fields $Y_1 = (1, 0, -y)$, $Y_2 = (0, 1, x)$ determine a global basis of the distribution attached to this Pfaff equation. Since $[Y_1, Y_2] = (0, 0, 2)$, it follows that Y_1, Y_2, $[Y_1, Y_2]$ are linearly independent at each point of R^3. Consequently, given any two points $M_i(x_i, y_i, z_i)$, $i = 1, 2$, there is a finite concatenation of field lines of Y_1, Y_2 that goes from M_1 to M_2. The orbits of Y_1 are the straight lines $y = c_1$, $z = -xc_1 + c_2$, and the orbits of Y_2 are the straight lines $x = c_1$, $z = yc_1 + c_2$.

4) Now we consider the Pfaff equation $x^2 dy - (1 - x)dz = 0$ on R^3. The vector fields $Y_1 = (1, 0, 0)$, $Y_2 = (0, 1 - x, x^2)$ form a global basis of the distribution attached to the given Pfaff equation. Since

$$[Y_1, Y_2] = (0, -1, 2x),\ [Y_1, [Y_1, Y_2]] = (0, 0, 2),$$

the vector fields Y_1, Y_2, $[Y_1, Y_2]$ are linearly independent everywhere except where $x = 0$ or $x = 2$, and Y_1, Y_2, $[Y_1, [Y_1, Y_2]]$ are linearly independent everywhere except where $x = 1$. It follows that for every point of R^3 the values of Y_1, Y_2, $[Y_1, Y_2]$ $[Y_1, [Y_1, Y_2]]$ span R^3. Consequently, given any two points $M_i(x_i, y_i, z_i)$, $i = 1, 2$, there is a finite concatenation of field lines of Y_1, Y_2 that join M_1 to M_2.

8.6. FIELD LINES AS INTERSECTIONS OF NONHOLONOMIC SPACES

Let $X = (X_1, \dots, X_n)$ be a C^1 vector field on an open and connected set $D \subset R^n$. The field lines of the vector field X are characterized by the symmetric differential system

$$\frac{dx_1}{X_1(x)} = \dots = \frac{dx_n}{X_n(x)}.$$

This differential system is equivalent to a system of $n - 1$ Pfaff equations, for example

$$-X_n(x)dx_1 + X_1(x)dx_n = 0, \dots, -X_n(x)dx_{n-1} + X_{n-1}(x)dx_n = 0,$$

and, for $n \geq 3$, each equation can be, or not, completely integrable. Therefore, through every field line of X can pass both usual hypersurfaces, and nonholonomic spaces.

The vector field X can be recovered from the vector fields

$$(-X_n, 0, \dots, 0, X_1), (0, -X_n, \dots, 0, X_2), \dots, (0, 0, \dots, -X_n, X_{n-1})$$

since the vector product of these is $X_n^{n-2} X$. The existence of the first integrals for the symmetric differential system shows that there exists a system of $n-1$ completely integrable Pfaff equations locally equivalent to the initial differential system.

Conversely, let us consider the Pfaff equation

$$\sum_{i=1}^{n} X_i(x)\,dx_i = 0$$

on D, which is supposed to be noncompletely integrable. To this Pfaff equation we attach $n-2$ arbitrary Pfaff equations

$$\sum_{i=1}^{n} X_i^\alpha(x)\,dx_i = 0, \quad \alpha = 1, \ldots, n-2,$$

such that the rank of the matrix

$$\begin{bmatrix} X_1 & \ldots & X_n \\ X_1^\alpha & \ldots & X_n^\alpha \end{bmatrix}$$

is $n-1$. The Pfaff system

$$X_1(x)\,dx_1 + \cdots + X_n(x)\,dx_n = 0,$$

$$X_1^\alpha(x)\,dx_1 + \cdots + X_n^\alpha(x)\,dx_n = 0, \quad \alpha = 1, \ldots, n-2,$$

is equivalent to the symmetric differential system

$$\frac{dx_1}{Y_1(x)} = \cdots = \frac{dx_n}{Y_n(x)},$$

where $Y = (Y_1, \ldots, Y_n)$ is a vector field collinear to the vector product of the vector fields X, X^α, $\alpha = 1, \ldots, n-2$. Taking into account the existence and uniqueness theorem for the lines of Y, we deduce that, being given a Pfaff equation, for every choice of the vectors X^α, $\alpha = 1, \ldots, n-2$ there exists a unique integral curve passing through the point $x_0 \in D$.

Examples. 1) Find the field lines of $X = yi + zj + xk$ and select two nonholonomic spaces (surfaces) which determine these curves.

Solution. The differential system with constant coefficients

$$\frac{dx}{dt} = y, \quad \frac{dy}{dt} = z, \quad \frac{dz}{dt} = x$$

admits the equilibrium point $(0, 0, 0)$ and the general solution

$$x = c_1 e^t + e^{-\frac{t}{2}} \left(c_2 \cos \frac{\sqrt{3}}{2} t + c_3 \sin \frac{\sqrt{3}}{2} t \right),$$

$$y = c_1 e^t + e^{-\frac{t}{2}} \left[\left(\frac{\sqrt{3}}{2} c_3 - \frac{1}{2} c_2 \right) \cos \frac{\sqrt{3}}{2} t - \left(\frac{\sqrt{3}}{2} c_2 - \frac{1}{2} c_3 \right) \sin \frac{\sqrt{3}}{2} t \right],$$

$$z = c_1 e^t + e^{-\frac{t}{2}} \left[-\frac{1}{2} c_2 \cos \frac{\sqrt{3}}{2} t + \left(\frac{\sqrt{3}}{2} c_2 - c_3 \right) \sin \frac{\sqrt{3}}{2} t \right], \quad t \in R.$$

The associated symmetric differential system $\frac{dx}{y} = \frac{dy}{z} = \frac{dz}{x}$ can be written as a Pfaff system

$$z dx - y dy = 0, \; x dy - z dz = 0.$$

These two Pfaff equations represent nonholonomic spaces (nonholonomic cylinders, see 8.7 and [96]) since they are not completely integrable. The intersection of these nonholonomic surfaces coincides with the family of all field lines of $\boldsymbol{X}$.

Obviously, through the field lines pass also constant level surfaces. For example

$$\frac{dx}{y} = \frac{dy}{z} = \frac{dz}{x} = \frac{(x^2 - yz)dx + (y^2 - zx)dy + (z^2 - xy)dz}{0}$$

implies $d(x^3 + y^3 + z^3 - 3xyz) = 0$ and therefore $x^3 + y^3 + z^3 - 3xyz = c_1$.

Remarks. 1) We have

$$\frac{dx}{y} = \frac{dy}{z} = \frac{dz}{x} = \frac{(z^2 - xy)dx + (x^2 - yz)dy + (y^2 - zx)dz}{0}.$$

Nevertheless the Pfaff form

$$(z^2 - xy)dx + (x^2 - yz)dy + (y^2 - zx)dz$$

is not an integrable combination, since

$$rot\,[(z^2 - xy)\boldsymbol{i} + (x^2 - yz)\boldsymbol{j} + (y^2 - zx)\boldsymbol{k}] = 3\boldsymbol{X} \neq 0.$$

However there exists an integrant factor for the Pfaff equation

$$(z^2 - xy)dx + (x^2 - yz)dy + (y^2 - zx)dz = 0,$$

but the difficulty of effective determination of that integrant factor is equivalent to the difficulty of finding integrable combinations for the symmetric differential system.

2) The vector field $X = (y, z, x)$ is solenoidal and so the flow generated by X conserves the volume.

8.7. DISTRIBUTION ORTHOGONAL TO AN AFFINE VECTOR FIELD

Let $X = (X_1, \ldots, X_n)$, $X_i(x) = \sum_{j=1}^{n} a_{ij} x_j + a_i$, be an affine vector field on R^n and

$$\sum_{i=1}^{n} \left(\sum_{j=1}^{n} a_{ij} x_j + a_i \right) dx_i = 0 \tag{4}$$

the Pfaff equation associated to X. This equation describes the distribution orthogonal to X.

Suppose that X is an irrotational vector field, i.e., $a_{ij} = a_{ji}$. Then and only then the Pfaff equation (4) is exact and its general solution is the family of hyperquadrics of R^n

$$0.5 \sum_{i,j=1}^{n} a_{ij} x_i x_j + \sum_{i=1}^{n} a_i x_i = c.$$

In other words, the hypersurfaces orthogonal to the field lines of an irrotational affine vector field are hyperquadrics.

Let us look for the conditions under which the Pfaff equation (4) is completely integrable (the distribution Ω defined by (4) is integrable).

Theorem. *Suppose that X is rotational, i.e., the matrix $[a_{ij}]$ is not symmetric.*

1) If $\mathrm{rank}[a_{ij}] = 1$, then the Pfaff equation (4) is completely integrable.

2) If $\mathrm{rank}[a_{ij}] = 2$, then the Pfaff equation (4) can be or not be completely integrable.

3) If $\mathrm{rank}[a_{ij}] \geq 3$, then the Pfaff equation (4) is not completely integrable.

Proof. According to the Frobenius theorem the Pfaff equation (4) is completely integrable if and only if

$$a_{il}(a_{kj} - a_{jk}) + a_{jl}(a_{ik} - a_{ki}) + a_{kl}(a_{ji} - a_{ij}) = 0, \; i, j, k, l = 1, \ldots, n. \tag{5}$$

1) It is known that a matrix $[a_{ij}]$ has the rank 1 if and only if there exist two vectors $[u_i]$, $[v_j]$ such that $a_{ij} = u_i v_j$. With this expression, the relations (5) are identically satisfied.

2) We consider the linear vector field

$$X = (x - y - z, x + y + z, x + y + z), \; (x, y, z) \in R^3,$$

whose associated matrix $\begin{bmatrix} 1 & -1 & -1 \\ 1 & 1 & 1 \\ 1 & 1 & 1 \end{bmatrix}$ has the rank 2. We find $\mathrm{rot} X = (0, -2, 2)$, hence

$(\boldsymbol{X}, \operatorname{rot} \boldsymbol{X}) = 0$, and so the condition of complete integrability (5) is satisfied.

For the linear vector field

$$\boldsymbol{X} = (x - y - z, x + y + 2z, x + y + 2z), \ (x, y, z) \in \boldsymbol{R}^3,$$

the associated matrix

$$\begin{bmatrix} 1 & -1 & -1 \\ 1 & 1 & 2 \\ 1 & 1 & 2 \end{bmatrix}$$

has the rank 2. We get $\operatorname{rot} \boldsymbol{X} = (-1, -2, 2)$, $(\boldsymbol{X}, \operatorname{rot} \boldsymbol{X}) = -x + y + z$ and so the condition of complete integrability (5) is not satisfied.

3) We prefer to prove the equivalent statement: under the hypothesis $\operatorname{rank}[a_{ij}] \geq 3$, the Pfaff equation (4) is completely integrable if and only if $a_{ij} = a_{ji}$.

Suppose that $\operatorname{rank}[a_{ij}]$ is 3. Then always we can admit that $|a_{\alpha\beta}|$, $\alpha, \beta = 1, 2, 3$ is the minor of order 3 different from zero (the reasoning with any other minor is analogous). Since $|a_{\alpha\beta}| \neq 0$, we can introduce the numbers $a^{\alpha\beta}$ such that

$$a^{\alpha\beta} a_{\alpha\gamma} = \delta^{\beta}_{\gamma}, \ a^{\alpha\beta} a_{\gamma\beta} = \delta^{\alpha}_{\gamma} \tag{6}$$

(The matrix $[a^{\alpha\beta}]$ is the inverse of the matrix $[a_{\alpha\beta}]$). Choose now from all the equations (5) those for which all the indices take the values $1, 2, 3$:

$$a_{\alpha\delta}(a_{\gamma\beta} - a_{\beta\gamma}) + a_{\beta\delta}(a_{\alpha\gamma} - a_{\gamma\alpha}) + a_{\gamma\delta}(a_{\beta\alpha} - a_{\alpha\beta}) = 0.$$

Multiplying by $a^{\alpha\beta}$, summing with respect to α, β and considering (6), we find $a_{\gamma\beta} = a_{\beta\gamma}$.

From the equations (5) we select now those for which the index i takes values from 1 to n, and all the other indices take the values $1, 2, 3$. If we use $a_{\gamma\beta} = a_{\beta\gamma}$, then these equations reduce to

$$a_{\beta\delta}(a_{i\gamma} - a_{\gamma i}) + a_{\gamma\delta}(a_{\beta i} - a_{i\beta}) = 0.$$

Multiplying by $a^{\beta\delta}$, summing and using (6), we find $a_{i\gamma} = a_{\gamma i}$.

With the preceding determinations, the equations (5) in which i and l run from 1 to n are identically satisfied, and those in which i, l, j run from 1 to n are reduced to $a_{\gamma l}(a_{ji} - a_{ij}) = 0$. As some numbers $a_{\gamma l}$ are different from zero, it follows that $a_{ij} = a_{ji}$, $i, j = 1, \ldots, n$.

The proof for the case $\operatorname{rank}[a_{ij}] = p$, $3 < p \leq n$, is analogous.

Suppose that $[a_{ij}]$ is not symmetric, but $0 < \operatorname{rank}[a_{ij}] \leq 2$. Because of the existence of the integrant factor μ for the Pfaff equation (4), the hypersurfaces orthogonal to field lines of the corresponding affine vector field are not hyperquadrics. For example, if $a_{ij} = u_i a_j$, and $(u_1, \ldots, u_n)$, $(a_1, \ldots, a_n)$ are not collinear, then the Pfaff equation (4) is written

$$\left(\sum_{i=1}^{n} u_i \, dx_i\right)\left(\sum_{j=1}^{n} a_j x_j\right) + \sum_{i=1}^{n} a_i \, dx_i = 0$$

and has the general solution

$$\sum_{i=1}^{n} u_i x_i + \ln \left| \sum_{i=1}^{n} a_i x_i \right| = c.$$

The linear vector field $X = (x - y - z, x + y + z, x + y + z)$ on R^3, associated to a given matrix of rank 2, satisfies the condition of complete integrability. The Bertrand algorithm shows that the surfaces orthogonal to the field lines of X are described by the Cartesian implicit equations

$$\operatorname{arc\,tg} \frac{y+z}{x} + \frac{1}{2} \ln [x^2 + (y+z)^2] = c.$$

The preceding facts lead to the following definition: The nonholonomic manifold defined by the Pfaff equation (4) in each of the following cases

1) $\operatorname{rank}[a_{ij}] = 2$ and the relations (5) are not satisfied,

2) $\operatorname{rank}[a_{ij}] \geq 3$, and the matrix $[a_{ij}]$ is not symmetric,

is called *nonholonomic hyperquadric*.

The case 1) of this definition, and the fact that any Pfaff equation on R^2 admits a local integrant factor, impose $n \geq 3$.

The nonholonomic hyperquadrics can be classified [96], [136], [137] after the type of set $Z(X)$ of zeros of the field X, whose elements are called *centres*.

Applications. 1) We consider the nonholonomic quadric described by the Pfaff equation $z dx - y dy = 0$. This equation admits a straight line of centres, $Ox : z = 0,\ y = 0$, and for that it represents a *nonholonomic cylinder* with axis Oz. This nonholonomic cylinder does not look like the family of cylinders with axis Oz, a fact which can be supported by the remark that it contains the axis Ox, the straight lines (Fig.102, $x_0 < y_0^2$)

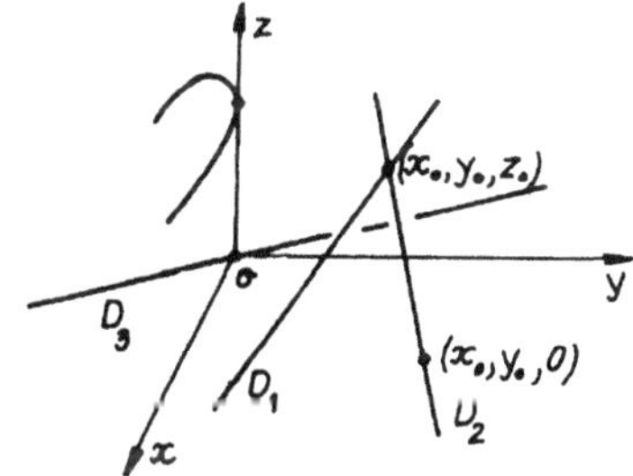

Fig. 102

$$D_1 : x = x_0 + \frac{y_0^2}{x_0} t,\ y = y_0 + \frac{y_0}{z_0} t,\ z = z_0 + t,\ t \in R,\ (x_0, y_0, z_0),\ z_0 \neq 0;$$

$$D_2 : x = x_0,\ y = y_0;\ D_3 : x = y = z$$

and the parabola

$$\Gamma : y^2 = 2x,\ z = 1.$$

2) A nonholonomic quadric without centres is called a *nonholonomic paraboloid*. For example, $\Sigma : dz = (x-y)dx + (x-2y)dy$. We remark that Σ contains the straight line

$$D : x = \sqrt{2}\,t,\ y = t,\ z = z_0,\ t \in R,$$

z_0 being fixed, and the intersection between Σ and the spiral

$$\Gamma : x = \cos t,\quad y = \sin t,\quad z = t,\quad t \in R,$$

consists of the points

$$A_k\left(0, \pm 1, \pm\frac{\pi}{2} + 2k\pi\right),\ k \in Z, \quad \text{and} \quad B_m(\pm 1, 0, m\pi),\ m \in Z.$$

The axis Oz is a symmetry axis of Σ (Fig.103).

3) The nonholonomic quadric $\Sigma : (x-y)dx + (x+y)dy + zdz = 0$ admits the centre $(0,0,0)$, the symmetry axis Oz and the symmetry plane xOy. The intersection of Σ with the plane xOz is the family of circles $y = 0,\ x^2 + z^2 = c_1$, the intersection with the plane yOz is the family of circles $x = 0,\ y^2 + z^2 = c_2$, and the intersection with the plane xOy is the family of curves (Fig.104)

$$z = 0,\ \operatorname{arctg}\frac{y}{x} + \frac{1}{2}\ln(x^2 + y^2) = c_3.$$

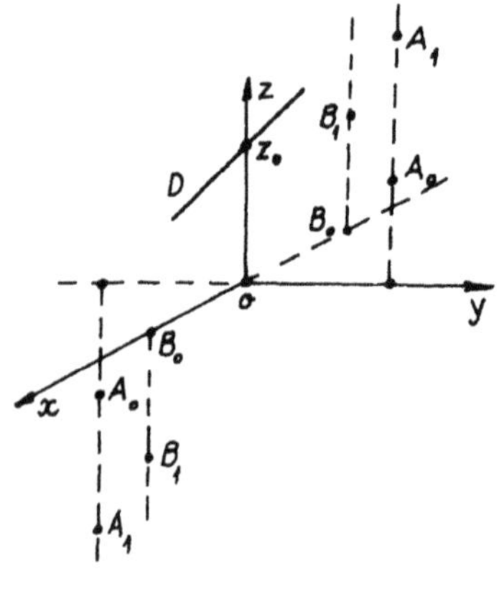

Fig. 103

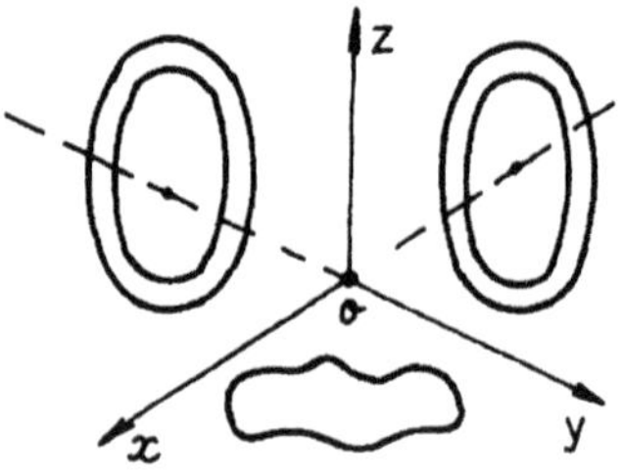

Fig. 104

8.8. PARAMETER DEPENDENCE OF SUBMANIFOLDS ORTHOGONAL TO FIELD LINES

Let us consider the C^∞ vector field

$$X(x,a) = (X_1(x,a),\dots,X_n(x,a)),\ x = (x_1,\dots,x_n) \in R^n,$$

which depends on the vector parameter $a = (a_1,\dots,a_m) \in R^m$. The submanifolds orthogonal to the field lines of X are solutions of the Pfaff equation

$$X_1(x,a)\,dx_1 + \cdots + X_n(x,a)\,dx_n = 0.$$

As in 8.3, to this Pfaff equation one can attach C_n^3 functions $f_{ijk}(x,a)$, $i<j<k$, by means of which we can decide the complete integrability in the following fashion:

1) If $f_{ijk}(x,a) = 0$, $\forall x \in R^n$, $\forall a \in R^m$, then the Pfaff equation is completely integrable and therefore X admits a family of hypersurfaces orthogonal to the field lines of X.

2) If $f_{ijk} \neq 0$, but there exists $a_0 \in R^m$ such that $f_{ijk}(x,a_0) = 0$, $\forall x \in R^n$, then the Pfaff equation is completely integrable only in the case $a = a_0$ and nonintegrable for $a \neq a_0$. Hence $X(x,a_0)$ admits a family of hypersurfaces orthogonal to the field lines, and $X(x,a)$ with $a \neq a_0$ admits only submanifolds of dimension at most $n-2$ orthogonal to field lines.

Generally, the flow generated by a vector field X conserves the set of submanifolds orthogonal to the field lines of X. That is why, the preceding remarks are strongly connected to the subclasses of the family after the vector parameter a of flows generated by the vector field $X(x,a)$.

To conclude, we point out again that the complete integrability of the Pfaff equation is equivalent to the fact that the vector field X is locally potential or locally biscalar. In this case, piecewise, the orbits of X are gradient lines or reparametrizations of gradient lines.

Examples. We consider the linear vector field

$$X = (X_1,\dots,X_n),\ X_i(x) = a_i\sum_{j=1}^{n} u_j x_j + u_i,\ u = {}^t[u_1,\dots,u_n],$$

which depends on the vector parameter $a = {}^t[a_1,\dots,a_n]$. The Pfaff equation associated to X

is

$$\left(\sum_{i=1}^{n} a_i\, dx_i\right)\left(\sum_{j=1}^{n} u_j x_j\right) + \sum_{i=1}^{n} u_i\, dx_i = 0.$$

If $a = 0$, then the general solution is the family of hyperplanes

$$H_c : \sum_{i=1}^{n} u_i x_i = c,$$

and if $a \neq 0$, then the general solution is the family of hypersurfaces

$$M_c : \sum_{i=1}^{n} a_i x_i + \ln\left|\sum_{i=1}^{n} u_i x_i\right| = c.$$

The division into two classes of the hypersurfaces orthogonal to the field lines of X corresponds to the two types of flows generated by X. Indeed, the differential system that describes the field lines

$$\frac{dx_i}{dt} = a_i \sum_{j=1}^{n} u_j x_j + u_i$$

has the general solution

$$x = e^{At}\left[x_0 + \left(\frac{t}{1!}I - \frac{t^2}{2!}A + \cdots + (-1)^n \frac{t^{n+1}}{(n+1)!}A^n + \cdots + \right)u\right],$$

$$t \in R, \quad x_0 \in R^n, \quad A = [a_i, u_j].$$

It follows the global flow (diffeomorphism) on R^n

$$x = e^{At}y + e^{At}\left[\frac{t}{1!}I - \frac{t^2}{2!}A + \cdots + (-1)^n \frac{t^{n+1}}{(n-1)!}A^n + \cdots\right]u$$

which consists of particular affine transformations. If $a = 0$, then the flow is reduced to translations, $x = y + tu, \quad t \in R$.

Remark. Since $\operatorname{div} X = (a, u)$, the flow generated by X conserves the volume only if the vectors a and u are orthogonal.

2) Let us now consider the linear vector field $X = (-x + \alpha y,\ \beta x - y + \alpha z,\ \beta y - z)$ on R^3, where α and β are real parameters. One finds $\operatorname{rot} X = (\beta - \alpha)(1, 0, 1)$. If $\beta = \alpha$, then X is a potential field and the quadrics $x^2 + y^2 + z^2 - 2\alpha xy - 2\alpha yz = c$ are orthogonal to the field lines of X. If $\beta \neq \alpha$, then

$$(X, \text{rot}X) = (\beta - \alpha)[-x + (\alpha + \beta)y - z]$$

and hence X admits only curves orthogonal to field lines.

Open problems. 1) Has the Hopf bifurcation of the flow generated by $X(x,a)$ any influence upon the set of submanifolds orthogonal to field lines?

2) For the set of submanifolds orthogonal to the field lines of $X(x,a)$, is there a bifurcation phenomenon?

8.9. EXTREMA WITH NONHOLONOMIC CONSTRAINTS

The study of problems of extrema subject to constraints has been from classical times a fertile field for the development of mathematical analysis [101], [111]. And it is well known that the submanifolds of R^p described by implicit Cartesian equations, which appear as constraints in an optimum problem, can be specified using the general solutions of a completely integrable Pfaff system and a point through which passes the respective submanifold. This remark suggests that we consider the extremum problems whose constraints are the integral manifolds of a Pfaff system (completely integrable or not) and give a sense to such problems in case that the Pfaff system is not completely integrable.

Some of our previous papers [112]-[116], [118]-[119] show that nonholonomic extrema can be characterized as constrained and uniformly constrained. Here we look from a new point of view on extrema constrained by a Pfaff system, establishing correlations between different notions and a dictionary between our previous ideas.

8.9.1. Extrema constrained by a Pfaff system

Let $D \subset R^p$ be an open set and let

$$\omega^j(x) = \sum_{i=1}^{p} \omega^j_i(x)dx^i = 0, \ j = \overline{1,q}, \ q < p \tag{S}$$

be a Pfaff system on D, where $\omega^j_i : D \to R$ are C^1 functions such that

$$\text{rank}\,[\omega^j_i(x)] = q, \ \forall x \in D.$$

Let I be a compact interval in R^m, $m \in \{1, 2, \dots, p-q\}$. An injective C^1 regular function $r : I \to D$, $r = (x^1, \dots, x^p)$, $x^i = x^i(u)$, $u = (u^1, \dots, u^m) \in I$, $i = \overline{1,q}$, for which we have

$$\sum_{i=1}^{p} \omega^j_i(r(u)) \frac{\partial x^i}{\partial u^k} = 0, \ \forall u \in I, \ k = \overline{1,m}, \ j = \overline{1,q},$$

is called an *integral manifold* of dimension m of the Pfaff system (S). We say that the integral manifold $r : I \to D$ passes through the point $x_0 \in D$ if there exists $u_0 \in I$ such that $r(u_0) = x_0$. For $m = 1$, the integral manifold is called an *integral curve*.

The Pfaff system (S) is called *completely integrable* if there exist the C^1 functions $g^j : D \to R$ with $dg^j = \omega^j$, $j = \overline{1,q}$. In this case through each point $x_0 \in D$ passes an integral manifold, whose dimension is $p-q$, which is described by the implicit Cartesian equations $g^j(x) = g^j(x_0)$, $j = \overline{1,q}$.

More about Pfaff systems, their geometry and applications, can be found, for instance, in [136], [137].

Definition. Let $f: D \to R$ be a C^1 function. We say that x_0 is a *point of minimum (maximum) for f constrained by the Pfaff system* (S) if for every integral manifold $r: I \to D$ of (S), which passes through x_0, there exists a neighborhood $V_{x_0} \subset D$ of x_0 such that

$$f(x) \geq f(x_0)\ (f(x) \leq f(x_0)),\ \forall\, x \in V_{x_0} \cap r(I).$$

If the preceding Definition refers only to the integral curves of the Pfaff system (S), then we use the name of *extremum constrained by the integral curves of a Pfaff system* [112]-[116].

Obviously, any point of extremum constrained by a Pfaff system is a point of extremum constrained by the integral curves of the system. The converse will be proved in section 8.9.3.

Theorem. *Let $f: D \to R$ be a C^1 function. The point $x_0 \in D$ is an extremum point of the function f constrained by the Pfaff system (S) iff, for every integral manifold $r: I \to D$, $r(u_0) = x_0$, there exists a neighborhood I_{u_0} of u_0 such that*

$$f(r(u)) \geq f(x_0) \quad (f(r(u)) \leq f(x_0)),\ \forall\, u \in I_{u_0}.$$

Proof. Let $r: I \to D$ be an integral manifold of (S) through x_0, and V_{x_0} a neighborhood of x_0 for which $f(x) \geq f(x_0)$, $\forall\, x \in r(I) \cap V_{x_0}$. Then $I_{u_0} = r^{-1}(V_{x_0})$. Conversely, the set $r(I_{u_0})$ is open in $r(I)$, whenever I_{u_0} is open, because r is a homeomorphism $I \to r(I)$. Consequently, we have a neighborhood V_{x_0} of x_0 with $V_{x_0} \cap r(I) = r(I_{u_0})$, and so $f(r(u)) \geq f(x_0)$, $\forall\, u \in I_{u_0}$ implies $f(x) \geq f(x_0)$, $\forall\, x \in V_{x_0} \cap r(I)$.

Since [112]-[113] show that the Lagrange multipliers rule survives for extrema constrained by the integral curves of a Pfaff system, we have

Theorem. *If $x_0 \in D$ is an extremum point of the C^1 function $f: D \to R$ constrained by the Pfaff system (S), then there exist $\lambda_1, \ldots, \lambda_q \in R$ such that*

$$df(x_0) + \sum_{j=1}^{q} \lambda_j\, \omega^j(x_0) = 0.$$

Definition. In the same hypotheses as in the preceding Definition, we say that $x_0 \in D$ is a *point of minimum (maximum) for f uniformly constrained by* (S) if there exists a neighborhood V of x_0 such that for every integral manifold $r: I \to D$ of (S), which passes through x_0, we have

$$f(x) \geq f(x_0)\ (f(x) \leq f(x_0)),\ \forall\, x \in V \cap r(I).$$

Obviously, any point of extremum uniformly constrained by (S) is an extremum point uniformly constrained by the integral curves of (S). The converse is not true.

For the main connections between the preceding notions we need some results about the C^1 curves, results that are important themselves. In this context we prefer the construction from the next paragraph though the subject exhibits several technicalities, which can be an annoyance or a source of fascination: depending upon one's point of view [19].

8.9.2. C^1 curves defined by sequences of points

The aim of this section is to show that certain conditions, which will appear in the main theorems, assure the existence of C^1 curves containing a given sequence of points. These ideas were developed in [19] for C^1 and C^2 curves, as tools for the connection between free extrema and extrema along a suitable family of curves.

Lemma. *Let* (a_n) *and* (b_n) *be two sequences of real numbers such that:*

1) $b_n \neq 0$ *and* $b_n \neq b_{n+1}$, $\forall\, n \in N$;

2) there exists $\lim\limits_{n\to\infty} \dfrac{a_n}{b_n} = r \in R$;

3) there exists $k > 0$ *such that* $\left|\dfrac{b_n}{b_{n+1}}\right| \geq k$ *for* $n \in N$.

Then there also exists

$$\lim_{n\to\infty} \frac{a_{n+1} - a_n}{b_{n+1} - b_n} = r\,.$$

Proof. For every $n \in N$, we have

$$\frac{a_{n+1}}{b_{n+1}} = \frac{a_{n+1} - a_n}{b_{n+1}} + \frac{a_n}{b_{n+1}} = \frac{a_{n+1} - a_n}{b_{n+1} - b_n} \cdot \frac{b_{n+1} - b_n}{b_{n+1}} + \frac{a_n}{b_n} \cdot \frac{b_n}{b_{n+1}}$$

$$= \frac{a_{n+1} - a_n}{b_{n+1} - b_n}\left(1 - \frac{b_n}{b_{n+1}}\right) + \left(\frac{a_n}{b_n} - \frac{a_{n+1}}{b_{n+1}}\right)\frac{b_n}{b_{n+1}} + \frac{a_{n+1}}{b_{n+1}}\frac{b_n}{b_{n+1}}\,.$$

We find

$$\frac{a_{n+1} - a_n}{b_{n+1} - b_n} = \frac{a_{n+1}}{b_{n+1}} - \left(\frac{a_n}{b_n} - \frac{a_{n+1}}{b_{n+1}}\right)\frac{\frac{b_n}{b_{n+1}}}{1 - \frac{b_n}{b_{n+1}}}.$$

From 2) it follows that $\lim_{n\to\infty}\left(\frac{a_n}{b_n} - \frac{a_{n+1}}{b_{n+1}}\right) = 0$, and, by 3), the quotient $\frac{\frac{b_n}{b_{n+1}}}{1 - \frac{b_n}{b_{n+1}}}$ is bounded.

So, passing to the limit the conclusion is obvious.

Lemma. *Let $a, b, c, d, \in R$, $a < b$, $c < d$. Then there exists an increasing C^1 function $f: [a,b] \to [c,d]$ that satisfies the conditions $f(a) = c$, $f(b) = d$, $f'(a) = f'(b) = 0$ and $0 \le f'(x) \le \frac{k(d-c)}{b-a}$, $\forall x \in [a,b]$, where k does not depend upon a, b, c, d.*

Proof. Such a function is, for instance,

$$f(x) = \frac{c-d}{(b-a)^3}(2x^3 - 3(a+b)x^2 + 6abx) + \frac{b^3c - 3ab^2c + 3a^2bd - a^3d}{(b-a)^3}$$

for which $k = \frac{3}{2}$.

Lemma. *Let (x_n), (y_n) be two sequences of real numbers such that $x_n \to 0$, $y_n \to 0$ and $\frac{y_n}{x_n} \to 0$. Then there exists a C^1 function $f: R \to R$ such that*

$$f(x_{n_k}) = y_{n_k}, \forall k \in N, f(0) = 0 \quad \textit{and} \quad f'(0) = 0,$$

for suitable subsequences (x_{n_k}), (y_{n_k}).

Proof. Suppose $x_n > 0$, $y_n > 0$ and choose (x_{n_k}) so that $2x_{n_{k+1}} \le x_{n_k}$. For each pair of intervals $[x_{n_{k+1}}, x_{n_k}]$, $[y_{n_{k+1}}, y_{n_k}]$ define the function f_k as in the preceding Lemma. Then the function

$$f(x) = \begin{cases} 0 & \text{if } x \le 0 \\ f_k(x) & \text{if } x \in [x_{n_{k+1}}, x_{n_k}], \forall k \in N \\ y_{n_1} & \text{if } x > x_{n_1} \end{cases}$$

is a suitable function because the subsequences (y_{n_k}) and (x_{n_k}) satisfy the conditions in the first Lemma.

Theorem. *Let* (x_n) *be a sequence of distinct points in* R^p *which converges to* $x \in R^p$. *Then there exist a subsequence* (x_{n_k}) *and a* C^1 *curve in* R^p *passing through each point* x_{n_k} *and* x.

Proof. By a translation, assume $x = (0, \dots, 0)$. Because $u_n = \dfrac{x_n}{\| x_n \|}$ is bounded, one may assume that it converges to $u \in R^p$. By a rotation we may consider $u = (1, 0, \dots, 0)$.

Then, if $x_n = (x_n^1, \dots, x_n^p)$, we have

$$\lim_{n \to \infty} \frac{x_n^1}{|x_n^1| \sqrt{1 + \left(\dfrac{x_n^2}{x_n^1}\right)^2 + \cdots + \left(\dfrac{x_n^p}{x_n^1}\right)^2}} = 1,$$

hence $\left(\dfrac{x_n^i}{x_n^1}\right) \to 0$ for $i \geq 2$.

Because $x_n^i \to 0$ for each $i = 1, \dots, p$, we may apply successively the last Lemma for each pair (x_n^i) and (x_n^1), $i \geq 2$. So we obtain a subsequence $x_{n_k} = (x_{n_k}^1, \dots, x_{n_k}^p)$ and C^1 functions $\varphi_i : R \to R$ so that $\varphi_i(x_{n_k}^1) = x_{n_k}^i$, $\forall k \in N$, and $\varphi_i(0) = 0$, $i = 2, \dots, p$. Then the curve $\alpha(t) = (t, \varphi_2(t), \dots, \varphi_p(t))$ has the required properties.

Theorem. *Let* $f : D \subset R^p \to R$ *be a function on the open set* D. *If* $x_0 \in D$ *is a minimum (maximum) point for the restriction of* f *to the image of any* C^1 *curve passing through* x_0, *then* x_0 *is a minimum (maximum) point for* f.

Proof. Without loss of generality suppose $f(x_0) = 0$. If x_0 would not be a minimum point of f, then we would have a sequence (x_n) with $x_n \to x_0$, $x_i \neq x_j$ for $i \neq j$ and $f(x_n) < 0$, $\forall n \in N$. From the above theorem, there would exist a C^1 curve passing through x_0 so that x_0 would not be a minimum point for the restriction of f to the image of this curve.

Remark. Obviously, the last Theorem remains valid on finite-dimensional differentiable manifolds.

8.9.3. Extrema constrained or uniformly constrained by a Pfaff system

Here we develop further the theory of 8.9.1 and we prove the existence of extremum points uniformly constrained by a Pfaff system.

Theorem. *A point $x_0 \in D$ is a point of extremum of a C^1 function $f: D \to R$ constrained by a Pfaff system (S) iff it is a point of extremum constrained by the integral curves of the system.*

Proof. We take into consideration the last Theorem in the preceding section, and the fact that each curve lying in an integral manifold of a Pfaff system is an integral curve of the system.

Theorem. *Suppose that the Pfaff system (S) is a completely integrable one and $\omega^j = dg^j$, $j = \overline{1,q}$. Let $x_0 \in D$ and $f: D \to R$ be a C^1 function. Then the following statements are equivalent.*

1) x_0 is an extremum point of f constrained by

$$g^j(x) = g^j(x_0),\ j = \overline{1,q}.$$

2) x_0 is an extremum point of f constrained by (S).

3) x_0 is an extremum point for f uniformly constrained by (S).

4) x_0 is an extremum point for f uniformly constrained by the integral curves of the system (S).

Proof. The assertion follows because the image of any integral manifold of (S) passing through x_0 is contained in the local maximal manifold of dimension $p - q$ defined by the system of equations

$$g^j(x) = g^j(x_0),\ j = \overline{1,q}.$$

Remark. This Theorem shows that complete integrability ensures the existence of uniformly constrained extrema points. We shall show that for a Pfaff system which is not completely integrable there also exist such points.

Theorem. *Let $x_0 \in D$ and M_{x_0} be the union of all integral curves of (S) which pass through x_0. If M_{x_0} is an integral manifold and $f: D \to R$ is a C^1 function, then the following statements are equivalent.*

1) x_0 is an extremum point for f constrained by (S).

2) x_0 is an extremum point for f uniformly constrained by (S).

3) x_0 is an extremum point for f uniformly constrained by the integral curves of the system (S).

Proof. First we remark that any integral manifold $r: I \subset R^m \to D$ passing through $x_0 \in D$ satisfies $r(I) \subset M_{x_0}$. If x_0 is an extremum point for f constrained by the Pfaff system (S), then x_0 is an extremum point for the restriction of f to the integral manifold M_{x_0}.

Consequently, there exists a neighborhood V of x_0 such that

$$f(x) \geq f(x_0) \quad (f(x) \leq f(x_0)),\ \forall\, x \in V \cap M_{x_0},$$

i.e., x_0 is an extremum point uniformly constrained by (S) since all the integral manifolds through x_0 are contained in M_{x_0}.

The implication 2) $\Rightarrow$ 3) is obvious.

Finally, if x_0 satisfies the condition 3), then x_0 is an extremum point constrained by the integral curves of the Pfaff system (S), and therefore, according to the first Theorem in this section, x_0 is an extremum point constrained by (S).

The preceding theorem can be generalized as follows.

Theorem. *Let $x_0 \in D$ and $f : D \to R$ be a C^1 function. Suppose there exist a finite number of integral manifolds of the Pfaff system (S) passing through x_0 whose union contains all the integral curves through x_0. Then the conclusion of the preceding Theorem holds true.*

Lemma. *Let $\eta(x) = \sum_{i=1}^{p} \eta_i(x) dx^i$ be a Pfaff form on D and $g : D \to R$ be a function of class C^1 without critical points. Then any integral curve of the Pfaff equation $dg + g\eta = 0$ (not necessarily completely integrable) which passes through a point of the integral hypersurface $M : g(x) = 0$ is contained in M.*

Proof. Let $\alpha : I \to D$, $\alpha(t) = (x^1(t), \ldots, x^p(t))$ be an integral curve of $dg + g\eta = 0$ and $\varphi(t) = g(\alpha(t))$. It follows that

$$\varphi'(t) + \varphi(t) \sum_{i=1}^{p} \eta_i(\alpha(t)) \frac{dx^i}{dt} = 0.$$

Therefore

$$\varphi(t) = C \exp\left(\int_{t_0}^{t} \sum_{i=1}^{p} \eta_i(\alpha(t)) \frac{dx^i}{dt} dt \right).$$

If α passes through a point of the integral hypersurface M, then there exists $t_0 \in I$ with $\varphi(t_0) = 0$. Hence $C = 0$, i.e., $\varphi(t) = 0, \forall\, t \in I$. Consequently $\alpha(I) \subset M$.

Examples. 1) Let

$$g : R^3 \to R,\ g(x, y, z) = z \text{ and } \omega = dg + g(z dx - dy) = z^2 dx - z dy + dz.$$

The Pfaff equation $\omega = 0$ is not completely integrable. On one hand the point $(0, 0, 0)$ is a minimum point for $f(x, y, z) = z + x^2 + y^2$ constrained by $\omega = 0$ and on the other hand, by the last Theorem in this section it is just a point of extremum uniformly constrained by $\omega = 0$.

Unfortunately the following question remains open [116], [119]: There exist points of constrained extrema that are not points of uniformly constrained extrema? Obviously, if these exist, they must be found for constraints described by the Pfaff systems which are not completely integrable (nonholonomic constraints).

2) Let $f : R^3 \to R$, $f(x, y, z) = z(y - x^2)(y - 3x^2)$. The point $(0, 0, 1)$ is a minimum point

for the restriction of f to any straight line passing by $(0,0,1)$ which is contained in the plane $z=1$. Indeed, if $\alpha(t)=(at,bt,1)$, $t\in R$ is such a straight line, then $f|_{\alpha(R)}$ is given by $\varphi(t)=t^2(b-a^2t)(b-3a^2t)$. Obviously $\varphi(t)\geq 0$ on a neighborhood of $t_0=0$. On the other hand $(0,0,1)$ is not a point of extremum for f with the constraint $z=1$; indeed for $\beta(t)=(t,2t^2,1)$, which is contained in the plane $z=1$, we find $\varphi(t)=f(\beta(t))=-t^4\leq 0$.

Generalization. Let M be a Riemannian manifold, let $x_0\in M$ and γ_{x_0x} a geodesic from $x_0=\gamma_{x_0x}(0)$ to $x=\gamma_{x_0x}(t)$. There exists a function $f:M\to R$ such that x_0 corresponds to the minimum point $t=0$, for every $f((\gamma_{x_0x}(t))$, but x_0 is not a minimum point for the function f.

3) The Pfaff equation $\omega=z^2dx-zdy+dz=0$ is not completely integrable. Let $f(x,y,z)=(y-x^2)(y-2x^2)+z$. Any integral curve of $\omega=0$, which passes through a point of the plane $z=0$, remains in this plane. Also any straight line through $(0,0,0)$ and included in the plane $z=0$ is an integrable curve of $\omega=0$. We remark that $(0,0,0)$ corresponds to the same point of minimum for the restriction of f to any straight line through $(0,0,0)$, and included in the plane $z=0$, but it is not a point of extremum for f constrained by $\omega=0$.

8.9.4. Extrema on star-shaped sets

Let Γ_{x_*} be the family of all integral curves $\gamma:[0,1]\to D$ of the Pfaff system (S) starting from the point $\gamma(0)=x_*$.

Definition. The set $D\subset R^p$ is called Γ_{x_*}- *star-shaped* at the point $x_*\in D$, if for any $x\in D$ there is $\gamma_x\in\Gamma_{x_*}$ with $\gamma_x(t)\in D$, for any $t\in[0,1)$, and $\gamma(1)=x$.

If any two points of D are joined by an integral curve of the Pfaff system (S), i.e., D is "convex" with respect to arcs of integral curves, then D is automatically star-shaped at each of its points. But there are examples of star-shaped sets that are not "convex."

Definition. Suppose D is Γ_{x_*}-star-shaped at $x_*\in D$. A function $f:D\to R$ is called *convex* at x_* with respect to the family Γ_{x_*}, briefly Γ_{x_*}*-convex*, if $f(\gamma(t))\leq tf(x)+(1-t)f(x_*)$, whenever $x\in D$ and $t\in[0,1]$.

Theorem. *Let $f:D\subset R^p\to R$ be a Γ_{x_*}-convex function, where D is Γ_{x_*}-star-shaped at $x_*\in D$. If x_* is a local minimum point for f constrained by the family Γ_{x_*}, then f has a global minimum at x_*.*

Proof. For any $x\in D$, $\gamma_x\in\Gamma_{x_*}$ and $t\in[0,1]$, the relations

$$f(\gamma_x(t))\geq f(\gamma_x(0))=f(x_*),\ f(\gamma_x(t))\leq tf(x)+(1-t)f(x_*)$$

imply

$$f(x_*)\leq f(x),\ \forall x\in D.$$

8.10. THERMODYNAMIC SYSTEMS AND THEIR INTERACTION

The aim of this section is to present certain features of thermodynamics, on a mathematical level that will emphasize the general and unifying aspects of the theory, rather than the specific physical details used in the standard text books [56].

8.10.1. Nonholonomic hypersurfaces determined by the Gibbs-Pfaff equation

Let R^5 be the real Euclidean space with 5 dimensions. For identification with the space of thermodynamic states, label the Cartesian coordinates on R^5 with U, T, S, P, V and adopt for them the following names:

U = *internal energy*, T = *temperature*, S = *entropy*, P = *pressure*, V = *volume*.

We consider the Gibbs-Pfaff equation

$$\theta = dU - TdS + PdV = 0. \tag{7}$$

Since

$$d\theta = -dT \wedge dS + dP \wedge dV,$$

it follows that

$$\theta \wedge d\theta = -dU \wedge dT \wedge dS + dU \wedge dP \wedge dV$$

$$- TdS \wedge dP \wedge dV - PdV \wedge dT \wedge dS \neq 0,$$

and hence the equation of Gibbs-Pfaff is not completely integrable (it does not admit an integrant factor). Consequently, even if we write

$$dS = \frac{1}{T}(dU + PdV),$$

the function $\frac{1}{T}$ is not an integrant factor for the Pfaff form $dU + PdV$ on R^5.

We remark that

$$\theta \wedge (d\theta)^2 = -2\,dU \wedge dT \wedge dS \wedge dP \wedge dV \neq 0$$

and hence the Gibbs-Pfaff form is a contact form. Therefore the integral submanifolds of the Gibbs-Pfaff equation are either curves or surfaces. Obviously, the integral curves are included in the integral surfaces.

An integral curve of the Gibbs-Pfaff equation is a C^2 regular function

$$\alpha : I \subset R \to R^5, \; \alpha(t) = (U(t), T(t), S(t), P(t), V(t))$$

whose components verify the ordinary differential equation of the first order

$$U' - TS' + PV' = 0, \tag{8}$$

where "$'$" means the derivative with respect to t. For a given point $M_0(U_0, T_0, S_0, P_0, V_0)$ and a nonzero vector $a = (a_1, a_2, a_3, a_4, a_5)$ fixed by the condition $a_1 - T_0 a_3 + P_0 a_5 = 0$, there exists an infinity of integral curves α (solutions of the differential equation (8)) which satisfy $\alpha(t_0) = M_0$, $\alpha'(t_0) = a$.

An integral surface of the Gibbs-Pfaff equation is a C^2 regular function

$$r : D \subset R^2 \to R^5, \; r(x,y) = (U(x,y), T(x,y), S(x,y), P(x,y), V(x,y))$$

whose components verify the system of equations with partial derivatives of the first order

$$\begin{cases} \dfrac{\partial U}{\partial x} - T\dfrac{\partial S}{\partial x} + P\dfrac{\partial V}{\partial x} = 0 \\ \dfrac{\partial U}{\partial y} - T\dfrac{\partial S}{\partial y} + P\dfrac{\partial V}{\partial y} = 0. \end{cases} \tag{9}$$

To this system we add the integrability conditions

$$\frac{\partial^2 U}{\partial x \partial y} = \frac{\partial^2 U}{\partial y \partial x}, \quad \frac{\partial^2 S}{\partial x \partial y} = \frac{\partial^2 S}{\partial y \partial x}, \quad \frac{\partial^2 V}{\partial x \partial y} = \frac{\partial^2 V}{\partial y \partial x}$$

which have as consequence the relation

$$\frac{\partial T}{\partial x}\frac{\partial S}{\partial y} - \frac{\partial S}{\partial x}\frac{\partial T}{\partial y} - \frac{\partial P}{\partial x}\frac{\partial V}{\partial y} + \frac{\partial V}{\partial x}\frac{\partial P}{\partial y} = 0. \tag{10}$$

For a given point $M_0(U_0, T_0, S_0, P_0, V_0)$ and two noncollinear vectors $a = (a_1, a_2, a_3, a_4, a_5)$, $b = (b_1, b_2, b_3, b_4, b_5)$ fixed by the conditions

$$a_1 - T_0 a_3 + P_0 a_5 = 0, \quad b_1 - T_0 b_3 + P_0 b_5 = 0, \quad a_2 b_3 - a_3 b_2 + a_5 b_4 - a_4 b_5 = 0,$$

there exists an infinity of integral surfaces r (solutions of system (9)) which satisfy

$$r(x_0, y_0) = M_0, \quad \frac{\partial r}{\partial x}(x_0, y_0) = a, \quad \frac{\partial r}{\partial y}(x_0, y_0) = b.$$

Remarks. 1) The general maximal integral surface of the Gibbs-Pfaff equation (7) is given by

$$U = f(S,V), \quad T = \frac{\partial f}{\partial S}, \quad P = -\frac{\partial f}{\partial V},$$

where f is an arbitrary C^2 function.

2) The Gibbs-Pfaff equation admits ruled integral surfaces, i.e., integral surfaces

of the form

$$r(x,y) = (u_1(x)+yu_2(x), t_1(x)+yt_2(x), s_1(x)+ys_2(x), \; p_1(x)+yp_2(x), v_1(x)+yv_2(x)).$$

Alternately,

1) an integral curve is characterized by a system of implicit Cartesian equations

$$f_i(U,T,S,P,V) = 0, \; i = 1, 2, 3, 4$$

attached to the submersion

$$f = (f_1, f_2, f_3, f_4) : R^5 \to R^4$$

with the property that the Gibbs-Pfaff equation (7) is a consequence of the equations

$$f_i(U,T,S,P,V) = 0, \; df_i(U,T,S,P,V) = 0, \; i = 1, 2, 3, 4;$$

2) an integral surface is characterized by a system of implicit Cartesian equations

$$g_j(U,T,S,P,V) = 0, \; j = 1, 2, 3$$

attached to the submersion

$$g = (g_1, g_2, g_3) : R^5 \to R^3$$

with the property that the Gibbs-Pfaff equation (7) is a consequence of the equations

$$g_j(U,T,S,P,V) = 0, \; dg_j(U,T,S,P,V) = 0, \; j = 1, 2, 3.$$

The set of all integral surfaces of the Gibbs-Pfaff equation (7) is a *nonholonomic hypersurface* in R^5 which will be denoted by $(R^5, \theta = 0)$. All these surfaces are orthogonal to the vector field $(1, 0, -T, 0, P)$ whose field lines are

$$U = t, \; T = c_1, \; S = -c_1 t + d_1, \; P = c_2, \; V = c_2 t + d_2, \; t \in R$$

$c_1, c_2, d_1, d_2 =$ arbitrary constants (family of straight lines).

The first fundamental form of the nonholonomic hypersurface $(R^5, \theta = 0)$ is obvious. The second fundamental form of the nonholonomic hypersurface $(R^5, \theta = 0)$ is

$$\Omega = \frac{1}{2\sqrt{1 + T^2 + P^2}}(dTdS - dPdV)$$

and consequently the Gauss-Kronecker curvature and the mean curvature of $(R^5, \theta = 0)$ vanish.

Remarks. 1) The Gibbs-Pfaff form determines on R^5 a contact structure. This induces an almost contact metric structure (ϕ, ξ, η, g) with

$$\phi = \begin{pmatrix} 0 & 0 & 1 & 0 & 0 \\ 0 & 0 & 0 & 1 & 0 \\ -1 & 0 & 0 & 0 & 0 \\ 0 & -1 & 0 & 0 & 0 \\ 0 & 0 & T & -P & 0 \end{pmatrix}, \quad \xi = \begin{pmatrix} 0 \\ 0 \\ 0 \\ 0 \\ 1 \end{pmatrix}, \quad \eta = (-T, P, 0, 0, 1)$$

$$g = \begin{pmatrix} 1+T^2 & -TP & 0 & 0 & -T \\ -TP & 1+P^2 & 0 & 0 & P \\ 0 & 0 & 1 & 0 & 0 \\ 0 & 0 & 0 & 1 & 0 \\ -T & P & 0 & 0 & 1 \end{pmatrix}$$

i.e.,

$$\phi^2 = -I + \xi\eta, \quad \eta\xi = 1, \quad \phi\xi = 0, \quad \eta\phi = 0, \quad {}^t\eta = g\xi,$$

$${}^t\phi g \phi = g - {}^t\eta\,\eta.$$

2) In a coming paper we shall refer to the Gibbs-Pfaff inequality

$$\theta = dU - TdS + PdV \leq 0.$$

8.10.2. Thermodynamic systems

Thermodynamics is an important model of a phenomenological theory that describes and unifies properties of different physical systems. Having in mind that the basis of this theory is the Gibbs-Pfaff equation (7), we accept the following mathematical point of view.

Definition. 1) An integral surface of the Gibbs-Pfaff equation (7) is called a *simple thermodynamic system.* The two variables x, y of the domain space R^2 are called the *states of the system.*

2) The nonholonomic hypersurface $(R^5, \theta = 0)$ is called a *thermodynamic system.*

Obviously a thermodynamic system is a collection of simple thermodynamic systems. In this context, the relation (10) is called the *Maxwell equation* attached to the thermodynamic system.

From the local point of view the states x, y of a simple thermodynamic system can be chosen as two of the five coordinates U, T, S, P, V. In this sense, the following 10 types of simple thermodynamic systems appear as naturally.

1) Let $x = U$, $y = T$, i.e.,

$$r(U,T) = (U, T, S(U,T), P(U,T), V(U,T)).$$

The system (9) becomes

$$1 - T\frac{\partial S}{\partial U} + P\frac{\partial V}{\partial U} = 0, \quad -T\frac{\partial S}{\partial T} + P\frac{\partial V}{\partial T} = 0.$$

The Maxwell equation is

$$-\frac{\partial S}{\partial U}-\frac{\partial P}{\partial U}\frac{\partial V}{\partial T}+\frac{\partial V}{\partial U}\frac{\partial P}{\partial T}=0.$$

2) Let $x=U,\ y=S$, i.e.,

$$r(U,S)=(U,T(U,S),S,P(U,S),V(U,S)).$$

The system (9) is written

$$1-T+P\frac{\partial V}{\partial U}=0,\quad -T+P\frac{\partial V}{\partial S}=0.$$

The Maxwell equation is

$$\frac{\partial T}{\partial U}-\frac{\partial P}{\partial U}\frac{\partial V}{\partial S}+\frac{\partial V}{\partial U}\frac{\partial P}{\partial S}=0.$$

3) Let $x=U,\ y=P$, i.e.,

$$r(U,P)=(U,T(U,P),S(U,P),P,V(U,P)).$$

The system (9) becomes

$$1-T\frac{\partial S}{\partial U}+P\frac{\partial V}{\partial U}=0,\quad -T\frac{\partial S}{\partial P}+P\frac{\partial V}{\partial P}=0.$$

The Maxwell equation is

$$\frac{\partial T}{\partial U}\frac{\partial S}{\partial P}-\frac{\partial S}{\partial U}\frac{\partial T}{\partial P}+\frac{\partial V}{\partial U}=0$$

4) Let $x=U,\ y=V$, i.e.,

$$r(U,V)=(U,T(U,V),S,(U,V),P(U,V),V).$$

The system (9) takes the form

$$1-T\frac{\partial S}{\partial U}=0,\quad -T\frac{\partial S}{\partial V}+P=0.$$

The Maxwell equation is

$$\frac{\partial T}{\partial U}\frac{\partial S}{\partial V}-\frac{\partial S}{\partial U}\frac{\partial T}{\partial V}-\frac{\partial P}{\partial U}=0.$$

5) Let $x=T,\ y=S$, i.e.,

$$r(T,S)=(U,(T,S),T,S,P(T,S),V(T,S)).$$

The system (9) takes the form

$$\frac{\partial U}{\partial T}+P\frac{\partial V}{\partial T}=0,\quad \frac{\partial U}{\partial S}-T+P\frac{\partial V}{\partial S}=0.$$

The Maxwell equation is

$$1-\frac{\partial P}{\partial T}\frac{\partial V}{\partial S}+\frac{\partial V}{\partial S}\frac{\partial P}{\partial S}=0.$$

6) Let $x=T,\ y=P$, i.e.,

$$r(T,P)=(U(T,P),T,S(T,P),P,V(T,P)).$$

The system (9) becomes

$$\frac{\partial U}{\partial T}-T\frac{\partial S}{\partial T}+P\frac{\partial V}{\partial T}=0,\quad \frac{\partial U}{\partial P}-T\frac{\partial S}{\partial P}+P\frac{\partial V}{\partial P}=0.$$

The Maxwell equation is

$$\frac{\partial S}{\partial P} + \frac{\partial V}{\partial T} = 0.$$

This is a basic case because T, P are measurable.

7) Let $x = T,\ y = V$, i.e.,

$$r(T,V) = (U(T,V), T, S(T,V), P(T,V), V).$$

The system (9) becomes

$$\frac{\partial U}{\partial T} - T\frac{\partial S}{\partial T} = 0,\quad \frac{\partial U}{\partial V} - T\frac{\partial S}{\partial V} + P = 0.$$

The Maxwell equation is

$$\frac{\partial S}{\partial V} - \frac{\partial P}{\partial T} = 0.$$

This is a basic case because T, V are measurable.

8) Let $x = S,\ y = P$, i.e.,

$$r(S,P) = (U(S,P), T(S,P), S, P, V(S,P)).$$

The system (9) is replaced by

$$\frac{\partial U}{\partial S} - T + P\frac{\partial V}{\partial S} = 0,\quad \frac{\partial U}{\partial P} + P\frac{\partial V}{\partial P} = 0.$$

The Maxwell equation is

$$-\frac{\partial T}{\partial P} + \frac{\partial V}{\partial P} = 0.$$

9) Let $x = S,\ y = V$, i.e.,

$$r(S,V) = (U(S,V), T(S,V), S, P(S,V), V).$$

The system (9) can be written

$$\frac{\partial U}{\partial S} - T = 0,\quad \frac{\partial U}{\partial V} + P = 0.$$

The Maxwell equation is

$$-\frac{\partial T}{\partial V} + \frac{\partial P}{\partial S} = 0.$$

10) Let $x = P,\ y = V$, i.e.,

$$r(P,V) = (U(P,V), T(P,V), S(P,V), P, V).$$

The system (9) becomes

$$\frac{\partial U}{\partial P} - T\frac{\partial S}{\partial P} = 0,\quad \frac{\partial U}{\partial V} - T\frac{\partial S}{\partial V} + P = 0. \tag{9'}$$

The Maxwell equation is

$$\frac{\partial T}{\partial P}\frac{\partial S}{\partial V} - \frac{\partial S}{\partial P}\frac{\partial T}{\partial V} - 1 = 0.$$

This is a basic case because P, V are measurable.

Definition. A simple thermodynamic system of type $r(P,V)$ is called an *ideal gas* if there exist a constant c and a function $f : I \subset R \to R$ such that

$$PV = cT,\ U = f(T) \quad \text{(Equations of state).}$$

For an ideal gas we have

$$S = \varphi(T) = c \ln V + d \quad \text{(Equation of state)}$$

as solution of (9′), where d is a constant and φ depends on f.

8.10.3. Minima of the energy of a thermodynamic system

Let $(R^5, \theta = 0)$ be the thermodynamic system. The function

$$f(U,T,S,P,V) = \frac{1}{2}(U^2 + T^2 + S^2 + P^2 + V^2)$$

is called the *kinetic energy* attached to the Riemannian structure δ_{ij} of R^5. The restriction of this function to $(R^5, \theta = 0)$ is called the *energy of the thermodynamic system.* We propose to find the minima of this energy, i.e., to find minima of f with the nonholonomic constraint $\theta = 0$. The constrained critical points are the solutions of the system

$$U + \lambda = 0, \; T = 0, \; S - \lambda T = 0, \; P = 0, \; V + \lambda P = 0,$$

which is obtained from the condition $df + \lambda\theta = 0$. We then have

$$M_0(U_0 = -\lambda, \, T_0 = 0, \, S_0 = 0, \, P_0 = 0, \, V_0 = 0).$$

The quadratic form

$$\varphi = dU^2 + dT^2 + dS^2 + dP^2 + dV^2 + \lambda(-dTdS + dPdV)$$

has the matrix

$$\begin{pmatrix} 1 & 0 & 0 & 0 & 0 \\ 0 & 1 & -\frac{\lambda}{2} & 0 & 0 \\ 0 & -\frac{\lambda}{2} & 1 & 0 & 0 \\ 0 & 0 & 0 & 1 & \frac{\lambda}{2} \\ 0 & 0 & 0 & \frac{\lambda}{2} & 1 \end{pmatrix}.$$

Therefore it is positive definite for $\lambda \in (-2, 2)$. Consequently all the points M_0, with

$\lambda \in (-2,2)$, are minimum points and $\min f = \dfrac{\lambda^2}{2}$.

8.10.4. Equilibrium states after interaction

Let there be the thermodynamic systems

$$(R^5, \theta_1 = dU_1 - T_1 dS_1 + P_1 dV_1 = 0),$$
$$(R^5, \theta_2 = dU_2 - T_2 dS_2 + P_2 dV_2 = 0).$$

In order to describe the interaction of these two systems we use the product manifold (with 10 dimensions)

$$M = R^5 + R^5 = \{(U_1, T_1, S_1, P_1, V_1, U_2, T_2, S_2, P_2, V_2)\}$$

and the product thermodynamic system

$$(M, \theta_1 = 0, \theta_2 = 0).$$

On M we consider the functions

$U = U_1 + U_2$, the *total internal energy*,
$S = S_1 + S_2$, the *total entropy*,
$V = V_1 + V_2$, the *total volume*.

In order to characterize the "equilibrium-after-interaction states" we can use the critical points of one of these functions constrained by the sets of constant level of the other two functions and by the Gibbs-Pfaff equations $\theta_1 = 0$, $\theta_2 = 0$ (see 8.9).

Theorem. *Critical points of* U *constrained by* $S = \text{const}$, $V = \text{const}$, $\theta_1 = 0$, $\theta_2 = 0$ *are the points of* $(M, \theta_1 = 0, \theta_2 = 0)$ *at which* $T_1 = T_2$ *(equal temperatures) and* $P_1 = P_2$ *(equal pressures).*

Proof. Let us find the critical points of $U = U_1 + U_2$ constrained by

$$S_1 + S_2 = \text{const}, \quad V_1 + V_2 = \text{const}$$
$$dU_1 - T_1\, dS_1 + P_1\, dV_1 = 0, \quad dU_2 - T_2\, dS_2 + P_2\, dV_2 = 0.$$

According to the theory in [112]-[116] these points are the solutions of the system

$$\lambda_1 + 1 = 0, \quad -\lambda_1 T_1 + \lambda_3 = 0, \quad \lambda_1 P_1 + \lambda_4 = 0$$
$$\lambda_2 + 1 = 0, \quad -\lambda_2 T_2 + \lambda_3 = 0, \quad \lambda_2 P_2 + \lambda_4 = 0$$

which is obtained by equalizing to zero the coefficients of the Pfaff form

$$\eta = dU_1 + dU_2 + \lambda_1\theta_1 + \lambda_2\theta_2 + \lambda_3(dS_1 + dS_2) + \lambda_4(dV_1 + dV_2).$$

Solving the system we find

$$\lambda_1 = -1,\ \lambda_2 = -1,\ \lambda_3 = -T_1 = -T_2,\ \lambda_4 = P_1 = P_2.$$

Theorem. *Critical points of* S *constrained by* $U = \text{const}$, $V = \text{const}$, $\theta_1 = 0$, $\theta_2 = 0$ *are the points of* $(M, \theta_1 = 0, \theta_2 = 0)$ *at which* $T_1 = T_2$ *and* $P_1 = P_2$.

Proof. Equalizing to zero the coefficients of the Pfaff form

$$\Omega = dS_1 + dS_2 + \lambda_1\theta_1 + \lambda_2\theta_2 + \lambda_3(dU_1 + dU_2) + \lambda_4(dV_1 + dV_2)$$

we find the system

$$1 - \lambda_1 T_1 = 0,\ 1 - \lambda_2 T_2 = 0,\ \lambda_1 + \lambda_3 = 0$$
$$\lambda_2 + \lambda_3 = 0,\ \lambda_1 P_1 + \lambda_4 = 0,\ \lambda_2 P_2 + \lambda_4 = 0.$$

It follows that

$$T_1 = T_2,\ P_1 = P_2.$$

Theorem. *Critical points of* V *constrained by* $U = \text{const}$, $S = \text{const}$, $\theta_1 = 0$, $\theta_2 = 0$ *are the points of* $(M, \theta_1 = 0, \theta_2 = 0)$ *for which* $T_1 = T_2$, $P_1 = P_2$.

Proof. Equalizing to zero the coefficients of the Pfaff form

$$\sigma = dV_1 + dV_2 + \lambda_1\theta_1 + \lambda_2\theta_2 + \lambda_3(dU_1 + dU_2) + \lambda_4(dS_1 + dS_2)$$

we find the system

$$1 - \lambda_1 P_1 = 0,\ 1 - \lambda_2 P_2 = 0,\ \lambda_1 + \lambda_3 = 0$$
$$\lambda_2 + \lambda_3 = 0,\ \lambda_1 T_1 + \lambda_4 = 0,\ \lambda_2 T_2 + \lambda_4 = 0.$$

It follows that $T_1 = T_2$, $P_1 = P_2$.

Remarks. 1) The constraints $T = T_1 + T_2 = \text{const}$, $P = P_1 + P_2 = \text{const}$ are not active.

2) We can find the extrema of the energy

$$F = \frac{1}{2}[(U_1 + U_2)^2 + (T_1 + T_2)^2 + (S_1 + S_2)^2 + (P_1 + P_2)^2 + (V_1 + V_2)^2]$$

constrained by

$$\theta_1 = 0,\ \theta_2 = 0.$$

3) The theory developed above can be extended naturally to the case of inequalities $\theta_1 \le 0$, $\theta_2 \le 0$.

8.11. PROPOSED PROBLEMS

1. Determine the general solutions for the following Pfaff equations:

$$(e^{x_1x_2}+1)\,dx_1 + \frac{x_1x_2-1}{x_2^2}e^{x_1x_2}dx_2 = 0 \quad (x_1, x_2) \in R^2 \setminus Ox_1,$$

$$dx_3 = \frac{x_3+a}{x_1}dx_1 + \frac{x_3+a}{x_2}dx_2, \; x_1 > 0, \; x_2 > 0, \; x_3+a > 0,$$

$$2x_1x_3dx_1 + 2x_2x_3dx_2 + (x_3^2 - x_2^2 - x_1^2)\,dx_3 = 0, \; x_3 > 0.$$

2. Analyse if the Pfaff equations associated to the conformal or projective vector fields (see 2.7, 2.8) are or are not completely integrable.

3. Solve the following systems:

$$\begin{cases} xzdx + z(2x-y)dy - x^2dz = 0 \\ x = y, \end{cases} \quad \begin{cases} (x^2-yz)dx + (y^2-zx)dy + (z^2-xy)dz = 0 \\ z = xy, \end{cases}$$

$$\begin{cases} (x^2-y^2-z^2)dx + 2xydy + 2xzdx = 0 \\ x^2+y^2+z^2 = 1, \end{cases} \quad \begin{cases} (x-y)dx + (x+y)dy + zdz = 0 \\ z = x^2+y^2. \end{cases}$$

4. Given the vector fields

1) $\boldsymbol{X}(x,y,z) = z(1-e^y)\boldsymbol{i} + xze^y\boldsymbol{j} + x(1-e^y)\boldsymbol{k}$,

2) $\boldsymbol{X}(x,y,z) = x^2yz\boldsymbol{i} + xy^2z\boldsymbol{j} + xyz^2\boldsymbol{k}$,

3) $\boldsymbol{X}(\boldsymbol{r}) = 2(\boldsymbol{a},\boldsymbol{r})\boldsymbol{a} + 2(\boldsymbol{b}\times\boldsymbol{r})\boldsymbol{b} - \dfrac{(\boldsymbol{a},\boldsymbol{r})^2 + (\boldsymbol{b},\boldsymbol{r})^2}{(\boldsymbol{a},\boldsymbol{b}\times\boldsymbol{r})}\boldsymbol{a}\times\boldsymbol{b}$.

Show that each $\boldsymbol{X}$ is a biscalar field and decide the functions f and λ such that $\boldsymbol{X} = \lambda\,\mathrm{grad} f$.

Answer.

1) $\boldsymbol{X}(x,y,z) = -x^2z^2\,\mathrm{grad}\,\dfrac{1-e^y}{xz}$,

2) $\boldsymbol{X}(x,y,z) = \dfrac{xyz}{2}\,\mathrm{grad}(x^2+y^2+z^2)$,

3) $\boldsymbol{X}(\boldsymbol{r}) = (\boldsymbol{a}\times\boldsymbol{b},\,\boldsymbol{r})\,\mathrm{grad}\dfrac{(\boldsymbol{a},\boldsymbol{r})^2 + (\boldsymbol{b},\boldsymbol{r})^2}{(\boldsymbol{a}\times\boldsymbol{b},\,\boldsymbol{r})}$.

5. We consider the vector field $\boldsymbol{V} = yz\boldsymbol{i} - xz\boldsymbol{j} + z\varphi(z,y)\boldsymbol{k}$, where φ is a function of

suitable class. Determine φ such that V is biscalar.

6. Let $V = \text{grad}\varphi(r) + \varphi(r)\text{grad}\psi(r)$, where $r = \sqrt{x^2+y^2+z^2}$, and φ, ψ are functions of suitable class.

1) Find the field lines of V.

2) Show that V is a potential vector field and determine the family of surfaces orthogonal to the field lines.

Hint. $V = (\exp(-\psi))\text{grad}(\varphi\exp\psi)$.

7. One considers the following vector fields:

1) $V = xzi + z(2x-y)j - x^2k$.
2) $V = x^2(y+z)i - y^2(z+x)j + z^2(y-x)k$,
3) $V = y^2z^2i + xyz^2j + xy^2zk$,
4) $V = xzi + yzj - (x^2+y^2)k$,
5) $V = (y-z)i + (z-x)j + (x-y)k$,
6) $V = x(y-z)i - y(x-z)j + z(x-y)k$.

Establish whether there exist families of surfaces orthogonal to the field lines. In case they exist, find the Cartesian implicit equations of the family of these surfaces. For the nonholonomic spaces, determine the intersections with axes and planes of coordinates (see also the problem 2 of 3.13).

8. Which of the following Pfaff equations defines nonholonomic quadrics:

$$(x+y)dx + (-x+z)dy - zdx = 0,$$
$$(5x-2y+4z)dx + (4x-y)dy + 2xdz = 0,$$
$$ydx + zdy - (6x+11y+6z)dz = 0,$$
$$ydx + (x+z)dy + (y+z)dz = 0\ ?$$

In the affirmative cases, determine the intersections of the nonholonomic quadrics with planes passing through axes of coordinates.

9. What kind of hypersurfaces are orthogonal to the field lines of a torse forming vector field?

Hint. Hypersurfaces for which all the points are umbilical points (parts of hyperplanes or of hyperspheres).

10. Let $D \subset R^n$, $n \geq 2$, an open and connected set and X be a C^∞ vector field on D, without zeros. Denote by Ω the distribution orthogonal to X. Show that the distribution Ω is involutive if and only if, for every local basis $\{Y_1, \ldots, Y_{n-1}\}$, there exist the C^∞ functions $C^\gamma_{\alpha\beta}$, $\alpha, \beta, \gamma = 1, \ldots, n-1$, such that

$$[Y_\alpha, Y_\beta] = \sum_{\gamma=1}^{n-1} C^\gamma_{\alpha\beta} Y_\gamma .$$

11. Analyse the dependence of parameters of the solutions of the following Pfaff equations:

$$x(x^2+y^2+a)dx + y(x^2+y^2-a)dy = 0,$$
$$(y-x^a)dx + xdy = 0,$$
$$bxy^2dx - ax^2dy + z(by^2-ax^2)dx = 0,$$
$$2(ay+z)dx + (x+3ay+3z)dy + (x-ay)dz = 0.$$

12. We consider the Lorenz vector field

$$\boldsymbol{X}(x,y,z) = (-\sigma x + \sigma y,\ -xz + rx - y,\ xy - bz),$$

where σ, r, b are real parameters. Has the Hopf bifurcation of the flow generated by $\boldsymbol{X}$ (see 3.6 and 7.4) any influence upon the curves orthogonal to the field lines?

13. On R^3 is given the vector field $\boldsymbol{V} = \varphi(r)[(\boldsymbol{a}\times\boldsymbol{r})\times\boldsymbol{r}]$, where $\boldsymbol{a}$ is a constant vector,

$$\boldsymbol{r} = x\boldsymbol{i} + y\boldsymbol{j} + z\boldsymbol{k},\ r = \sqrt{x^2+y^2+z^2},$$

and φ is a C^1 function.

1) Compute $\mathrm{rot}\boldsymbol{V}$ and $\mathrm{div}\boldsymbol{V}$.

2) Determine the surfaces orthogonal to the field lines of $\boldsymbol{V}$.

3) Find φ such that the circulation of $\boldsymbol{V}$ along any closed curve is zero. Then compute the flux of $\boldsymbol{V}$ by the sphere $r^2 - 2(\boldsymbol{a},\boldsymbol{r}) = 0$.

Hint. $\mathrm{rot}\,\boldsymbol{V} = 3\varphi(r)(\boldsymbol{a}\times\boldsymbol{r}) - \varphi'(r)(\boldsymbol{a}\times\boldsymbol{r})\times\dfrac{\boldsymbol{r}}{r'}$, $\mathrm{div}\,\boldsymbol{V} = 2(\boldsymbol{a},\boldsymbol{r})\varphi(r)$.

14. Minimize $f(x,y,z) = x^2 - 10x - yz$ subject to $dz = xdy - ydx$.

15. Maximize $f(x,y,z) = x^2 - xyz$ subject to $x^2dy - (1-x)dz = 0$.

9. DYNAMICS INDUCED BY A VECTOR FIELD

The energy of a vector field X *is the scalar field defined by* $f = \frac{1}{2}\|X\|^2$. *Thus the energy of a vector field is created by the vector field and by the Euclidean structure* δ_{ij} *of* R^n. *The energy* f *has interesting properties imposed either by the behavior of the gradient, Hessian or Laplacian of* f, *or by the behavior of* f *along field lines.*

Study of the energy of a vector field and of the geometric dynamics induced by a vector field is now fashionable. Particularly, investigation of the variation of energy along field lines is a new idea that deserves the attention of specialists, because it leads to supplementary information about the phenomenon whose local evolution is described by the vector field. An interesting result of this discovery [110] is the criterion of 9.1, which states a condition under which field lines cannot be closed curves. At the same time it is fitting to recall that the energy of X *can be used in problems of completeness and in problems of stability such as the Lyapunov function.*

Section 9.2 refers to differential equations of motion in Lagrange and Hamiltonian forms. Section 9.3 shows that any kinematic differential system on the Riemannian manifold (R^n, δ_{ij}) *induces a Lorentz-Udriste world-force law, i.e., it induces a nonclassical dynamics of the given vector field or of an associated particle. This kind of dynamics is called geometric dynamics, since its formulation requires a new geometric structure on* R^n: *either Riemann-Jacobi, or Riemann-Jacobi-Lagrange, or Finsler-Jacobi [132]. The cases of Riemann-Jacobi or Riemann-Jacobi-Lagrange structure are imposed by the behavior of an external tensor field of type (1,1). The case of the Finsler-Jacobi structure appears when the initial metric is chosen such that the energy of the given vector field is constant. Sections 9.4 - 9.10 study the energies of particular vector fields with geometrical and physical significance and describe the geometric dynamics induced by these vector fields.*

Section 9.11 presents the connection between the theory of Bobbio-Marrucci and the Monge representation, and analyses the behavior of thermodynamical potentials along field lines of the Bobbio-Marrucci vector field.

9.1. ENERGY AND FLOW OF A VECTOR FIELD

Let D be an open and connected set of R^n and X be a vector field of class C^2 on D. The vector field X and the Euclidean structure give the real function $f: D \to R$, $f(x) = \frac{1}{2}\|X(x)\|^2$. Since a vector field X represents locally the velocity of variation of a physical process, half of the square of the vector field length will represent the density of the kinetic energy of a medium in movement. The function f is called the *energy* of the vector field X.

One remarks that zeros of f coincide with zeros of X (if they exist!). These zeros, i.e., the equilibrium positions of the process, are global minimum points and hence critical points of the energy f, but the converse is not true without supplementary conditions. Since

$$\frac{\partial f}{\partial x_j} = \sum_{i=1}^{n} X_i \frac{\partial X_i}{\partial x_j},$$

the hypothesis $\frac{D(X_1, \ldots, X_n)}{D(x_1, \ldots, x_n)} \neq 0$, on D, implies that critical points of the energy f are equilibrium positions and therefore global minimum points; however, there can exist critical points of f which are not zeros of X.

If the energy f is a convex function, then its critical points coincide with the global minimum points (particularly, with zeros of X, if those zeros exist).

Let us investigate the variation of the energy f along the field lines of X. For this we shall use

$$df(X) = D_X f = (D_X X, X)$$

$$|D_X f| \leq \|D_X X\| \|X\| = \sqrt{2} \|D_X X\| \sqrt{f}$$

$$|D_X f| \leq \|D_X X\| \|X\| \leq 2 \|DX\| f,$$

where DX is the Jacobian matrix of X.

We denote by $\alpha : I \to D$ a field line of X. If $D_X X \circ \alpha = 0$, then α is a straight line. Also $(D_X X, X) \circ \alpha = (\|D_X X\| \circ \alpha)(\|X\| \circ \alpha)$ if and only if along $\alpha(t)$ we have $D_X X = \frac{\mu}{2} X$, i.e., α is a straight line reparametrized by $s = h(t)$, $t \in J$, where

$$h(t) = a + b \int_{t_0}^{t} \exp\left(\frac{1}{2} \int_{t_0}^{r} \mu(\alpha(u))du \right) dr, \quad a, b = \text{const}$$

Theorem. *Let f be the energy of the vector field X on D and $\alpha : I \to D$ be a field line of X.*

1) The restriction of f to $\alpha(I)$ is given by

i) $f \circ \alpha(t) = f \circ \alpha(t_0)$ if α is a straight line,

ii) $f \circ \alpha(t) = f \circ \alpha(t_0) \exp \int_{t_0}^{t} \mu(\alpha(u))du$ if α is a straight line reparametrized by $s = h(t)$;

iii) $f\circ\alpha(t) = f\circ\alpha(t_0) + \int_{t_0}^{t}(D_X X, X)\circ\alpha(u)\,du$ *otherwise,*

and it satisfies

$$f\circ\alpha(t_0)\exp(-v(t)) \le f(\alpha(t)) \le f\circ\alpha(t_0)\exp v(t),$$

where $v(t) = 2\int_{t_0}^{t}\|DX\|\circ\alpha(u)\,du$.

2) If X *has no zero on* D, *and* α *is neither a straight line nor a straight line reparametrized by* $s = h(t)$, *then the restriction* $f\circ\alpha$ *satisfies*

$$\left|\sqrt{f\circ\alpha(t)} - \sqrt{f\circ\alpha(t_0)}\right| \le \frac{\sqrt{2}}{2}\int_{t_0}^{t}\|D_X X\|\circ\alpha(u)\,du,\ t \ge t_0.$$

Proof. 1) The first part is a direct consequence of the relations

$$\frac{d}{dt}f\circ\alpha = D_X f\circ\alpha,\ D_X f = (D_X X, X).$$

For the second part we remark that the relation $|D_X f| \le \|DX\|\|X\|^2$ implies $\left|\frac{d}{dt}f\circ\alpha\right| \le 2(\|DX\|\circ\alpha)f\circ\alpha$. This allows to prove that the function

$$\varphi(t) = f\circ\alpha(t)\exp\left(-2\int_{t_0}^{t}\|DX\|\circ\alpha(u)\,du\right)$$

is decreasing on $[t_0, t]\subset I$. Indeed,

$$\frac{d\varphi}{dt} = \left[\frac{d}{dt}f\circ\alpha(t) - 2(\|DX\|\circ\alpha(t))(f\circ\alpha(t))\right]\exp\left(-2\int_{t_0}^{t}\|DX\|\circ\alpha(u)\,du\right) \le 0.$$

The relation $\varphi(t) \le \varphi(t_0)$ implies

$$f\circ\alpha(t) \le f\circ\alpha(t_0)\exp\left(2\int_{t_0}^{t}\|DX\|\circ\alpha(u)\,du\right).$$

Anologously, since the function

$$\psi(t) = f\circ\alpha(t)\exp\left(2\int_{t_0}^{t}\|DX\|\circ\alpha(u)\right)du$$

is increasing, it follows the left-hand part of the double inequality written in the theorem.

2) The relation

$$|D_X f\circ\alpha| \le \sqrt{2}(\|D_X X\|\circ\alpha)\sqrt{f\circ\alpha}$$

is written as

$$\left|\frac{d}{dt}f\circ\alpha\right| \le \sqrt{2}(\|D_X X\|\circ\alpha)\sqrt{f\circ\alpha}$$

and in the hypotheses of the theorem it remains a strict inequality.

The function

$$\varphi(t) = \sqrt{f\circ\alpha(t)} - \frac{\sqrt{2}}{2}\int_{t_0}^{t}\|D_X X\|\circ\alpha(u)\,du$$

satisfies

$$\frac{d\varphi}{dt}(t) = \frac{1}{2\sqrt{f\circ\alpha(t)}}\frac{d}{dt}f\circ\alpha(t) - \frac{\sqrt{2}}{2}\|D_X X\|\circ\alpha(t) < 0$$

on any interval $[t_0, t]\subset I$. Therefore φ is strictly decreasing, and therefore $\varphi(t) \le \varphi(t_0) = \sqrt{f\circ(t_0)}$.

Analogously, one shows that the function

$$\psi(t) = \sqrt{f\circ\alpha(t)} + \frac{\sqrt{2}}{2}\int_{t_0}^{t}\|D_X X\|\circ\alpha(u)\,du$$

is strictly increasing, and hence

$$\psi(t) \ge \psi(t_0) = \sqrt{f\circ\alpha(t_0)}.$$

Remarks. 1) $D_X f = (D_X X, X)$ gives at every point x the initial rate of change of the energy f as the point x moves in the $X(x)$ direction, i.e., (initially) along the field line starting at x tangent to $X(x)$. The zeros of the $(D_X X, X)$ are either zeros of X, zeros of $D_X X$, or points at which $D_X X$ and X are orthogonal vectors.

2) If $D_X f \ge 0$ and α is a field line of X, then $f\circ\alpha$ is an increasing function.

Theorem. *If $(D_X X, X)$ is different from zero at any point of D, then the field lines of X cannot be closed (and therefore nor periodic) curves.*

Proof. Let $\alpha : I\to D$ be a field line of X. Suppose there exist $t_1, t_2 \in I$, $t_1 < t_2$ such that $\alpha(t_1) = \alpha(t_2)$. It follows that $f\circ\alpha(t_1) = f\circ\alpha(t_2)$ and the preceding theorem implies

$$\int_{t_1}^{t_2}\mu(\alpha(u))\,du = 0 \quad\text{or}\quad \int_{t_1}^{t_2}(D_X X, X)\circ\alpha(u)\,du = 0.$$

The Mean Value theorem on $[t_1, t_2]$ implies $(D_X X, X)\circ\alpha(u_0) = 0$, which contradicts the hypothesis.

Theorem. *Let $\alpha : I\to D$ be a field line of X. If α is a straight line reparametrized by $s = h(t)$, $t\in I$, and $\mu\circ\alpha$ is increasing, then $f\circ\alpha : I\to R$ is a convex function. If α is neither a straight line, nor a straight line reparametrized by $s = h(t)$, $t\in I$, and $(D_X X, X)\circ\alpha$ is increasing, then $f\circ\alpha : I\to R$ is convex.*

Proof. We refer to the last part. The hypotheses give

$$\frac{d^2}{dt^2} f \circ \alpha(t) = \frac{d}{dt}(D_X X, X) \circ \alpha(t) \geq 0, \ \forall t \in I.$$

Suppose that X has no zero on D, a hypothesis that permits the construction of the unit vector field $U = \dfrac{X}{\|X\|}$. The field lines of the versor field U are normal representations of the field lines of the vector field X. Knowledge of the nonconstant orbits of a vector field X is equivalent to knowledge of the direction of X. On the other hand, the direction of X is described by the associated versor field.

Suppose that X is a vector field of class C^1 and denote by $Z(X)$ the set of zeros of X on D. Of course the C^1 unit vector field $U = \dfrac{X}{\|X\|}$ is defined on $D \setminus Z(X)$.

Let us show that the restriction of the energy $f = \dfrac{1}{2}\|X\|^2$ to a field line of U is well determined by the restrictions of the scalar fields $\operatorname{div} U$ and $\operatorname{div} X$ to the respective field line. For these we denote by $\beta(s)$, $s \in I$, a field line of U, the parameter s being the curvilinear abscissa.

Theorem. *Set* $l = \|X\| \circ \beta$, $\varphi = \operatorname{div} U \circ \beta$, $\psi = \operatorname{div} X \circ \beta$. *Then*

$$l(s) = \left(l_0 + \int_{s_0}^{s} \psi(r) \exp\left(\int_{s_0}^{s} \varphi(t)dt \right) dr \right) \exp\left(-\int_{s_0}^{s} \varphi(t)dt \right),$$

with $l(s_0) = l_0 > 0$ *arbitrarily given.*

Proof. The relations

$$X = \|X\| U, \ \operatorname{div} X = D_U \|X\| + \|X\| \operatorname{div} U$$

show that

$$\frac{dl}{ds} = -l\varphi + \psi,$$

i.e., the length $l = \sqrt{2f}$ is determined by φ and ψ as a general solution of a linear differential equation of order one. Imposing the initial condition, $l(s_0) = l_0$, we find the solution in the theorem.

If $\varphi(s) > 0$, $\forall s \in I$, then l is uniformly continuous with respect to $l(s_0) = l_0 > 0$. If $s = s_1$ is a critical point of l, then

$$0 = \frac{dl}{ds}(s_1) = -l(s_1)\varphi(s_1) + \psi(s_1).$$

The sign of the derivative

$$\frac{d^2 l}{ds^2}(s_1) = -l(s_1)\frac{d\varphi}{ds}(s_1) + \frac{d\psi}{ds}(s_1)$$

can decide the type of critical point.

Corollary. *If X is a solenoidal vector field, then*

$$l(s) = l(s_0)\exp\left(-\int_{s_0}^{s}\varphi(t)\,dt\right),$$

with $l(s_0) = l_0$ arbitrarily given only if β is not a closed curve.

Proof. Taking into account the relation $0 = \operatorname{div} X = D_U\|X\| + \|X\|\operatorname{div} U$, we find

$$\frac{dl}{ds} = -l\varphi.$$

Consequently, the function in the theorem is the solution of this differential equation.

If $D\setminus Z(X)$ contains a closed field line β of U, then the scalar field defined by $l = \|X\| > 0$ cannot be given arbitrarily on the neighborhood of $\beta(s_0)$ in $\beta(I)$. Indeed, the hypothesis $\beta(a) = \beta(b)$ implies

$$\oint_{\beta}(\operatorname{div} U)\,ds = \int_a^b \varphi(t)\,dt = 0.$$

Corollary. *Let X be a C^1 solenoidal vector field. If* $\operatorname{div} U$ *has no zero in $D\setminus Z(X)$, then the field lines of U cannot be closed.*

Proof. The hypothesis $\beta(a) = \beta(b)$ implies

$$\int_a^b \varphi(t)\,dt = 0.$$

Therefore, there exists $t_0 \in [a,b]$ such that $\varphi(t_0) = 0$, which is contradictory.

If X is a C^1 solenoidal vector field, and $s = s_1$ is a critical point of l, then

$$0 = \frac{dl}{ds}(s_1) = -\,l(s_1)\,\varphi(s_1)$$

and hence $\varphi(s_1) = 0$. Since

$$\frac{d^2 l}{ds^2}(s_1) = -\,l(s_1)\,\frac{d\varphi}{ds}(s_1),$$

the sign of $\dfrac{d\varphi}{ds}(s_1)$ decides the type of the critical point.

9.2. DIFFERENTIAL EQUATIONS OF MOTION IN LAGRANGIAN AND HAMILTONIAN FORM

Let R^n be as a manifold and $TR^n \approx R^{2n}$ be its tangent bundle. The coordinates x^i on R^n induce the coordinates $(x^i, \dot{x}^j)$, $i, j = 1, \ldots, n$ on TR^n, called *tangent coordinates*.

Any function $L : TR^n \to R$ of C^2 class is called a *Lagrangian*, but in motion problems we choose L to be given by the formula

$$L(x,\dot{x}) = \frac{1}{2}\delta_{ij}\dot{x}^i\dot{x}^j - V(x),$$

where $E(x,\dot{x}) = \frac{1}{2}\delta_{ij}\dot{x}^i\dot{x}^j$ is the kinetic energy, and $V(x)$ is the potential energy.

Definition. The variational principle

$$\delta\int_a^b L(x(t),\dot{x}(t))\,dt = 0,$$

where the variation is over smooth curves in R^n with fixed endpoints, is called the *principle of critical action.*

The principle of critical action is unchanged if we replace the integrand $L(x(t),\dot{x}(t))$ by $L(x(t),\dot{x}(t)) - \frac{d}{dt}S(x(t),t)$, for any function $S(x,t)$. This reflects the gauge invariance of classical mechanics and is closely related to Hamilton-Jacobi theory.

Theorem. *The principle of critical action is equivalent to the Euler-Lagrange equations*

$$\frac{d}{dt}\frac{\partial L}{\partial \dot{x}^i} = \frac{\partial L}{\partial x^i}, \quad i = 1, \dots, n,$$

whose solutions are the extremals of the Lagrangian L.

Let $L: TR^n \to R$ be a Lagrangian. Denote by $T^*R^n \approx R^{2n}$ the dual tangent bundle. The mapping

$$\varphi : TR^n \to T^*R^n, \ (x^i,\dot{x}^j) \to (x^i,p_j), \ \ p_j = \frac{\partial L}{\partial \dot{x}^j}$$

is called the *Legendre transformation.*

Definition. The Lagrangian L is called *hyperregular* if φ is a diffeomorphism.

If L is a hyperregular Lagrangian, then the function

$$H : T^*R^n \to R, \ H(x^i,p_j) = \sum p_j\dot{x}^j - L(x^i,\dot{x}^j)$$

is called *Hamiltonian (total mechanical energy).*

Remark. Different Lagrangians can produce the same Hamiltonian.

Theorem. *The Euler-Lagrange equations for L are equivalent to the Hamilton equations*

$$\frac{dp_i}{dt} = -\frac{\partial H}{\partial x^i}, \quad \frac{dx^i}{dt} = \frac{\partial H}{\partial p_i}, \quad i = 1, \dots, n.$$

Finally, we remark that TR^n can be identified with T^*R^n, via the Riemannian metric δ_{ij}, and in this sense we can use throughout the coordinates (x,y).

9.3. NEW GEOMETRICAL MODEL OF PARTICLE DYNAMICS

Now we shall show that any autonomous differential system of order one can be prolonged to a conservative differential system of order two. Equivalently, any flow induces a dynamics of the given vector field or of an associated particle [132]. In geometric dynamics, any nonconstant field line (with chaotic behaviour or not) is a geodesic of a Riemann-Jacobi-Lagrange structure. This new geometric structure blows up at equilibrium points.

Theorem. *Let f be the energy of a C^2 vector field $X = (X_1, \dots, X_n)$ on D. Any orbit of X is a trajectory of a dynamical system (either potential or nonpotential) with n degrees of freedom for which the total energy*

$$H(x,y) = \frac{1}{2}\sum_{i=1}^{n}(y^i)^2 - f(x)$$

is conserved.

Proof. Let

$$\frac{dx^i}{dt} = X_i(x), \quad i = 1, \dots, n, \quad x = (x^1, \dots, x^n)$$

be the differential system that describes the orbits of X. Differentiating along a fixed orbit and denoting

$$\Omega_{ji} = \frac{\partial X_i}{\partial x^j} - \frac{\partial X_j}{\partial x^i} \quad \text{(see rot}X\text{ like a matrix)}$$

we obtain the prolongation

$$\frac{d^2x^i}{dt^2} = \sum_{j=1}^{n}\frac{\partial X_i}{\partial x^j}(x)\frac{dx^j}{dt} = \sum_{j=1}^{n}\frac{\partial X_j}{\partial x^i}(x)\frac{dx^j}{dt} + \sum_{j=1}^{n}\Omega_{ji}\frac{dx^j}{dt}.$$

This can be changed into the conservative prolongation

$$\frac{d^2x^i}{dt^2} = \frac{\partial f}{\partial x^i} + \sum_{j=1}^{n}\Omega_{ji}(x)\frac{dx^j}{dt}. \tag{*}$$

Indeed, multiplying each equation of the system (*) by $\frac{dx^i}{dt}$, summing with respect to i from 1 to n, and taking into account that the matrix $[\Omega_{ji}(x)]$ is skew-symmetric, we find

$$\frac{d}{dt}\left(\frac{1}{2}\sum_{i=1}^{n}\left(\frac{dx^i}{dt}\right)^2 - f(x)\right) = 0.$$

Theorem (Lorentz-Udrişte world-force law). *Every nonconstant trajectory of the dynamical system (*) which corresponds to the total energy H (constant) is a reparametrized horizontal geodesic of the Riemann-Jacobi-Lagrange structure*

$$g_{ij} = (H+f)\,\delta_{ij}, \quad N^i{}_j = \Gamma^i_{jk}y^k + \Omega^i{}_j, \quad i,j,k = 1,2,3.$$

Proof. We shall use the tensorial notations, the Einstein convention for the sum and the Lagrangian

$$L = \frac{1}{2}\delta_{ij}\frac{dx^i}{dt}\frac{dx^j}{dt} - X_i\frac{dx^i}{dt} + f$$

which produces the Hamiltonian

$$H = \frac{1}{2}\delta_{ij}\frac{dx^i}{dt}\frac{dx^j}{dt} - f.$$

The equations of the extremals of L are just the equations (*).

Now we introduce a reparametrization $s = \varphi(t)$, denoting the derivative with respect to s by a dot. We find

$$L = \frac{1}{2}\delta_{ij}\dot{x}^i\dot{x}^j\varphi'^2 - X_j\dot{x}^j\varphi' + f$$

$$\frac{\partial L}{\partial x^j} = -\frac{\partial X_j}{\partial x^i}\dot{x}^j\varphi' + \frac{\partial f}{\partial x^i}, \qquad \frac{\partial L}{\partial\left(\frac{dx^i}{dt}\right)} = \delta_{ij}\dot{x}^j\varphi' - X_i$$

$$\frac{d}{dt}\frac{\partial L}{\partial\left(\frac{dx^i}{dt}\right)} = \delta_{ij}\ddot{x}^j\varphi'^2 + \delta_{ij}\dot{x}^j\varphi'' - \frac{\partial X_i}{\partial x^j}\dot{x}^j\varphi',$$

and consequently the equations of extremals are written

$$\delta_{ij}\ddot{x}^j\varphi'^2 + \delta_{ij}\dot{x}^j\varphi'' = \frac{\partial f}{\partial x^i} + \left(\frac{\partial X_i}{\partial x^j} - \frac{\partial X_j}{\partial x^i}\right)\dot{x}^j\varphi'.$$

Now we use the Riemann-Jacobi metric $g_{ij} = (H+f)\delta_{ij}$, with $H = \text{const} > -f$, and its connection Γ^i_{jk}. If X_i are the components of the vector field X, then $\Omega_{ij} = \partial_i X_j - \partial_j X_i = X_{j,i} - X_{i,j}$ are the components of $\mathrm{rot}X$, where the comma means the covariant derivative with respect to Γ^i_{jk}. If $D_* \subset D$, $u \in TD_*$ and $x = \pi(u)$, then the fields

$$\omega = X_i(\pi(u))dx^i, \ \Omega = \Omega_{ij}(\pi(u))dx^i \wedge dx^j$$

are globally defined on the tangent bundle TD_*.

We denote $\Omega^i{}_j = g^{ih}\Omega_{hj}$, $\Omega^{ij} = g^{jk}\Omega^i{}_k$. The tensor Ω^{ij} is the external tensor field for the following structure.

The functions $\Gamma^i_{jk}y^k$ define a global nonlinear connection [41] on TD_*. We change this nonlinear connection into the nonlinear connection

$$N^i{}_j(x,y) = \Gamma^i_{jk}(x)y^k + \Omega^i{}_j(x), \ x = (x^i), \ y = (y^k).$$

There appears the Riemann-Jacobi-Lagrange manifold $(D_*, g_{ij}, N^i{}_j)$ with the properties:

- the nonlinear connection $N^i{}_j$ is determined by the gravitational potentials $g_{ij}(x)$ and the vector field components $X_i(x)$,

- the horizontal geodesics of the manifold $(D_*, g_{ij}, N^i{}_j)$ are characterized by the equations of Lorentz-Udriste world force

$$\ddot{x}^i + \Gamma^i_{jk}\dot{x}^j\dot{x}^k = -\Omega^i{}_j\dot{x}^j \quad \text{or shortly} \quad \ddot{x}^i + N^i{}_j(x,\dot{x})\dot{x}^j = 0.$$

Reparametrizing the horizontal geodesics by $s = \varphi(t)$, it follows that

$$\delta_{ij}\ddot{x}^j\varphi'^2 + \delta_{ij}\dot{x}^j\frac{df}{dt}\frac{\varphi'}{H+f} = \frac{\partial f}{\partial x^i} - \Omega_{ij}\dot{x}^j\frac{\varphi'}{H+f}.$$

Identifying the differential equations of the extremals with the equations of the horizontal geodesics we find

$$\frac{\varphi''}{\varphi'} = \frac{\frac{df}{dt}}{H+f} \quad \text{or} \quad \varphi' = k(H+f).$$

The condition $k^2 = 2$ is equivalent to

$$g_{ij}\dot{x}^i\dot{x}^j = (H+f)\,\delta_{ij}\frac{dx^i}{dt}\frac{dx^j}{dt}\varphi'^{-2} = 2\,(H+f)^2\varphi'^{-2} = 1.$$

Of course a field hypersurface of **X** is a ruled hypersurface in the Riemann-Jacobi-Lagrange manifold $(D_*, g_{ij}, N^i_{\ j})$. But other properties of such hypersurfaces are still open problems.

Remarks. 1) The trajectories (solutions) of the dynamical system (*) group into three classes: the set of original field lines corresponding to the energy $H = 0$; a set of trajectories for the energy $H = \text{const} < 0$; a set of trajectories for the energy $H = \text{const} > 0$.

2) The connection Γ^i_{jk} blows up at equilibrium points.

3) If $\text{rot}X = 0$, then the dynamical system (*) reduces to a potential one, and the associated geometrical structure is Riemann-Jacobi. If X is a unit vector field, then the naturally associated geometric dynamics is described by a Finsler-Jacobi structure [132].

4) The change of the vector field **X** into **-X** produces the change of $\text{rot}X$ into $-\text{rot}X$.

5) Another prolongation is the nonpotential, nonconservative, dynamical system

$$\frac{d^2x^i}{dt^2} = \frac{\partial f}{\partial x^i} + \sum_{j=1}^n \Omega_{ji}(x)X_j(x),$$

which is similar to the differential system describing a geostrophic wind. The vector field $Y = (Y_1, \ldots, Y_n)$, $Y_i = \sum_{j=1}^n \Omega_{ij}(x)X_j(x)$ corresponds to a dissipation of energy along the solutions α that are not orthogonal to Y.

Open problem. The preceding theory shows that every dynamical system of order one can be prolonged to a suitable dynamical system of order two whose trajectories are geodesics of a Lagrangian defined by the velocity vector field (Lagrange structure of order one). In a similar way every dynamical system of order two can be prolonged to a suitable dynamical system of order four whose trajectories are geodesics of a Lagrangian defined by velocity and acceleration vector fields (Lagrange structure of order two). This point of view can create better examples for higher order Lagrange spaces [42].

9.4. DYNAMICS INDUCED BY AN IRROTATIONAL VECTOR FIELD

Let $X = (X_1, \dots, X_n)$ be a C^2 irrotational vector field on $D \subset R^n$, i.e.,

$$\frac{\partial X_i}{\partial x_j}(x) = \frac{\partial X_j}{\partial x_i}(x), \ \forall x = (x_1, \dots, x_n) \in D, \ i, j = 1, \dots, n.$$

The relations of the definition are equivalent to the fact that for any $x \in D$ the matrix $\left[\frac{\partial X_i}{\partial x_j}(x)\right]$ is symmetric. Also it is known that X is an irrotational vector field on D if and only if it is locally potential.

Let

$$f = \frac{1}{2}\|X\|^2 = \frac{1}{2}\sum_{i=1}^{n} X_i^2$$

be the energy of X. Since

$$\frac{\partial f}{\partial x_j} = \sum_{i=1}^{n} X_i \frac{\partial X_i}{\partial x_j} = \sum_{i=1}^{n} X_i \frac{\partial X_j}{\partial x_i},$$

it follows that $\operatorname{grad} f = D_X X$. Evidently zeros of X are critical points of the energy f, and the set of critical points of f contains the orbits of X which are straight lines. The existence of a field line α of X which is a straight line (equivalent $D_X X = 0$) imposes

$$\operatorname{rank}\left[\frac{\partial X_i}{\partial x_j}(\alpha(t))\right] \le n - 1.$$

If $x_0 \in D$ is a critical point of the energy f and $\operatorname{rank}\left[\frac{\partial X_i}{\partial x_j}(x_0)\right] = n$, then x_0 is a zero of X.

If the quadratic form $Y_x \to (D_{Y_x} X, Y_x)$, $Y_x \in T_x D$ is positive definite for any $x \in D$, then the critical points of f are zeros of X. Indeed, the relation $(\operatorname{grad} f, X) = D_X f = (D_X X, X)$ confirms this statement.

The matrix of the Hessian $d^2 f$ has the elements

$$\frac{\partial^2 f}{\partial x_j \partial x_k} = \sum_{i=1}^{n} \frac{\partial X_i}{\partial x_j}\frac{\partial X_i}{\partial x_k} + \sum_{i=1}^{n} X_i \frac{\partial^2 X_i}{\partial x_j \partial x_k},$$

and the matrix of elements $\sum_{i=1}^{n} \frac{\partial X_i}{\partial x_j} \frac{\partial X_i}{\partial x_k}$ is positive semidefinite. If the matrix of elements $\sum_{i=1}^{n} X_i \frac{\partial^2 X_i}{\partial x_j \partial x_k}$ is also positive semidefinite, then the energy f is convex on D.

Computing the trace of the Hessian, we find the Laplacian

$$\Delta f = \sum_{i,j=1}^{n} \frac{\partial X_i}{\partial x_j} \frac{\partial X_i}{\partial x_j} + \sum_{i,j=1}^{n} X_i \frac{\partial^2 X_j}{\partial x_i \partial x_j} = \sum_{i,j=1}^{n} \left(\frac{\partial X_i}{\partial x_j} \right)^2 + D_X(\operatorname{div} X).$$

Theorem. *Let X be a C^2 irrotational vector field on D. If $\operatorname{div} X$ is an increasing function along the field lines of X, then the critical points of the energy f can be only minimum or saddle points.*

Proof. Let $\alpha : I \to D$ be a field line of X. The hypothesis that $\operatorname{div} X \circ \alpha$ is an increasing function is equivalent to $D_X(\operatorname{div} X) \geq 0$. It follows that $\Delta f \geq 0$, i.e., f is a subharmonic function.

Corollary. *Let X be a C^2 irrotational vector field on D. If any nonzero vector $X(x)$ satisfies $D_{X(x)}(\operatorname{div} X) > 0$ and the energy f attains a local maximum at a point $x_0 \in D$, then X vanishes identically on a neighborhood of x_0.*

Proof. Suppose that x_0 is a local maximum point (necessarily a critical point) of the energy f and $X(x_0) \neq 0$. It follows that the Hessian $d^2 f(x_0)$ is negative semidefinite and hence $\Delta f(x_0) \leq 0$. On the other hand, $\Delta f > 0$ at any point x with $X(x) \neq 0$ which is a contradiction. It remains that $X(x_0) = 0$. Since $f(x_0) = 0$ is a maximum, the energy f and therefore the vector field X must vanish identically on a neighborhood of x_0.

Remark. The condition $D_X(\operatorname{div} X) > 0$ implies the fact that $\operatorname{div} X$ is a strictly increasing function on the field lines of X.

Corollary. *Let X be a C^2 irrotational and solenoidal ($\Rightarrow$ harmonic) vector field on D. The critical points of the energy f can be only minimum or saddle points.*

Remarks. 1) The theory of magnetic traps requires the investigation of the point at which the energy of the magnetic field is a minimum, without these points being zeros of the field (see Chapter 10).

2) Let $X = (X_1, \ldots, X_n)$ be a harmonic vector field on D. Obviously each component X_i is a harmonic function. On the other hand a nonconstant harmonic function on D (open and connected set) has no extrema on D (hence it can have only saddle points on D). If the domain D is bounded and the harmonic function on D is continuous on ∂D, then the minimum and maximum of the function are attained on ∂D.

Considering the general relation

$$\Delta f = \sum_{i,j=1}^{n} \left(\frac{\partial X_i}{\partial x_j} \right)^2 + \sum_{i=1}^{n} X_i \Delta X_i ,$$

we deduce that for a harmonic vector field X, the critical points of the energy f and of partial energies $\frac{1}{2} X_1^2, \ldots, \frac{1}{2} X_n^2$ can be minimum or saddle points only.

The irrotational vector fields are local potential fields, i.e., for every $x_0 \in D$ there exists an open set $U \subset D$ that contains x_0 and a real function $\varphi : U \to R$ such that $X = \text{grad}\varphi$ on U. Thus $f|_U = \frac{1}{2} \|\text{grad}\varphi\|^2$. The constant level sets (hypersurfaces) $\varphi(x) = c$ are orthogonal to the field lines of X.

Theorem. *Let X be a C^2 irrotational vector field on D, and $f = \frac{1}{2} \|X\|^2$ be its energy. Any orbit of X is a trajectory of the potential dynamical system with n degrees of freedom*

$$\frac{d^2 x}{dt^2} = \text{grad} f.$$

Every nonconstant trajectory of this dynamical system, which correspond to a constant value H of the Hamiltonian, is a reparametrized geodesic of the Riemann-Jacobi manifold

$$(D \setminus Z(X),\ g_{ij} = (H+f)\delta_{ij},\ i,j=1,2,3),$$

where $Z(\mathbf{X})$ is the set of zeros of the irrotational vector field.

9.5. DYNAMICS INDUCED BY A KILLING VECTOR FIELD

Let $X = (X_1, \ldots, X_n)$ be a C^∞ vector field on R^n. The vector field X is a Killing vector field on R^n, i.e.,

$$\frac{\partial X_i}{\partial x_j} + \frac{\partial X_j}{\partial x_i} = 0,\ i,j = 1, \ldots, n$$

if and only if

$$X(x) = Ax + b, \; x \in R^n,$$

where $A = [a_{ij}]$ is a skew-symmetric matrix of order n. The rank of A is an even number (see 2.6).

The energy of the Killing vector field X is the real function defined by

$$f(x) = \frac{1}{2} \|Ax + b\|^2.$$

Because

$$\frac{\partial f}{\partial x_j} = \sum_{i=1}^{n} X_i \frac{\partial X_i}{\partial x_j} = -\sum_{i=1}^{n} X_i \frac{\partial X_j}{\partial x_i},$$

it follows that

$$\mathrm{grad} f = -D_X X, \; D_X f = 0.$$

These relations make obvious the assertions that zeros of X (if they exist!) are critical points of f, and that the set of critical points includes all the orbits of X, inclusive those that are straight lines (i.e., the energy f is a constant along each orbit).

Since

$$\frac{\partial^2 f}{\partial x_j \partial x_k} = \sum_{i=1}^{n} \frac{\partial X_i}{\partial x_j} \frac{\partial X_i}{\partial x_k}$$

is a positive semidefinite matrix, the energy f is a convex function on R^n. Therefore its critical points (if they exist!) are global minimum points, and hence they coincide with zeros of X. The constant level sets of the energy f are hyperquadrics, and the global flow generated on R^n by $\mathrm{grad} f$ (a complete vector field) increases the volume excepting the case in which X is parallel.

The convexity of f and the preceding remarks show that there are exactly three mutually exclusive possibilities:

1) the set of zeros of X is a hyperplane of even codimension;

2) the union of the orbits of X, which are (nonconstant) straight lines, is a nonvoid, closed and convex set;

3) the energy f has no minimum points.

Theorem. *Let $X(x) = Ax + b$ be a Killing vector field on R^n and f be its energy. Any orbit of X is a trajectory of the potential dynamical system with n degrees of freedom*

$$\frac{d^2 x}{dt^2} = -\mathrm{grad} f.$$

The geometric dynamics (see 9.3) described by this second order differential system is induced by a Killing vector field.

9.6. DYNAMICS INDUCED BY A CONFORMAL VECTOR FIELD

Let $X = (X_1, \dots, X_n)$ be a vector field of class C^∞ on R^n, $n > 2$. Suppose that X is a conformal vector field, i.e.,

$$\frac{\partial X_i}{\partial x_j} + \frac{\partial X_j}{\partial x_i} = \psi\, \delta_{ij}, \quad \psi = \frac{2}{n}\,\mathrm{div}X, \quad i, j = 1, \dots, n.$$

The general solution of this system of partial differential equations is (see 2.7)

$$X_j(x) = \frac{1}{2} x_j \sum_{k=1}^{n} c_k x_k - \frac{1}{4} c_j \sum_{i=1}^{n} x_i^2 + \sum_{k=1}^{n} c_{jk} x_k + d_j,$$

$$c_{ij} + c_{ji} = c\,\delta_{ij}, \quad \psi(x) = \sum_{k=1}^{n} c_k x_k + c.$$

Let $f = \frac{1}{2}\|X\|^2$ be the energy of the conformal vector field X. We find

$$\frac{\partial f}{\partial x_j} = \sum_{i=1}^{n} X_i \frac{\partial X_i}{\partial x_j} = -\sum_{i=1}^{n} X_i \frac{\partial X_j}{\partial x_i} + \psi X_j,$$

i.e.,

$$\mathrm{grad} f = -D_X X + \psi X, \; D_X f = \psi f.$$

These relations imply:

1) Zeros of X (if they exist!) are critical points of the energy f.

2) Critical points of the energy f are either zeros of the energy f or zeros of $\mathrm{div}X$.

3) The set of critical points of the energy f includes the orbits of X which are straight lines reparametrized by

$$s = a + b\int_{t_0}^{t} \exp\left(\int_{t_0}^{r} \psi(\alpha(u))du\right) dr.$$

The matrix of the Hessian $d^2 f$ of the energy f has the components

$$\frac{\partial^2 f}{\partial x_j \partial x_k} = \sum_{i=1}^{n} \frac{\partial X_i}{\partial x_j}\frac{\partial X_i}{\partial x_k} + \sum_{i=1}^{n} X_i \frac{\partial^2 X_i}{\partial x_j \partial x_k} = \sum_{i=1}^{n} \frac{\partial X_i}{\partial x_j}\frac{\partial X_i}{\partial x_k}$$

$$+ \frac{1}{2}\left(X_j c_k + X_k c_j - \delta_{jk}\sum_{i=1}^{n} c_j X_i\right).$$

It follows that the Laplacian

$$\Delta f = \sum_{i,j=1}^{n}\left(\frac{\partial X_i}{\partial x_j}\right)^2 + \frac{2-n}{2}\sum_{i=1}^{n} c_i X_i.$$

Theorem. *Let X be a conformal vector field on R^n and f be its energy. If $\alpha : I \to R^n$ is a field line of X, then*

$$f \circ \alpha(t) = f \circ \alpha(t_0) \exp\left(\int_{t_0}^{t} \psi(\alpha(u))du\right).$$

Proof. Consequence of the relations

$$\frac{d}{dt} f \circ \alpha = D_X f \circ \alpha, \; D_X f = \psi f.$$

Remark. Zeros of the vector field X coincide with zeros of the energy f.

Particularly, let $X = (X_1, \ldots, X_n)$ be a homothetic vector field on R^n, with $\psi = c \neq 0$, i.e.,

$$X_i(x) = \sum_{k=1}^{n} c_{jk} x_h + d_j, \; c_{11} + \cdots + c_{nn} = \frac{n}{2} c \neq 0.$$

If $f = \frac{1}{2}\|X\|^2$ is the energy of the homothetic vector field X, then:

1) critical points of f are zeros of X,

2) the energy f is a proper function of the operator X with respect to the proper value c,

3) the energy f is convex,

4) the field lines of X cannot be closed.

Theorem. *Let X be a conformal vector field on R^n, $n \geq 3$, and f be its energy. Every orbit of X is a trajectory of the conservative (nonpotential) dynamical system with n*

degrees of freedom

$$\frac{d^2 x_i}{dt^2} = \frac{\partial f}{\partial x_i} + \sum_j (c_j x_i - c_i x_j + c_{ij} - c_{ji}) \frac{dx_j}{dt}.$$

This second order differential system describes the geometric dynamics (see 9.3) induced by a conformal vector field.

9.7. DYNAMICS INDUCED BY AN AFFINE VECTOR FIELD

Let $X = (X_1, \ldots, X_n)$ be a vector field of class C^∞ on R^n. The vector field X is affine, i.e.,

$$\frac{\partial^2 X_i}{\partial x_j \partial x_k} = 0, \quad i, j, k = 1, \ldots, n$$

if and only if $X(x) = Ax + b$, $x \in R^n$, where $A = [a_{ij}]$ is a constant quadratic matrix, and b is a constant (parallel) column vector.

Let $f(x) = \frac{1}{2} \|Ax + b\|^2$ be the energy of the affine vector field X. One finds

$$D_Y f = (AY, Ax + b), \ \forall\, Y \in \mathcal{X}(R^n),$$

and therefore zeros of X (if they exist!) are critical points of the energy f. Particularly, the relations

$$D_X X = A(Ax + b), \ D_X f = (A(Ax + b), Ax + b)$$

show that the set of critical points of the energy f contains the field lines of X which are straight lines. The existence of a field line α of X which is a straight line of R^n imposes $\operatorname{rank} A \le n - 1$. If $x_0 \in R^n$ is a critical point of the energy f and $\operatorname{rank} A = n$, then x_0 is a zero of X.

The gradient of the energy f has the components

$$\frac{\partial f}{\partial x_j} = \sum_{i=1}^n \frac{\partial X_i}{\partial x_j} X_i = \sum_{i=1}^n a_{ij} X_i .$$

The matrix of the Hessian $d^2 f$ of the energy f has the components

$$\frac{\partial^2 f}{\partial x_j \partial x_k} = \sum_{i=1}^n \frac{\partial X_i}{\partial x_j} \frac{\partial X_i}{\partial x_k} = \sum_{i=1}^n a_{ij} a_{ik} .$$

Thus $d^2f \geq 0$ and hence the energy f is a convex function on R^n. This result implies the fact that critical points of f (if they exist!) coincide with global minimum points of f, and therefore with zeros of X. Also, the flow determined on R^n by $\text{grad} f$ (complete vector field) increases the volume excepting the case in which X is a parallel vector field.

The geometric dynamics (see 9.3) induced by an affine vector field is described by the second order differential system in the next

Theorem. *Let X be an affine vector field on R^n and f be its energy. Every orbit of X is a trajectory of the conservative (nonpotential) dynamical system with n degrees of freedom*

$$\frac{d^2x_i}{dt^2} = \frac{\partial f}{\partial x_i} + \sum_j (a_{ij} - a_{ji}) \frac{dx_j}{dt}.$$

9.8. DYNAMICS INDUCED BY A PROJECTIVE VECTOR FIELD

Let $X = (X_1, \ldots, X_n)$ be a C^∞ vector field on R^n, $n \geq 2$. The vector field X is projective, i.e.,

$$\frac{\partial^2 X_i}{\partial x_j \partial x_k} = c_j \delta_{ik} + c_k \delta_{ij}, \; i, j, k = 1, \ldots, n,$$

if and only if

$$X_i(x) = x_i \sum_{j=1}^n c_j x_j + \sum_{j=1}^n a_{ij} x_j + d_i.$$

The gradient of the energy $f = \frac{1}{2} \|X\|^2$ has the components

$$\frac{\partial f}{\partial x^j} = X_j \sum_{k=1}^n c_k x_k + c_j \sum_{i=1}^n X_i x_i + \sum_{i=1}^n a_{ij} X_i.$$

Obviously, zeros of the vector field X (if they exist!) are critical points of f. Computing the second partial derivatives, we find

$$\frac{\partial^2 f}{\partial x_j \partial x_k} = \sum_{i=1}^n \frac{\partial X_i}{\partial x_j} \frac{\partial X_i}{\partial x_k} + \sum_{i=1}^n X_i \frac{\partial^2 X_i}{\partial x_j \partial x_k}$$

$$= \sum_{i=1}^n \frac{\partial X_i}{\partial x_j} \frac{\partial X_i}{\partial x_k} + \sum_{i=1}^n X_i (c_j \delta_{ik} + c_k \delta_{ij}) = \sum_{i=1}^n \frac{\partial X_i}{\partial x_j} \frac{\partial X_i}{\partial x_k} + X_k c_j + X_j c_k$$

and

$$\Delta f = \sum_{i,j=1}^n \left(\frac{\partial X_i}{\partial x_j} \right)^2 + 2 \sum_{i=1}^n c_i X_i = \sum_{i,j=1}^n \left(\frac{\partial X_i}{\partial x_j} \right)^2 + \frac{2}{n+1} D_X(\text{div} X).$$

The geometric dynamics (see 9.3) induced by a projective vector field is described by the dynamical system in the following

Theorem. *Let X be a projective vector field on R^n, $n \geq 2$, and f be its energy. Any orbit of X is a trajectory of the conservative (nonpotential) dynamical system with n degrees of freedom*

$$\frac{d^2 x_i}{dt^2} = \frac{\partial f}{\partial x_i} + \sum_j (c_j x_i - c_i x_j + a_{ij} - a_{ji}) \frac{dx_j}{dt}.$$

9.9. DYNAMICS INDUCED BY A TORSE FORMING VECTOR FIELD

Let $X = (X_1, \dots, X_n)$ be a torse forming vector field on $D \subset R^n$, i.e., X is of class C^∞ and

$$\frac{\partial X_i}{\partial x_j} = a\delta_{ij} + X_i Y_j,\ i, j = 1, \dots, n,$$

where a is a C^∞ scalar field on D and $Y = (Y_1, \dots, Y_n)$ is a C^∞ vector field on D. The energy

$$f = \frac{1}{2} \|X\|^2$$

satisfies

$$\frac{\partial f}{\partial x_j} = \sum_{i=1}^n X_i \frac{\partial X_i}{\partial x_j} = aX_j + 2fY_j.$$

It follows that

$$\mathrm{grad} f = aX + 2fY,\ D_X f = 2(a + (X, Y))f.$$

Thus:

1) Zeros of X (zeros of f, global minimum points of f) are critical points of f.

2) Critical points of the energy f are critical points of f or zeros of $a + (X, Y)$.

By direct calculation we find

$$\frac{\partial^2 f}{\partial x_i \partial x_k} = X_j \frac{\partial a}{\partial x_k} + 2f \frac{\partial Y_j}{\partial x_k} + a^2 \delta_{jk} + aX_j Y_k + 2aX_k Y_j + 4f Y_j Y_k,$$

$$\Delta f = D_X a + 2f \mathrm{div}\, Y + na^2 + 3(X, Y)a + 4f\|Y\|^2.$$

Theorem. *Let X be a torse forming vector field on $D \subset R^n$. If x_0 is a local maximum point of the energy f and $a(x_0) \neq 0$, then x_0 is a zero of $a + (X, Y)$.*

Proof. Let x_0 be a local maximum point of the energy f. Then x_0 is a critical point of f (and therefore either a zero of f or a zero of $a + (X, Y)$), and $\Delta f(x_0) \leq 0$. Suppose $X(x_0) = 0$. It follows that $\Delta f(x_0) = na^2(x_0) > 0$, a contradiction! It remains that $X(x_0) \neq 0$ and hence x_0 is a zero of $a + (X, Y)$.

The field lines of a torse forming vector field X are reparametrized straight lines. The expression of the energy f of X along a field line $\alpha : I \to D$ is

$$f \circ \alpha(t) = f \circ \alpha(t_0) \exp\left(2\int_{t_0}^{t} (a + (X, Y)) \circ \alpha(u)\right) du.$$

This formula shows that f is either a constant or has an exponential variation on the field lines of X. If $(a + (X, Y)) \circ \alpha$ is increasing, then $f \circ \alpha$ is convex.

The geometric dynamics (see 9.3) induced by a torse forming vector field is realized by the following dynamical system.

Theorem. *Let X be a torse forming vector field on $D \subset R^n$, and f be its energy. Every orbit of X is a trajectory of the conservative (nonpotential) dynamical system with n degrees of freedom*

$$\frac{d^2 x_i}{dt^2} = \frac{\partial f}{\partial x_i} + \sum_j (X_i Y_j - X_j Y_i) \frac{dx_j}{dt}.$$

9.10. ENERGY OF THE HAMILTONIAN VECTOR FIELD

Let us consider the Hamiltonian $H : R^{2n} \to R$, $(x,y) \to H(x,y)$ of class C^3 and the Hamiltonian vector field

$$X = (X_i, X_{n+i}),\ X_i = -\frac{\partial H}{\partial y_i},\ X_{n+i} = \frac{\partial H}{\partial x_i},\ i = 1, \dots, n.$$

Of course the Hamiltonian vector field X is solenoidal, i.e., $\mathrm{div} X = 0$. We denote

$$Y = \mathrm{grad}\, H = \left(\frac{\partial H}{\partial x_i}, \frac{\partial H}{\partial y_i}\right)$$

and we remark that $X = JY$, where

$$J = \begin{bmatrix} 0 & -I \\ I & 0 \end{bmatrix}$$

is the matrix of the canonical complex structure of R^{2n}.

The energy $f = \frac{1}{2}\|X\|^2$ of the Hamiltonian vector field X can be written as

$$f = \frac{1}{2}\|\mathrm{grad} H\|^2.$$

This result is not accidental. It is a consequence of the fact that X is obtained from $\mathrm{grad} H$ by the rotation given by the matrix J (X and $\mathrm{grad} H$ are orthogonal vector fields, i.e., X is a vector field tangent to the constant level hypersurfaces attached to the function H), and shows that zeros of f are critical points of H.

Let $\alpha : I \to R^{2n}$ be a gradient line of H. The function $f \circ \alpha$ is monotonically increasing. If $I = [t_0, \infty)$ and there exists $\lim_{t \to \infty} \alpha(t) = x_1$, then x_1 is a critical point of H (a zero of X) and therefore a zero of f (see 5.1).

The vector field $Y = \operatorname{grad} H$ is irrotational and hence

$$\operatorname{grad} f = D_Y Y = D_{-JX}(-JX) = D_{JX} JX.$$

Thus one observes that zeros of X are critical points of f and that the set of critical points of f contains the orbits of JX which are straight lines.

We denote $x_{n+i} = y_i$ and we use the indices $\alpha, \beta, \gamma = i, n+i$. The matrix of the Hessian of f has the elements

$$\frac{\partial^2 f}{\partial x_\alpha \partial x_\beta} = \sum_{\gamma=1}^{2n} \frac{\partial Y_\gamma}{\partial x_\alpha} \frac{\partial Y_\gamma}{\partial x_\beta} + \sum_{\gamma=1}^{2n} Y_\gamma \frac{\partial^2 Y_\gamma}{\partial x_\alpha \partial x_\beta} = \sum_{\gamma=1}^{2n} \frac{\partial X_\gamma}{\partial x_\alpha} \frac{\partial X_\gamma}{\partial x_\beta} + \sum_{\gamma=1}^{2n} X_\gamma \frac{\partial^2 X_\gamma}{\partial x_\alpha \partial x_\beta}.$$

Considering that $\dfrac{\partial Y_\gamma}{\partial x_\alpha} = \dfrac{\partial Y_\alpha}{\partial x_\gamma}$, we find the Laplacian

$$\Delta f = \sum_{\alpha,\gamma=1}^{2n} \left(\frac{\partial Y_\gamma}{\partial x_\alpha} \right)^2 + D_Y(\operatorname{div} Y) = \sum_{\alpha,\gamma=1}^{2n} \left(\frac{\partial X_\gamma}{\partial x_\alpha} \right)^2 + D_{JX}(\operatorname{div} JX).$$

Also, we have $\operatorname{div} JX = -\Delta H$. Consequently, the following statements are true:

1) JX is a solenoidal vector field if and only if H is a harmonic scalar field;

2) If H is a harmonic scalar field, then f is a subharmonic scalar field.

Theorem. *Let X be a Hamiltonian vector field on R^{2n}. If every nonzero vector $X(x)$ satisfies $D_{JX(x)}(\operatorname{div} JX) > 0$ and the energy f attains a local maximum at a point x_0, then X vanishes identically on a neighborhood of x_0.*

Proof. Suppose that x_0 is a local maximum point of f (necessarily a critical point of f) and $X(x_0) \neq 0$. It follows that the Hessian $d^2 f(x_0)$ is negative semidefinite and hence $\Delta f(x_0) \leq 0$. On the other hand, $\Delta f > 0$ at any point at which X is not zero, a contradiction. It remains that $X(x_0) = 0$. Because $f(x_0) = 0$ is a maximum, the function f and therefore X must vanish identically on a neighborhood of x_0.

At the end let us consider the Hamiltonian

$$H(x,y) = \frac{1}{2} y^2 + V(x), \; x \in I \subset R, \; y \in R$$

which is attached to a potential dynamical system with one degree of freedom, with V as a function of class C^3. Here, the Hamiltonian vector field is $(-y, V'(x))$ and has the energy $f(x,y) = \frac{1}{2}(V'^2(x) + y^2)$. The energy f is lower bounded, but it is not upper bounded. Also, any critical point x_0 of V produces a global minimum point $(x_0, 0)$ of f.

Since $df(x,y) = V'(x)V''(x)dx + ydy$, the critical points of the energy are the solutions of the system $V'(x)V''(x) = 0$, $y = 0$. Between these points are found $(x_0, 0)$, where x_0 is an extremum or inflexion point for the function V.

Using the Hessian $d^2f(x,y) = (V'(x)V''(x))'dx^2 + dy^2$ we deduce that f is convex if and only if the function $V'V''$ is increasing. Also, $\Delta f = 1 + (V'V'')'$ and hence $f: I \times R \to R$ can be harmonic. Indeed, the differential equation $1 + (V'V'')' = 0$ admits the solutions

$$V(x) = \pm\left(\frac{x-b}{2}\sqrt{-x^2+2bx+c} - \frac{b^2+c}{2}\arcsin\frac{b-x}{\sqrt{b^2+c}} + d\right),$$

which are of class C^3.

We consider the differential system

$$\frac{dx}{dt} = -y, \quad \frac{dy}{dt} = V'(x)$$

which describes the field lines of the vector field $(-y, V'(x))$ and suppose that $(x_0, 0)$ is an equilibrium point. Using the linear approximation

$$\frac{dx}{dt} = -y, \quad \frac{dy}{dt} = V''(x_0)(x-x_0),$$

we find the following conclusions:

1) if $V''(x_0) \geq 0$, then the equilibrium point $(x_0, 0)$ is stable;

2) if $V''(x_0) < 0$ (it follows that x_0 is a maximum point of V), then the equilibrium point $(x_0, 0)$ is unstable.

9.11. KINEMATIC SYSTEMS OF CLASSICAL THERMODYNAMICS

The first goal is to analyse some properties of the Bobbio-Marrucci kinematic systems of thermodynamics, insisting on the behaviour of the fundamental scalar fields of thermodynamics along the field lines. The second goal is to find the Monge representations of Lorenz, Goodwin and Euler vector fields [134].

9.11.1. Monge representation and Bobbio-Marrucci result

In the theory of vector fields on R^3, the Monge Theorem is wellknown (see 2.4): *If F is a C^∞ vector field on an open connected subset $D \subset R^3$, then for any $x_0 \in D$ with $\mathrm{rot}F(x_0) \neq 0$ there exists an open subset $U \subset D$ that contains x_0 and three scalar fields h, f, g of class C^∞ on U, such that*

$$F|_U = f\nabla g + \nabla h,$$

where ∇ *is the gradient operator.*

The scalar fields f, g, h are called *Monge potentials* of the vector field F. They are not unique.

On spaces R^n, with $n > 3$, there exist vector fields that do not admit a Monge representation.

Let R^n, $n \le 8$, be the representative space of the classical thermodynamics. A point in this space will be denoted by $x = (x_1, \dots, x_n)$.

We consider the fundamental C^∞ scalar fields

$$U, T, S : R^n \to R$$

which represent the *internal energy*, the *absolute temperature* and the *entropy* respectively. The scalar field $A = U - TS$ is called the *Helmholtz free energy*.

Bobbio and Marrucci [6] have shown that the classical equations of thermodynamics can be transcribed in the language of the theory of vector fields on R^n using the vector field (Monge representation) $F = T\nabla S - \nabla U$ or, equivalently, $F = -S\nabla T - \nabla A$. Obviously the result is meaningful for $n > 3$.

Let $\alpha_x : I \to R^n$ be the maximal field line of F that satisfies the initial conditions $\alpha_x(0) = x$. The flow T_t generated by F is defined by $T_t(x) = \alpha_x(t)$.

9.11.2. Behavior of U, T, S, A along field lines of the vector field $F = T\nabla S - \nabla U$

In this section, suppose $\alpha(t)$, $t \in I$ is a maximal nonconstant field line of the C^∞ vector field $F = T\nabla S - \nabla U$ at $x \in R^n$. Let there be the scalar fields

$$\varphi = T\|\nabla S\| - \|\nabla U\|, \quad \psi = T\|\nabla S\| + \|\nabla U\|.$$

Theorem. *0) Suppose* $\nabla U \perp \nabla S$ *along* α. *If* $T \circ \alpha \ge 0$, *then the function* $S \circ \alpha$ *is increasing. If* $T \circ \alpha \le 0$, *then the function* $S \circ \alpha$ *is decreasing.*

1) If $\varphi \circ \alpha \ge 0$, *then* $T \circ \alpha \ge 0$ *and the function* $S \circ \alpha$ *is increasing. In this case the critical points of* $S \circ \alpha$ *(if any) are minimum points, and the curve* α *cannot be closed excepting the case when it is included in the critical set of* S.

2) If $\varphi \circ \alpha \le 0$, *then* $T \circ \alpha \le 0$ *and the function* $S \circ \alpha$ *is decreasing. In this case the critical points of* $S \circ \alpha$ *(if any) are maximum points, and the curve* α *can be closed only if it is included in the critical set of* S.

Proof. Using the chain rule for derivatives and the Cauchy-Schwarz inequality for the scalar product, we obtain

$$\frac{d(S \circ \alpha)}{dt} = (\nabla S, T\nabla S - \nabla U)(\alpha(t)) = T\|\nabla S\|^2 - (\nabla S, \nabla U)|_{\alpha(t)}.$$

It follows that the zeros of F are critical points of $S \circ \alpha$. Also

$$\|\nabla S\|(T\|\nabla S\| - \|\nabla U\|)\,|_{\alpha(t)} \le \frac{d(S\circ\alpha)}{dt} \le \|\nabla S\|(T\|\nabla S\| + \|\nabla U\|)\,|_{\alpha(t)}.$$

1) $\dfrac{d(S\circ\alpha)}{dt}(t) \ge 0, \forall t \in I$, i.e., $S\circ\alpha$ is increasing.

Suppose that α is closed, i.e., $\alpha(t_1) = \alpha(t_2)$ for $t_1 < t_2$, and $\alpha(I)$ is not included in the set of critical points of S. There follows the contradiction

$$0 = S(\alpha(t))\Big|_{t_1}^{t_2} = \int_{t_1}^{t_2} \frac{d(S\circ\alpha)}{dt}\,dt > 0.$$

Theorem. *0) If $\nabla U \perp \nabla S$ along α, then $U\circ\alpha$ is decreasing.*

1) Let $T\circ\alpha \ge 0$, and $\varphi\circ\alpha \le 0$ or $T\circ\alpha \le 0$ and $\psi\circ\alpha \ge 0$. Then $U\circ\alpha$ is decreasing. In these cases the critical points of $U\circ\alpha$ (if any) are maximum points, and the curve α can be closed only if it is included in the critical set of U.

Proof. First we use the chain rule for derivatives,

$$\frac{d(U\circ\alpha)}{dt} = (\nabla U, T\nabla S - \nabla U)(\alpha(t)) = T(\nabla U, \nabla S) - \|\nabla U\|^2\,|_{\alpha(t)}.$$

Now we take into account the Cauchy-Schwarz inequality for the scalar product. For $T\circ\alpha \ge 0$ we find

$$-\|\nabla U\|(T\|\nabla S\| + \|\nabla U\|) \le \frac{d(U\circ\alpha)}{dt} \le \|\nabla U\|(T\|\nabla S\| - \|\nabla U\|).$$

For $T\circ\alpha \le 0$ we obtain

$$-\|\nabla U\|(T\|\nabla S\| + \|\nabla U\|) \le \frac{d(U\circ\alpha)}{dt} \le -\|\nabla U\|(T\|\nabla S\| + \|\nabla U\|)$$

and the final part of the proof is similar to those of the preceding theorem.

Suppose $\alpha(t)$, $t \in I$ is included in a constant level set of T. If this set is described by the equation $T(x) = T_0$, then it follows that

$$\frac{d\alpha}{dt} = \nabla(T_0 S - U)$$

and therefore α is a gradient line of $T_0 S - U$. So the following theorem is valid (see 5.1).

Theorem. *Let $I = (\omega_-(x), \omega_+(x))$ and $\alpha : I \to R^n$ be a maximal gradient line of $T_0 S - U$. Denote by $T_t(x)$ the gradient flow. Then the following assertions hold true.*

1) α is a curve of maximal local increase of $T_0 S - U$; consequently there exist the limits

$$\lim_{t\downarrow\omega_-(x)} (T_0 S - U)(T_t(x)), \qquad \lim_{t\uparrow\omega_+(x)} (T_0 S - U)(T_t(x)).$$

2) α is a closed curve only in the case when it reduces to a critical point of $T_0 S - U$.

3) If $\omega_+(x)$ *is finite, then* $\lim_{t \uparrow \omega_+(x)} (T_0 S - U)(T_t(x)) = \infty$.

4) If $\omega_+(x) = \infty$, *and there exists* $\lim_{t \to \infty} \alpha(t) = x_0$, *then* x_0 *is a critical point of* $T_0 S - U$.

The preceding theorems have the following

Corollary. *If* α *is a nonconstant closed field line of* F, *then it must pass from the region of* R^n *described by* $T(x) < 0$ *to the region described by* $T(x) > 0$, *transversal to the "hypersurface" described by* $T(x) = 0$.

Now we consider the functions $A = U - TS$ and $A \circ \alpha$. It follows that

$$\frac{d(A \circ \alpha)}{dt} = (\nabla A, T\nabla S - \nabla U)(\alpha(t)) = -\|T\nabla S - \nabla U\|^2 - S(\nabla T, T\nabla S - \nabla U)\big|_{\alpha(t)}.$$

Theorem. *If* ∇T *and* $F = T\nabla S - \nabla U$ *are orthogonal vector fields, then* $A \circ \alpha$ *is decreasing. In this case the critical points of* $A \circ \alpha$ *(if any) are maximum points, and the curve* α *cannot be closed.*

Proof.

$$\frac{d(A \circ \alpha)}{dt} = -\|T\nabla S - \nabla U\|^2(\alpha(t)) \leq 0.$$

Remark. Particularly, this theorem is true when the level "hypersurfaces" attached to the fundamental scalar fields U, T, S are mutually orthogonal.

Examples. 1) Suppose U, T, S are linear forms on R^n, i.e.,

$$U = \sum_{i=1}^{n} u_i x_i, \quad T = \sum_{i=1}^{n} t_i x_i, \quad S = \sum_{i=1}^{n} s_i x_i,$$

where u_i, t_i, s_i are constants and $x = {}^t(x_1, \ldots, x_n) \in R^n$.

The differential system (kinematic system)

$$\frac{dx_i}{dt} = s_i \sum_{j=1}^{n} t_j x_j - u_i, \; i = 1, \ldots, n$$

admits the general solution

$$x = e^{At}\left[x_0 - \left(\frac{t}{1!}I - \frac{t^2}{2!}A + \cdots + (-1)^n \frac{t^{n+1}}{(n+1)!}A^n + \cdots\right)u\right], \; t \in R, \; x_0 \in R^n,$$

$$A = [s_i t_j], \; u = {}^t(u_1, \ldots, u_n).$$

This generates a global flow (diffeomorphism) on R^n,

$$x = e^{At}\left[y - \left(\frac{t}{1!}I - \frac{t^2}{2!}A + \cdots + (-1)^n \frac{t^{n+1}}{(n+1)!}A^n + \cdots\right)u\right],$$

which consists of particular affine transformations.

Since

$$\operatorname{div} \boldsymbol{F} = (\nabla S, \nabla T) = \sum_{i=1}^{n} s_i t_i,$$

the flow conserves (contracts, expands) the volume if the angle between ∇S and ∇T is right (obtuse, acute). If $S = 0$, then the flow reduces to translations, $x = y - tu$, $t \in R$.

2) Suppose $T(x) = T_0$, and U, S are quadratic forms on R^n, i.e.,

$$U = \frac{1}{2}\sum_{i,j=1}^{n} u_{ij} x_i x_j, \quad S = \frac{1}{2}\sum_{i,j=1}^{n} s_{ij} x_i x_j,$$

where u_{ij}, s_{ij} are constants and $x = {}^t(x_1, \ldots, x_n) \in R^n$.

The differential system (kinematic system)

$$\frac{dx_i}{dt} = \sum_{j=1}^{n} (T_0 s_{ij} - u_{ij}) x_j, \quad i = 1, \ldots, n$$

admits the general solution

$$x = e^{At} x_0, \quad A = [T_0 s_{ij} - u_{ij}].$$

This generates a global flow (diffeomorphism) on R^n, $x = e^{At} y$, which consists of particular affine transformations.

9.11.3. Behavior of U, T, S, A along field lines of the vector field $F = - S\nabla T - \nabla A$

Suppose again $\alpha(t)$, $t \in I$, is a maximal nonconstant field line of the C^∞ vector field $F = - S\nabla T - \nabla A$ (same field as in §2, but another expression) at $x \in R^n$.

We consider the functions $U = A + TS$ and $U \circ \alpha$. It follows that

$$\frac{d(U \circ \alpha)}{dt} = (\nabla U, -S\nabla T - \nabla A)(\alpha(t)) = -\|S\nabla T + \nabla A\|^2 - T(\nabla S, S\nabla T + \nabla A)|_{\alpha(t)}.$$

Theorem. *If ∇S and $F = - S\nabla T - \nabla A$ are orthogonal vector fields, then $U \circ \alpha$ is decreasing. In this case the critical points of $U \circ \alpha$ (if any) are maximum points, and the curve α cannot be closed.*

Proof. We use the relation

$$\frac{d(U \circ \alpha)}{dt} = -\| S\nabla T + \nabla A\|^2 (\alpha(t)) < 0$$

Remark. Particularly, the theorem works when the level "hypersufaces" attached to fundamental scalar fields T, S, A are mutually orthogonal.

Let there be

$$\lambda = S\|\nabla T\| + \|\nabla A\|, \ \mu = S\|\nabla T\| - \|\nabla A\|.$$

Theorem. *0) Suppose* $\nabla T \perp \nabla A$ *along* α. *If* $S \circ \alpha \le 0$, *then* $T \circ \alpha$ *is increasing. If* $S \circ \alpha \ge 0$, *then* $T \circ \alpha$ *is decreasing.*

1) If $\lambda \circ \alpha \le 0$, *then* $S \circ \alpha \le 0$ *and the function* $T \circ \alpha$ *is increasing. In this case the critical points of* $T \circ \alpha$ *(if any) are minimum points, and the curve* α *can be closed only if it is included in the critical set of* T.

2) If $\mu \circ \alpha \ge 0$, *then* $S \circ \alpha \ge 0$ *and the function* $T \circ \alpha$ *is decreasing. In this case the critical points of* $T \circ \alpha$ *(if any) are maximum points, and the curve* α *can be closed only if it is included in the critical set of* T.

Proof. We use the chain rule for derivatives and the Cauchy-Schwarz inequality for the scalar product. If follows that

$$\frac{d(U \circ \alpha)}{dt} = (\nabla T, -S\nabla T - \nabla A)(\alpha(t)) = -S\|\nabla T\|^2 - (\nabla T, \nabla A)|_{\alpha(t)}$$

and

$$-\|\nabla T\|(S\|\nabla T\| + \|\nabla A\|)|_{\alpha(t)} \le \frac{d(T \circ \alpha)}{dt} \le \|\nabla T\|(-S\|\nabla T\| + \|\nabla A\|)|_{\alpha(t)}.$$

Theorem. 0) *If* $\nabla T \perp \nabla A$ *along* α, *then* $A \circ \alpha$ *is decreasing.*

1) *Let* $S \circ \alpha \le 0$, *and* $\lambda \circ \alpha \le 0$ *or* $S \circ \alpha \ge 0$, *and* $\mu \circ \alpha \le 0$. *Then* $A \circ \alpha$ *is decreasing. In this case the critical points of* $A \circ \alpha$ *(if any) are maximum points, and the curve* α *can be closed only if it is included in the critical set of* A.

Proof.

$$\frac{d(A \circ \alpha)}{dt} = (\nabla A, -S\nabla T - \nabla A)(\alpha(t)) = -S(\nabla T, \nabla A) - \|\nabla A\|^2|_{\alpha(t)}.$$

For $S \circ \alpha \le 0$, we find

$$\|\nabla A\|(S\|\nabla T\| - \|\nabla A\|)|_{\alpha(t)} \le \frac{d(A \circ \alpha)}{dt} \le -\|\nabla A\|(S\|\nabla T\| + \|\nabla A\|)|_{\alpha(t)},$$

and for $S \circ \alpha \ge 0$, we obtain

$$-\|\nabla A\|(S\|\nabla T\| + \|\nabla A\|)|_{\alpha(t)} \le \frac{d(A \circ \alpha)}{dt} \le \|\nabla A\|(S\|\nabla T\| - \|\nabla A\|)|_{\alpha(t)}.$$

Using these relations, we get the desired result.

Suppose $\alpha(t)$, $t \in I$ is included in the "hypersurface" of R^n described by the equation $S(x) = S_0$. It follows that $\frac{d\alpha}{dt} = -\nabla(S_0 T + A)$ and therefore α is a minus gradient line of $S_0 T + A$.

The preceding theorems imply

Corollary. *If there exists a closed nonconstant field line of* F, *then it must pass from the region of* R^n *described by* $S(x) < 0$, *to the region described by* $S(x) > 0$, *transversal to the "hypersurface" described by* $S(x) = 0$.

9.11.4. Monge representation of some classical vector fields

1) **The Lorenz vector field.** The system of equations

$$\frac{dx}{dt} = \sigma(y-x), \quad \frac{dy}{dt} = rx - y - xz, \quad \frac{dz}{dt} = xy - bz$$

discovered by Lorenz [37], where σ, r, b are positive parameters, has chaotic behaviour, by practically any definition of that term. The geometric dynamics determined by this system has not yet been studied.

The Lorenz vector field is not biscalar, but there exist the functions U, T, S such that the Lorenz vector field $(\sigma(y-x), rx-y-xz, xy-bz)$ is the Bobbio-Marrucci vector field

$$F = T\nabla S - \nabla U.$$

Theorem. *A* C^∞ *vector field* $F = T\nabla S - \nabla U$ *is the Lorenz vector field if and only if*

$$U(x,y,z) = \sigma\left(\frac{x^2}{2} - xy\right) + \frac{y^2}{2} + \frac{bz^2}{2} + \varphi(xy^2, (r-\sigma-z)y^{-1}),$$

where φ *is a* C^∞ *function.*

Proof. A vector field $F = T\nabla S - \nabla U$ is the Lorenz vector field if and only if

$$V = \left(\frac{\partial U}{\partial x} + \sigma(y-x), \frac{\partial U}{\partial y} + rx - y - xz, \frac{\partial U}{\partial z} + xy - bz\right)$$

is a biscalar vector field, i.e., $(V, \operatorname{rot} V) = 0$. Since $\operatorname{rot} V = (2x, -y, r-\sigma-z)$, the biscalarity condition is equivalent to the equation with partial derivatives

$$2x\frac{\partial U}{\partial x} - y\frac{\partial U}{\partial y} + (r-z-\sigma)\frac{\partial U}{\partial z} + \sigma xy - 2\sigma x^2 + y^2 + bz(-r+z+\sigma) = 0.$$

This equation has a general solution in the theorem.

2) **The Goodwin vector field.** Some biochemical processes with negative feedback can be modeled by the differential system of Goodwin [59]

$$\frac{dx}{dt} = \frac{1}{1+z^n} - ax, \quad \frac{dy}{dt} = x - by, \quad \frac{dz}{dt} = y - cz,$$

where a, b, c are strictly positive parameters, n is a natural number, and x, y, z are *concentration functions.*

The Goodwin vector field is not biscalar. Let us find the function U such that the Bobbio-Marrucci vector field $F = T\nabla S - \nabla U$ is the Goodwin vector field

$$\left(\frac{1}{1+z^n} - ax, x - by, y - cz\right).$$

Theorem. *The vector field* $F = T\nabla S - \nabla U$ *is Goodwin if and only if*

$$U(x,y,z) = ax^2 - xy + by^2 - \frac{c}{2}z^2 + \int_0^z \frac{dz}{1+z^n} + \varphi\left(x-z,\, y-\frac{1}{1+z^n}\right),$$

where φ *is a* C^∞ *function.*

3) **The Euler vector field.** The motion of a rigid body around a fixed point is characterized by the differential system of Euler [2]

$$\frac{dx}{dt} = ayz, \quad \frac{dy}{dt} = bzx, \quad \frac{dz}{dt} = cxy,$$

where a, b, c are constants determined by the principal moments of inertia. The Euler vector field (ayz, bzx, cxy) is biscalar and therefore it is a Bobbio-Marrucci field with $U = 0$.

Theorem. *The* C^∞ *vector field* $F = T\nabla S - \nabla U$ *is the Euler vector field if and only if* $U(x,y,z) = \varphi(x^{a-c}y^{b-c}, x^{b-a}z^{b-c})$, *where* φ *is a* C^∞ *function.*

10. MAGNETIC DYNAMICAL SYSTEMS AND SABBA ŞTEFĂNESCU CONJECTURES

10.1. BIOT-SAVART-LAPLACE DYNAMICAL SYSTEMS

Section 10.1.1 recalls known facts about the magnetic field $\boldsymbol{H}$ *produced by the Biot-Savart-Laplace law for a massive conductor* $\overline{D}$. *Section 10.1.2 proves that, generally, the part of a magnetic line that lies in* ext $\overline{D}$ *is a trajectory of a potential dynamical system of order two (a geodesic of the Riemann-Jacobi structure), and the part that lies in* int $\overline{D}$ *is a trajectory of a nonpotential dynamical system of order two (a geodesic of a Riemann-Jacobi-Lagrange structure). Consequently, we have discovered new variants of Lorentz world-force laws describing nonclassical magnetic dynamics. This section presents also some properties of magnetic traps, two significant examples, and formulates an open problem. Section 10.1.3 describes the magnetic dynamical systems that can be reduced to 2-dimensional Hamiltonian systems. Section 10.1.4 analyses the magnetic fields to determine which ones are symmetric or antisymmetric with respect to some symmetries.*

The theory in this paragraph was published in [133].

10.1.1. The Biot-Savart-Laplace vector field

Let D be an open connected set of R^3, with a piecewise smooth boundary ∂D. Denote by $\boldsymbol{J}$ a C^∞ vector field on $\overline{D} = D \cup \partial D$.

The vector field

$$\boldsymbol{H}(M) = \frac{1}{4\pi} \int_D \frac{\boldsymbol{J}(P) \times \boldsymbol{PM}}{PM^3} \, dv_P, \quad M \in R^3$$

is called *the Biot-Savart-Laplace vector field*. The name comes from the situation in which $\overline{D}$ is a domain with a current density $\boldsymbol{J}(P)$, $P \in \overline{D}$, when the magnetic field $\boldsymbol{H}$ generated on R^3 by the electric current is approximated by the preceding formula due to J.B. Biot, F.Savart, P.S.Laplace [16], [43].

Remarks. 1) Since the measure (volume) of ∂D is zero, the preceding integral can be considered on $\overline{D} = D \cup \partial D$.

2) The integral defining $\boldsymbol{H}(M)$, $M \in \overline{D}$ is an improper integral of the first type (both of the first and of the second type) if the domain D is bounded (unbounded).

3) The Biot-Savart-Laplace vector field $\boldsymbol{H}$ is of class C^∞ on $R^3 \setminus \partial D$ and of class C^0 on ∂D.

4) The vector field J can have zeros on $\overline{D}$.

The vector field H is solenoidal. Hence it admits a vector potential

$$A(M) = \frac{1}{4\pi}\int_D \frac{J(P)}{PM}\,dv_P.$$

Indeed,

$$\mathrm{rot}A(M) = \nabla_M \times A(M) = \nabla_M \times \frac{1}{4\pi}\int_D \frac{J(P)}{PM}\,dv_P$$

$$= \frac{1}{4\pi}\int_D \nabla_M \times \frac{J(P)}{PM}\,dv_P = -\frac{1}{4\pi}\int_D J(P)\times\nabla_M \frac{1}{PM}\,dv_P$$

$$= \frac{1}{4\pi}\int_D J(P)\times\frac{PM}{PM^3}\,dv_P = H(M).$$

On the other hand,

$$\mathrm{div}\,A(M) = (\nabla_M, A(M)) = \frac{1}{4\pi}\int_D \left(\nabla_M, \frac{J(P)}{PM}\right)dv_P$$

$$= \frac{1}{4\pi}\int_D \left(J(P), \nabla_M\frac{1}{PM}\right)dv_P = -\frac{1}{4\pi}\int_D \left(J(P), \nabla_P\frac{1}{PM}\right)dv_P$$

$$= -\frac{1}{4\pi}\int_D \left(\nabla_P, \frac{J(P)}{PM}\right)dv_P + \frac{1}{4\pi}\int_D \frac{1}{PM}(\nabla_P, J(P))\,dv_P$$

$$= -\frac{1}{4\pi}\int_{\partial D} \frac{(n(P), J(P))}{PM}\,dv_P + \frac{1}{4\pi}\int_D \frac{\mathrm{div}J(P)}{PM}\,dv_P,$$

where $n(P)$ is the unit normal vector field of the surface ∂D. If J is a solenoidal vector field (a stationary electrokinetic field), and ∂D is a field surface of J, i.e., $(n(P), J(P)) = 0$, then $\mathrm{div}\,A(M) = 0$, and so A is a solenoidal vector field.

Under the hypothesis $\mathrm{div}A(M) = 0$, we compute

$$\mathrm{rot}H(M) = \nabla_M \times (\nabla_M \times A(M)) = \nabla_M(\nabla_M, A(M)) - (\nabla_M, \nabla_M)A(M)$$

$$= \nabla_M \mathrm{div}A(M) - \nabla_M^2 A(M) = -\nabla_M^2 A(M) = -\Delta_M A(M),$$

so that $\mathrm{rot}H(M) = 0$ for $M \in R^3 \setminus D$, and $\mathrm{rot}H(M) = J(M)$ for $M \in D$; also, we have

$$\mathrm{div}\,H(M) = \mathrm{div}\,\mathrm{rot}A(M) = 0.$$

Consequently, the vector field H is not irrotational, but the restriction of H to $R^3 \setminus \overline{D}$ is an irrotational vector field. This restriction admits a local scalar potential. Also, the vector field H is solenoidal.

Remarks. 1) We notice that

$$\nabla_M F(PM) = F'(PM)\frac{PM}{PM} = -\nabla_P F(PM),\ \forall F: R \to R,\ \text{differentiable}.$$

2) If the point M has the coordinates (x,y,z) and the point P has the coordinates (ξ,η,ζ), then

$$\frac{\partial}{\partial x} A(M) = -\int_D \frac{\partial}{\partial \xi}\left(\frac{J(P)}{PM}\right) dv_P, \text{ etc.}$$

3) If J is a constant vector field on D, then the magnetic field H generated on R^3 by J is a biscalar field, i.e., $(H, \text{rot}H) = 0$.

4) The domain D can be replaced by a surface or a curve. In case of a curve, the current density J must be nonzero everywhere along the curve.

10.1.2. Dynamics induced by the Biot-Savart-Laplace vector field

Let $H = H_x i + H_y j + H_z k$ be a C^∞ magnetic field defined on R^3. Denote by $r = xi + yj + zk$ the position vector of the point $M(x,y,z)$.

The *magnetic line* α starting from $M_0(x_0, y_0, z_0)$ at moment $t = 0$ is the oriented curve $r = r(t)$, $t \in (-\varepsilon, \varepsilon)$ that satisfies the Cauchy problem

$$\frac{dr}{dt} = H(r),\ r(0) = r_0.$$

The *magnetic surface* $\Sigma : h(x,y,z) = c$ relying on a curve $\beta : (a,b) \to R^3$ is the solution of the Cauchy problem

$$(H, \nabla h) = 0,\ h(\beta(u)) = h(\beta(0)),\ \forall u \in (a,b).$$

A magnetic surface is generated by magnetic lines, and, in the absence of symmetries, a magnetic line is an open curve. Sometimes the image of an open field line is dense in the magnetic surface.

Open problem. Let A be a subdomain of D, and H_A, H_D be the Biot-Savart-Laplace vector field on A, respectively D. Do there exist domains $A \subset D$ with the property that H_A and H_D have the same phase portrait on $R^3 - \bar{D}$? See also [98].

Let U be an open connected set of R^3 with a piecewise smooth boundary ∂U, and T_t the flow generated by the magnetic vector field H. The flow T_t conserves the volume, since $\text{div}H = 0$. The set U or its closure $\bar{U}$ is called a *trap region* of the magnetic field H *(magnetic trap)* if $T_t(\bar{U}) \subset \bar{U}$, $\forall t \geq 0$. Particularly, any T_t - invariant set is a trap region. A magnetic trap is characterized by the fact that a magnetic line starting inside cannot leave it (because such a line cannot attain the boundary ∂U). The magnetic line starting in the exterior of the magnetic trap can enter or not into the trap.

Suppose that the unit normal vector field n of the surface ∂U is oriented toward ext$U$. If U is a magnetic trap, then on the boundary ∂U we have $(n, H) \leq 0$. Conversely, if $(n, H) = 0$ on ∂U, then ∂U is a magnetic surface; if $(n, H) > 0$ on ∂U, then $R^3 \setminus U$ is a trap region of the magnetic field H, and if $(n,H) < 0$ on ∂U, then U is a trap region of the magnetic field H.

Suppose there exist two magnetic traps U_1 and U_2 such that their boundaries $\partial U_1, \partial U_2$ have a common part, which is a surface Σ or a curve γ. Then Σ is a magnetic surface, and γ is a magnetic line, respectively.

Theorem. *Let U be an open connected set of R^3 with a piecewise smooth boundary ∂U. If U is a magnetic trap and $\overline{U} = U \cup \partial U$ is compact, then the closed surface ∂U is a magnetic surface and $T_t(\overline{U}) = \overline{U}$.*

Proof. Suppose that the unit normal vector field n of the surface ∂U is oriented toward ext$U$. Since $\operatorname{div} H = 0$, by Gauss' Theorem we obtain $\int_{\partial U} (n,H)\,d\sigma = 0$. If ∂U is not a magnetic surface, i.e., $(n,H) \neq 0$, then (n,H) must change sign on the closed surface ∂U and consequently U is not a magnetic trap.

The last assertion of the Theorem is a consequence of the conservation of volume.

Remark. If H is a magnetic field and $\overline{U}$ is not a compact set, then it is possible that U is a magnetic trap for H without ∂U being a magnetic surface. For example, the magnetic field $H(x,y,z) = i$, the region $U : x + y + z + 1 > 0$, the boundary $\partial U : x + y + z + 1 = 0$, the unit normal $n = \dfrac{-i-j-k}{\sqrt{3}}$ all imply $(n,H) < 0$; therefore U is a magnetic trap. Also, this example shows that in the preceding context the T_t - invariant set $\bigcap_{t \geq 0} T_t(U)$ can be the void set.

In the following part of this section we refer only to the Biot-Savart-Laplace vector field. Is the region D in the Biot-Savart-Laplace formula a magnetic trap or not? A possible answer was given in the preceding theorem. The next theorem presents another alternative.

Theorem. *Suppose that the unit normal vector field n of the surface ∂D is oriented toward ext$D$. Let*

$$\varphi : \overline{D} \times \partial D \to R, \quad \varphi(P,M) = (n(M), J(P) \times PM).$$

1) If $\varphi(P,M) = 0$, $\forall P \in \overline{D}$, $\forall M \in \partial D$, i.e., the vector fields $n(M), J(P), PM$ are coplanar on $\overline{D} \times \partial D$, then ∂D is a magnetic surface, and $R^3 \setminus D$ and D are magnetic traps.

2) If $\varphi(P,M) > 0$, $\forall P \in \dot{D}$, $\forall M \in \partial D$, then $R^3 \setminus D$ is a magnetic trap.

3) If $\varphi(P,M) < 0$, $\forall P \in \overline{D}$, $\forall M \in \partial D$, then D is a magnetic trap.

Proof. Consequences of the relation

$$(n(M), H(M)) = \int_D \frac{(n(M), J(P) \times PM)}{PM^3}\, dv_P, \quad \forall M \in \partial D.$$

Remark. In the case 1) the vector fields J and H are tangent to ∂D. In the cases 2)-3), the vector field J is tangent to ∂D and the vector field H is transversal to ∂D.

Let

$$f: R^3 \to R,\ f = \frac{1}{2}(H_x^2 + H_y^2 + H_z^2)$$

be the energy of $\boldsymbol{H}$, leaving aside the multiplicative factor μ (see [130]).

Theorem. *Any magnetic line in* $\mathrm{int}(R^3 \setminus D)$ *is a trajectory of a potential dynamical system with three degrees of freedom associated to the potential* $-f$ *on* $\mathrm{int}(R^3 \setminus D)$.

Proof. Let α be a magnetic line included in $\mathrm{int}(R^3 \setminus D)$. Differentiating $\frac{d\boldsymbol{r}}{dt} = \boldsymbol{H}$ along α, considering that $\mathrm{rot}\,H = 0$, and replacing $\frac{d\boldsymbol{r}}{dt}$ by $\boldsymbol{H}$, we find the prolongation

$$\frac{d^2\boldsymbol{r}}{dt^2} = \nabla f,$$

which is a potential dynamical system of order two.

Remark. If α contains at least one point of ∂D, then the previous assertion fails.

Denoting $\frac{d\boldsymbol{r}}{dt} = -\boldsymbol{v}$, the differential system of order two

$$\frac{d^2\boldsymbol{r}}{dt^2} = \nabla f$$

can be written as a Hamiltonian system

$$\frac{d\boldsymbol{r}}{dt} = -\boldsymbol{v},\ \frac{d\boldsymbol{v}}{dt} = -\nabla f,$$

on the phase space $\boldsymbol{R}^6$, with the Hamiltonian

$$\mathcal{H}(\boldsymbol{r}, \boldsymbol{v}) = \frac{1}{2}\|\boldsymbol{v}\|^2 - f(\boldsymbol{r}).$$

The Hamiltonian flow conserves the phase space volume. The Hamiltonian $\mathcal{H}$ is a first integral of the Hamiltonian dynamical system. The theory of Hamiltonian systems shows that the preceding prolongation is a new Lorentz law based on a geometrical structure that incorporates the magnetic field.

Theorem. *The trajectory of the dynamical system*

$$\frac{d^2\boldsymbol{r}}{dt^2} = \nabla f,\ \boldsymbol{r}(0) = \boldsymbol{r}_0 \in R^3 \setminus \overline{D},$$

having $\mathcal{H} > -f$ *as constant total energy and staying in* $R^3 \setminus \overline{D}$ *is a reparametrized geodesic of the Riemann-Jacobi metric*

$$g_{ij} = (\mathcal{H} + f)\,\delta_{ij},\ i, j, = 1, 2, 3$$

Remark. If the domain D is reduced to a curve γ, then the theorems hold true on $R^3 \setminus \gamma$.

Theorem. *Any magnetic line included in* D *is a trajectory of a nonpotential dynamical system with three degrees of freedom for which the energy* $\mathcal{H} = \frac{1}{2}\|\boldsymbol{v}\|^2 - f(x, y, z)$ *is conserved.*

Proof. If $r(0) = r_0 \in D$ and α rests in D, then differentiating $\frac{dr}{dt} = H$ along α, and replacing $\frac{dr}{dt}$ by H in the convenient terms, we get a prolongation

$$\frac{d^2 r}{dt^2} = \nabla f + J \times \frac{dr}{dt},$$

which is a nonpotential dynamical system of order two. If we take the scalar product with $\frac{dr}{dt}$, we find $\frac{d}{dt}\mathcal{H} = 0$, i.e., the energy $\mathcal{H}$ is conserved.

Recently [99], [130], [132] we have discovered a suitable geometrical structure (see 3.9) showing that the preceding conservative nonpotential dynamical system of order two describes a new Lorentz world-force law (nonclassical magnetic dynamics).

Theorem (Lorentz-Udrişte world-force law). *The trajectory of the dynamical system*

$$\frac{d^2 r}{dt^2} = \nabla f + J \times \frac{dr}{dt}, \quad r(0) = r_0 \in D$$

having $\mathcal{H} > -f$ as constant total energy and staying in D is a reparametrized horizontal geodesic of the Riemann-Jacobi-Lagrange structure

$$g_{ij} = (\mathcal{H} + f)\delta_{ij}, \quad N^i{}_j = \Gamma^i_{jk} y^k + F^i{}_j, \quad i, j, k = 1, 2, 3,$$

where

Γ^i_{jk} *is the Riemann connection determined by the metric* g_{ij},

$N^i_j = \Gamma^i_{jk} y^k + F^i_j$ *is a nonlinear connection, and* $F_{ij} = (\mathrm{rot}\, H)_{ij}$, $F^i{}_j = g^{ih} F_{hj}$.

Obviously the Riemann-Jacobi-Lagrange structure incorporates the magnetic field both by the Riemann-Jacobi metric and by the nonlinear connection.

Remarks. 1) The vector field $J \times \frac{dr}{dt}$ does not produce a dissipation of energy along the solution α since it is orthogonal to the curve α.

2) The trajectories of the preceding conservative (potential or nonpotential) dynamical systems of order two divide into three classes:

- the set of original magnetic lines that correspond to the energy $\mathcal{H} = 0$;
- a set of trajectories for the energy $\mathcal{H} = \mathrm{const} < 0$;
- a set of trajectories for the energy $\mathcal{H} = \mathrm{const} > 0$.

3) The geometric magnetic dynamics is altered by changing the magnetic field **H** into -**H**. Can we explain the migration of the earth's magnetic poles in the context of geometric magnetic dynamics?

4) Another prolongation is the nonpotential nonconservative dynamical system

$$\frac{d^2 \boldsymbol{r}}{dt^2} = \nabla f + \boldsymbol{J} \times \boldsymbol{H}.$$

Since $\operatorname{rot}(\boldsymbol{J} \times \boldsymbol{H}) \neq 0$, the vector field $\boldsymbol{J} \times \boldsymbol{H}$ corresponds to a dissipation of energy along the solutions α that are not orthogonal to $\boldsymbol{J} \times \boldsymbol{H}$.

5) In both cases the projection of the acceleration $\frac{d^2 \boldsymbol{r}}{dt^2}$ on $\boldsymbol{J}$ depends only on the projection of ∇f on $\boldsymbol{J}$.

Open problem. What is the physical significance for trajectories of the preceding conservative differential systems, which correspond to positive or negative constant energy?

If the magnetic line α traverses ∂D, then its part contained in D is a trajectory of a nonpotential dynamical system of order two, and its part in $R^3 \setminus \bar{D}$ is a trajectory of a potential dynamical system of order two. Obviously, α can be smooth or not at the traversing point of ∂D, being a field line of the vector field $\boldsymbol{H}$ which is of class C^∞ on $R^3 \setminus \partial D$ and of class C^0 on ∂D.

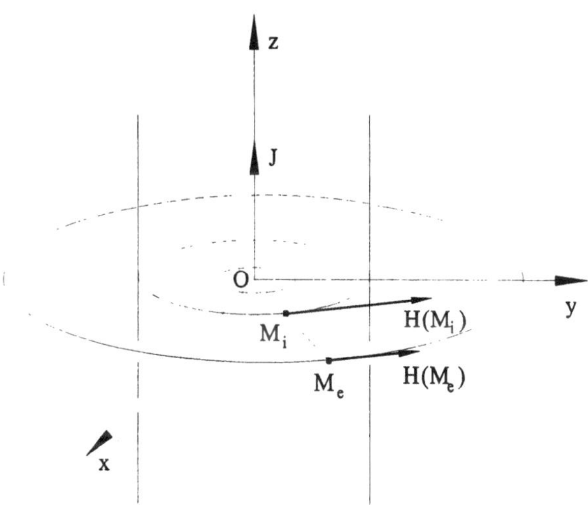

Fig. 105

Examples.

1) Suppose that $\bar{D} = D \cup \partial D$ is a circular cylinder of radius a carrying a steady current I. We fix the Cartesian frame $Oxyz$ such that Oz is the axis of the cylinder, and $\boldsymbol{J} = \frac{I}{\pi a^2} \boldsymbol{k}$ is the current density. The electric current generates the magnetic field (Fig. 27, 105) given by [16]

$$\boldsymbol{H}(M) = \frac{-y\boldsymbol{i} + x\boldsymbol{j}}{2\pi a^2} I, \quad \text{for} \quad M(x,y,z) \in \bar{D},$$

and

$$H(M) = \frac{-yi + xj}{2\pi(x^2+y^2)} I, \quad \text{for} \quad M(x,y,z) \in R^3 \setminus \bar{D}.$$

The Oz - axis consists of zeros of H. The nonconstant magnetic lines are circles with centers on Oz, and situated in planes orthogonal to Oz. The boundary ∂D is a magnetic surface, though H is only continuous on ∂D. The regions D and $R^3 \setminus \bar{D}$ are magnetic traps. Even in this simple case, we have no answer for the preceding open problem, though the trajectories of the associated conservative differential systems of order two are cylindrical helices around Oz.

2) Suppose that $\bar{D} = D \cup \partial D$ is an infinite prism of rectangular section $[-a, a] \times [-b, b]$ carrying a steady current I. We choose a Cartesian frame $Oxyz$ such that Oz is the axis of the prism, and $J = \frac{I}{4ab} k$ is the current density (Fig.106).

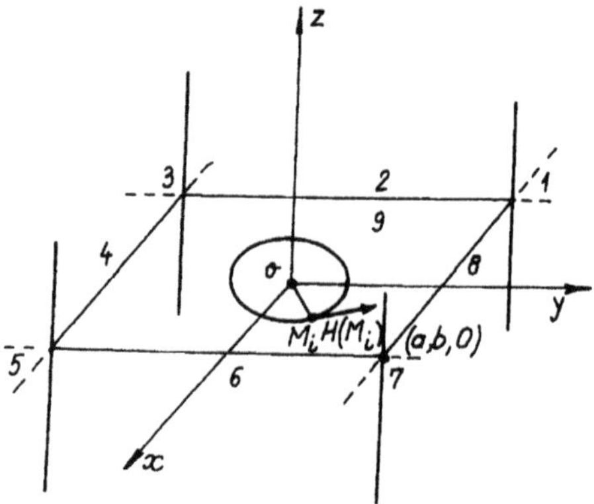

Fig, 106

The magnetic field generated by J on R^3 has the components $(H_x, H_y, 0)$, where [43]

$$H_x = -\frac{I}{2ab}[(y-b)(\arctan\frac{x-a}{y-b} - \arctan\frac{x+a}{y-b}) - (y+b)(\arctan\frac{x-a}{y+b}$$

$$-\arctan\frac{x+a}{y+b}) - \frac{x+a}{2}\ln\frac{(x+a)^2+(y-b)^2}{(x+a)^2+(y+b)^2} + \frac{x-a}{2}\ln\frac{(x-a)^2+(y-b)^2}{(x-a)^2+(y+b)^2}],$$

$$H_y = -\frac{I}{2ab}[(x-a)(\arctan\frac{y+b}{x-a} - \arctan\frac{y-b}{x-a}) - (x+a)(\arctan\frac{y+b}{x+a}$$

$$-\arctan\frac{y-b}{x+a}) - \frac{y-b}{2}\ln\frac{(x-a)^2+(y-b)^2}{(x+a)^2+(y-b)^2} + \frac{y+b}{2}\ln\frac{(x-a)^2+(y+b)^2}{(x+a)^2+(y+b)^2}].$$

The field H is defined on D and $R^3 \setminus D$ by the same formulas and can be extended by continuity to ∂D. The boundary ∂D is piecewise smooth, and is not a magnetic surface.

The field $\boldsymbol{H}$ is continuous on ∂D. If $S : R^3 \to R^3$ is the symmetry with respect to Oz, and $\boldsymbol{H}$ is regarded as $\boldsymbol{H} : R^3 \to R^3$, then $\boldsymbol{H} \circ S = S \circ \boldsymbol{H}$.

The Oz -axis consists of zeros of $\boldsymbol{H}$. The field lines are closed curves (symmetrical with respect to Oz) included in the family of curves

$$\int_{x_0}^{x} H_y(x,y)\,dx - \int_{y_0}^{y} H_x(x_0,y)\,dy = b_k, \quad z = c.$$

Computing the integrals, the first equation becomes

$$\begin{aligned}
&\frac{(x-a)^2+(y+b)^2}{2}\arctan\frac{y+b}{x-a} + (y+b)^2\arctan\frac{x-a}{y+b}\\
&-\frac{(x-a)^2+(y-b)^2}{2}\arctan\frac{y-b}{x-a} - (y-b)^2\arctan\frac{x-a}{y-b}\\
&+\frac{(x+a)^2+(y-b)^2}{2}\arctan\frac{y-b}{x+a} + (y-b)^2\arctan\frac{x+a}{y-b}\\
&-\frac{(x-a)^2+(y+b)^2}{2}\arctan\frac{y+b}{x+a} - (y+b)^2\arctan\frac{x+a}{y+b}\\
&-\frac{(x-a)(y-b)}{2}\ln((x-a)^2+(y-b)^2 + \frac{(x+a)(y-b)}{2}\ln((x+a)^2+(y-b)^2)\\
&+\frac{(x-a)(y+b)}{2}\ln((x-a)^2+(y+b)^2) - \frac{(x+a)(y+b)}{2}\ln((x+a)^2+(y+b)^2)\\
&+\frac{(y+b)^2}{2}\left(\arctan\frac{y+b}{x_0+a} + \arctan\frac{x_0+a}{y+b} - \arctan\frac{y+b}{x_0-a} - \arctan\frac{x_0-a}{y+b}\right)\\
&+\frac{(y-b)^2}{2}\left(\arctan\frac{y-b}{x_0-a} + \arctan\frac{x_0-a}{y-b} - \arctan\frac{y-b}{x_0+a} - \arctan\frac{x_0+a}{y-b}\right) = c_k.
\end{aligned}$$

The parameters b_k, c_k are constants depending on the regions $k = 1,2,\ldots,9$ in the Fig.106, containing the fixed point $(x_0, y_0, 0)$. Also, we must have in mind that

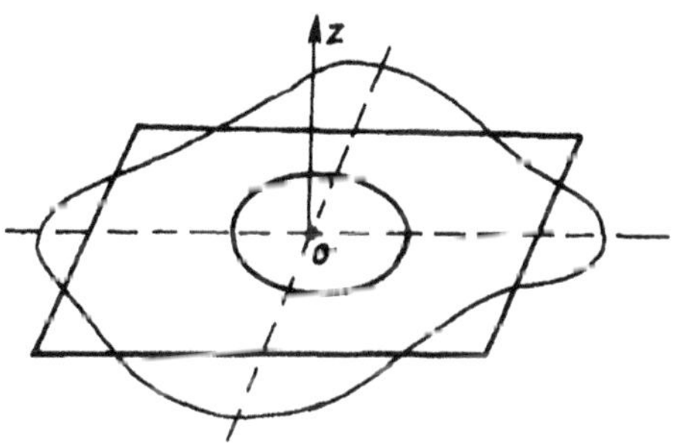

Fig. 107

$$\arctan u + \arctan\frac{1}{u} = (signu)\,\frac{\pi}{2}.$$

Some of these field lines traverse the boundary of the rectangle $[-a, a] \times [-b, b]$, Fig.107.

Let us consider the Runge-Kutta approximations of Cauchy problems

$$\frac{dx}{dt} = H_x, \quad \frac{dy}{dt} = H_y, \quad \frac{dy}{dt} = 0,$$

$$x(0) = x_0, \; y(0) = 0, \; z_0 = 0,$$

obtained by using a personal computer, referring to the case $a = 1$, $b = 2$, the step $p = 0.02$ and the following table

Initial points x_0	0.6	0.9	1.2	1.5	1.8	2.00	2.5
Number of Interations	220	220	220	275	350	520	900

We remark that Runge-Kutta approximations of magnetic lines through points corresponding to $x_0 \in (0;0.9)$ have a shape similar to those of an ellipse, and the curvature of the magnetic lines corresponding to $x_0 \in (1.2;2.5)$ has non-constant sign (Fig.107).

Generally, the sign of the curvature of a magnetic line α coincides with the sign of the function

$$H_x^2 \frac{\partial H_y}{\partial x} + H_x H_y \left(\frac{\partial H_y}{\partial y} - \frac{\partial H_x}{\partial x} \right) - H_y^2 \frac{\partial H_x}{\partial y} = H_x^2 \frac{\partial H_y}{\partial x} + 2 H_x H_y \frac{\partial H_y}{\partial y} - H_y^2 \frac{\partial H_x}{\partial y}$$

along $\alpha(I)$, but this sign cannot be constant throughout the plane xOy.

The shape of the preceding magnetic lines around the points on xOy (yOz) becomes obvious if we take into account that the component $H_x(x,y)$ vanishes for $y = 0$ (the component $H_y(x,y)$ vanishes for $x = 0$).

In fact, if $\alpha(t) = (x(t), y(t), 0)$, $t \in R$ is the maximal solution of the preceding Cauchy problem, then $x_0 \neq 0$ is an extremum value of the function $x(t)$, $t \in R$.

10.1.3. Magnetic dynamical systems that are bidimensional Hamiltonian systems

Let $H = H_x i + H_y j + H_z k$ be the magnetic field of Biot-Savart-Laplace and

$$\frac{dx}{dt} = H_x, \quad \frac{dy}{dt} = H_y, \quad \frac{dz}{dt} = H_z$$

the associated magnetic dynamical system. Suppose $H_z = 0$, $H_x = H_x(x,y)$, $H_y = H_y(x,y)$. Since

$$0 = \operatorname{div} H = \frac{\partial H_x}{\partial x} + \frac{\partial H_y}{\partial y},$$

there exists a function $\mathcal{H} : R^2 \to R$ such that

$$\frac{\partial \mathcal{H}}{\partial y} = H_x, \quad \frac{\partial \mathcal{H}}{\partial x} = -H_y$$

and therefore the magnetic dynamical system reduces to the bidimensional Hamiltonian system

$$\frac{dx}{dt} = \frac{\partial \mathcal{H}}{\partial y}, \quad \frac{dy}{dt} = -\frac{\partial \mathcal{H}}{\partial x}.$$

(see the examples of 10.1.2).

Suppose that H_z is a nonzero function and that $\frac{H_x}{H_z}$, $\frac{H_y}{H_z}$ are functions of x and y only. The magnetic dynamical system transcribes

$$\frac{dx}{dz} = \frac{H_x}{H_z}, \quad \frac{dy}{dz} = \frac{H_y}{H_z}.$$

If there exists $\mathcal{H} : R^2 \to R$ such that

$$\frac{\partial \mathcal{H}}{\partial y} = \frac{H_x}{H_z}, \quad \frac{\partial \mathcal{H}}{\partial x} = -\frac{H_y}{H_z},$$

then

$$0 = \frac{\partial}{\partial x}\left(\frac{H_x}{H_z}\right) + \frac{\partial}{\partial y}\left(\frac{H_y}{H_z}\right) = \operatorname{div}\frac{H}{H_z} = \frac{1}{H_z}\operatorname{div}H + \left(H, \operatorname{grad}\frac{1}{H_z}\right) = -\frac{(H, \operatorname{grad}H_z)}{H_z^2},$$

and hence H_z is either a constant function or a first integral of the magnetic dynamical system (i.e., $H_z(x,y,z) = c$ are field surfaces of H).

Conversely, if H_z is either a first integral of the magnetic dynamical system or a constant function and the ratios $\frac{H_x}{H_z}$, $\frac{H_y}{H_z}$ are functions of x, y only, then the Hamiltonian $\mathcal{H}$ does exist. Consequently, the following theorem is true.

Theorem. *Suppose that none of the components (H_x, H_y, H_z) is the function zero. The corresponding magnetic dynamical system is reducible to a bidimensional Hamiltonian system if at least one of the components (H_x, H_y, H_z) is either a constant or a first integral of the magnetic dynamical system, and the ratios of the other two by this component depend effectively only on the variables that index them.*

Remark. Suppose that the magnetic dynamical system reduces to a Hamiltonian system on xOy. Then the magnetic lines are geodesics of a Riemann-Jacobi structure which is conformal to the Euclidean structure on R^2.

10.1.4. Symmetric and antisymmetric magnetic fields

The examples in 10.1.2 suggest the following considerations.

Let $S : R^3 \to R^3$ be an arbitrary symmetry and H be the Biot-Savart-Laplace field regarded as a function of the type $H : R^3 \to R^3$.

If $H \circ S = S \circ H$, then the magnetic field H is called *symmetric*. If $H \circ S = -S \circ H$, then the magnetic field H is called *antisymmetric*.

Theorem. *Let D, J, H be the mathematical entities from the Biot-Savart-Laplace formula, and S be the symmetry of R^3 with respect to the origin. Suppose $S(D) = D$.*

1) If $J \circ S = S \circ J$, then $H \circ S = -S \circ H$.

2) If $J \circ S = -S \circ J$, then $H \circ S = S \circ H$.

Proof. 1) We consider the change of variables in the triple integral, and the action of an orthogonal transformation upon the vector product. Since $S(x,y,z) = (-x,-y,-z)$, successively we have

$$H \circ S(M) = \int_{S(D)} \frac{J \circ S(P) \times S(P)S(M)}{S(P)S(M)^3} dv_{S(P)} = \int_D \frac{S \circ J(P) \times S \circ PM}{PM^3} dv_P$$

$$= (\operatorname{sign} S) S \circ \int_D \frac{J(P) \times PM}{PM^3} dv_P = -S \circ H(M).$$

Theorem. *Let D, J, H be the mathematical entities from the Biot-Savart-Laplace formula, and S be the symmetry of R^3 with respect to Oz. Suppose $S(D) = D$.*

1) If $J \circ S = S \circ J$, then $H \circ S = S \circ H$.

2) If $J \circ S = -S \circ J$, then $H \circ S = -S \circ H$.

Proof. 1) The symmetry with respect to Oz is $S(x,y,z) = (-x,-y,z)$. It follows that

$$H \circ S(M) = \int_{S(D)} \frac{J \circ S(P) \times PM}{S(P)S(M)^3} dv_{S(P)} = \int_D \frac{S \circ J(P) \times S \circ PM}{PM^3} dv_P$$

$$= \int_D (\operatorname{sign} S) S \circ \frac{J(P) \times PM}{PM^3} dv_P = S \circ \int_D \frac{J(P) \times PM}{PM^3} dv_P = S \circ H(M).$$

Remark. The theory in this section can be extended to any isometry.

10.2. SABBA ŞTEFĂNESCU CONJECTURES

Section 10.2.1 presents the history of magnetic lines. Section 10.2.2 refers to contributions of Sabba Ştefănescu to the theory of lines of magnetic fields generated by the filiform electric circuits and recall the following conjecture [63]-[88]: **the differential system that describes the field lines of the magnetic field generated by a union of piecewise rectilinear electric circuits admits an algebraic first integral.**

10.2.1. History of magnetic lines

Let $H = H_x i + H_y j + H_z k$ be a stationary C^∞ magnetic field. Some real geophysics and plasma confinement problems are based on properties of H derived from:

(a) the geometry-topology of the field lines (magnetic lines), oriented curves, which are solutions of the differential system

$$\frac{dx}{dt} = H_x, \quad \frac{dy}{dt} = H_y, \quad \frac{dz}{dt} = H_z; \tag{1}$$

(b) the geometry-topology of the field surfaces (magnetic surfaces) which are constant level sets attached to the solutions of the partial differential equation

$$H_x \frac{\partial f}{\partial x} + H_y \frac{\partial f}{\partial y} + H_z \frac{\partial f}{\partial z} = 0. \tag{2}$$

The field lines and surfaces are integral characteristics of the magnetic vector field.

In the beginning, physicists considered the simplest configurations that can produce magnetic fields: rectilinear circuits, plane circuits and permanent magnets. The study of such fields inclined to spread the wrong idea that the hypothesis $\operatorname{div} H = 0$ implies close magnetic field lines or lines going to infinity. But, in 1928, using an example of a magnetic field produced by a circular current and a rectilinear one, Tamm showed that there are magnetic systems where the field lines do not close and do not go to infinity. In the current language, this was the first example of magnetic lines with ergodic behaviour: an open field line that fills densely a torus (Fig. 108).

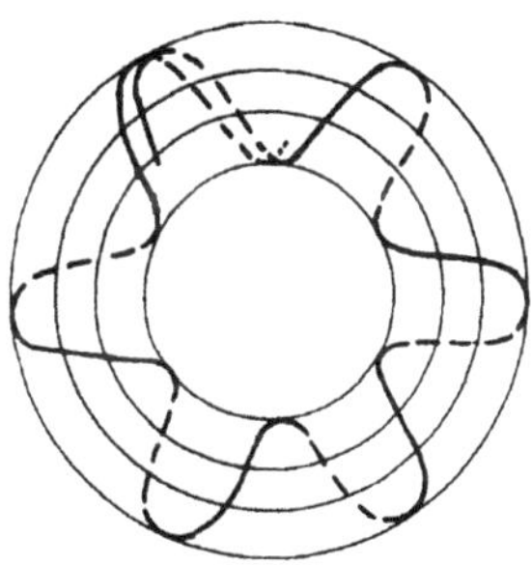

Fig. 108

As early as 1925 Sabba Ştefănescu drew attention to the fact that the morphology of the magnetic fields generated by currents through union of piecewise rectilinear electric circuits is not yet well understood or applied. These magnetic fields generate mathematical surprises, as important as Tamm's. For example, a current ramification can generate algebraic magnetic lines.

The isolated equilibrium points of the differential system (1), that is the isolated zeros of field H, are points near which there appear bifurcations, being saddle type points; some lines come toward the point, without touching it, others start from a neighborhood of the respective point, while others pass near the respective point. If a field line does not "come or start," as compared to an isolated equilibrium point, then, it cannot have a beginning or an end dictated by the morphology of the respective point. This observation leads us to postulate the existence of three types of magnetic lines that "come or start" as compared to an isolated equilibrium point [5], [104]:

(1) field lines that start at infinity and end at infinity;

(2) (open or close) field lines that remain in a bounded set;

(3) field lines that begin at infinity, but are caught by a trap in a bounded set.

The mathematical problems regarding magnetic fields are peculiar examples of the general theory of dynamical systems with integral invariants ($\text{div}\,\boldsymbol{H} = 0$) and from this point of view the papers of the mathematicians Poincare, Birkhoff, Kolmogorov, Arnold, Barbu, Halanay, etc are interesting.

The specialists in plasma theory dealt with the exact structure of symmetrical fields. They succeeded in obtaining magnetic lines by quadratures and they put into evidence the magnetic surfaces distortion.

10.2.2. Some results and conjectures of Sabba Ştefănescu

The results of Sabba Ştefănescu, regarding the lines of the magnetic field generated by piecewise rectilinear electric circuits, are exposed in more than 25 published papers and in a series of manuscripts that are still unpublished. The theme of these papers was imposed on one hand by electrical prospecting of the underground, building nuclear reactors (fusion of the atomic nucleus), guidance of charge particles in the terrestrial magnetic field, and on the other hand, by mathematical peculiarities. These are the reasons to study the phase portraits of magnetic fields produced by elementary configurations.

Chronologically the ideas of Sabba Ştefănescu are the following [63]-[89]:

(1) In the paper [63], regarding the lines of the magnetic field around a ramification of currents, there appeared for the first time the idea of the importance of algebraic field lines: "if the intensities running over the beams of a current ramification can be represented by integer numbers, then the field lines are algebraic."

(2) The previous idea was studied again in 1928 [65], [66], finding the lines of the Schlumberger electromagnetic field, used for underground electrical prospecting.

(3) Between 1935 and 1936 [67], [68], there were found the magnetic lines generated by the currents configuration in Fig.109 and it was emphasized that these lines are curves expressed by elementary transcendental functions, drawn on the family of algebraic magnetic surfaces.

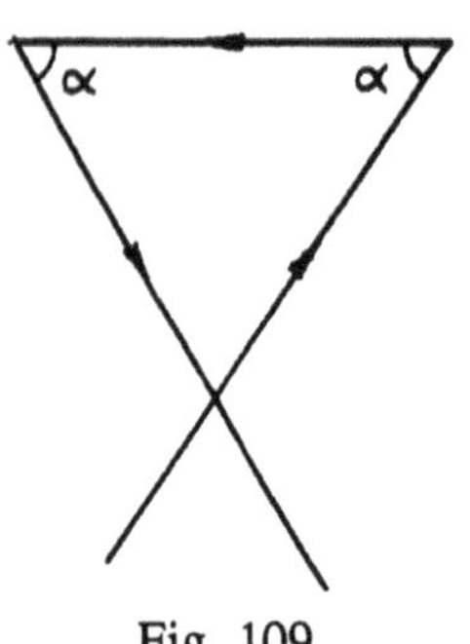

Fig. 109

For example, the paper [67] studies the phase portrait of the magnetic field around a symmetric twice-bent electric circuit. Results: explicit formulas of the components of the magnetic field, the set of equilibrium points is an ellipse, explicit formulas for the field lines and an algebraic first integral, homoclinic behaviour of the magnetic field.

(4) Between 1937 and 1938 [69], the case in Fig.110 was solved showing that the magnetic lines are algebraic curves

of order 16.

(5) The general case of the plane two-times curved filiform current (Fig.111) was solved in 1951 [70], by putting into evidence again an algebraic first integral.

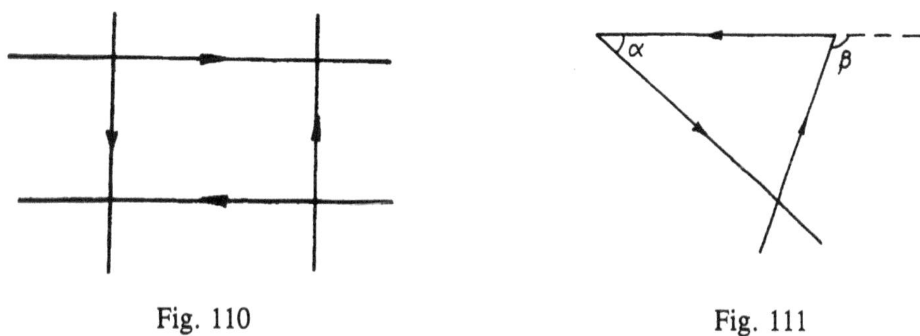

Fig. 110 Fig. 111

(6) Between 1951 and 1955, the techniques of underground electrical prospecting, suggested also the study of the magnetic lines of a triangle of rectilinear currents. These lines proved to be situated on a family of algebraic magnetic surfaces of orders 6 [71], [72].

For an equilateral triangle of rectilinear currents, it was noticed that an algebraic magnetic surface is the geometrical locus for which the ratio between the product of distances at the planes of symmetry of the triangle, and the product of distances to its three sides, is constant. This physical and geometrical significance carries over to a more general case (1953): the magnetic lines of a regular polygon of n rectilinear equal intensity currents are situated on an algebraic surface of order $2n$, which is the geometrical locus of the points for which the ratio between the product of distances at the n symmetry planes of the regular polygon, and product of distances at its n sides, is constant [71], [72].

(7) In 1956 [73], [74] emphasis was again on the theory of electrical prospecting by A.C. methods that call for research on magnetic lines around straight line currents, and the idea of a single algebraic first integral was clearly underlined. Also a procedure was given for obtaining the second first integral, using the notion of integral invariant (the method of invariant flow).

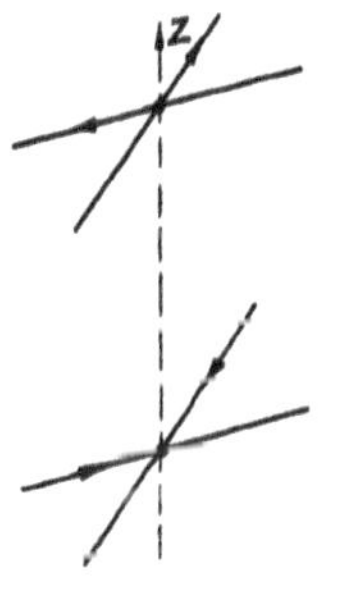

Fig. 112

(8) Between 1957 and 1958 [68], Sabba Ştefănescu analysed magnetic lines around two pairs of rectilinear electric circuits in parallel planes, the currents having the sense in Fig 112. Results: explicit computation of a family of algebraic magnetic surfaces of degree 8, the magnetic lines in the plane $z = 0$ are open curves, the magnetic lines with open helicoidal shape are defined on the magnetic algebraic surfaces by Abelian integrals, an example of a magnetic line that can be everywhere dense in a magnetic surface.

These ideas were developed in 1956 [76] for the magnetic lines around a directilinear dicurrent.

(9) Between 1960 and 1961 there were considered thoroughly the magnetic field lines investigations of two rectilinear electric currents and

the magnetic field lines of *AB* transmitter, by written papers in cooperation with Misac Nabighian. These papers draw the attention by more computing power and more geometrical-topological aspects of the studied field lines and maintain the idea of an algebraic first integral [76], [77]. Also in this period, the magnetic field lines around a ground socket in a parallel stratification ground were found [78].

Results: the differential system of the magnetic lines admits a family of algebraic ruled magnetic surfaces, the magnetic lines are open helicoidal curves that can be defined on the ruled magnetic surfaces by elliptical integrals of the first and second kind (the step of these helices, measured on an arbitrary generator of an algebraic magnetic surface, is constant and characteristic for the considered surface).

(10) Between 1967 and 1969 there were studied the lines of the magnetic field, determined by a rectangle of equal intensity rectilinear electric currents [79].

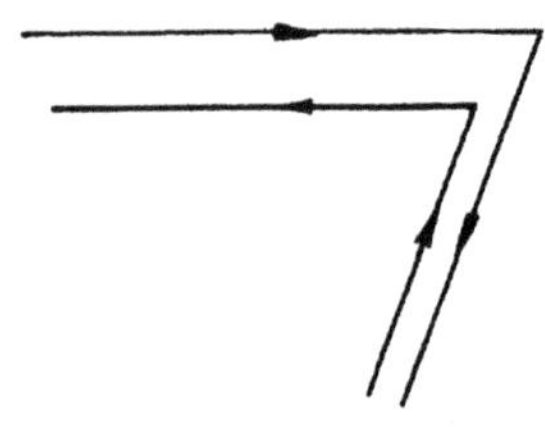

Fig. 113

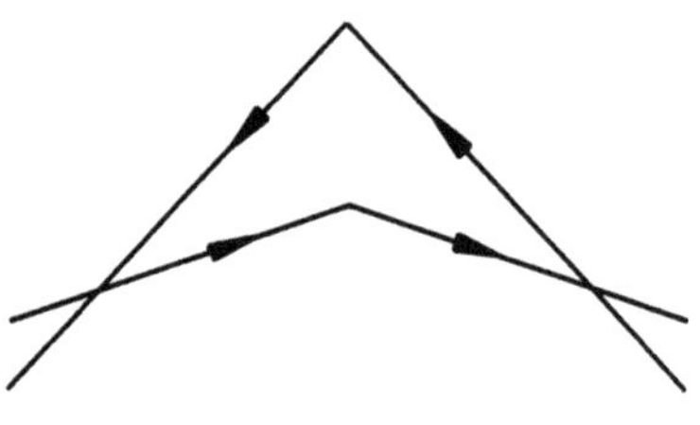

Fig. 114

In 1970, the case in Fig.113 was solved emphasizing new examples of open magnetic lines [80]. This paper discusses some configurations that are strongly connected with circuits feasible in the laboratories, but with open magnetic lines. Two new ideas are introduced: 1) the needle-current as the limit of an angular current whose angle tends to zero, while the current intensity tends toward infinity; 2) the U-dicurrent, as the limit of a piecewise rectilinear U-shaped current, with two vertices, in which the distance between the parallel sides tends toward zero, while the current intensity tends to infinity. In this case the phase portrait contains open helicoidal magnetic lines.

The case of magnetic field lines of equal rectilinear currents distributed on a centred parallelogram was discussed in 1972 [81] and 1973 [82], with conclusions and solution techniques similar to those from the preceding papers.

(11) For a plane rhombus, complete integration of the differential system describing magnetic lines was performed using elementary transcendental functions and errors function [83].

The case of the bifilar, plane, symmetrically bent electric line (Fig.114) was solved in 1977 [84] again emphasizing the existence of an algebraic first integral.

(12) The papers [85]-[87] deal with open magnetic lines and particularly with the ergodicity behaviour of these lines. Also, these papers list open problems, point again to the method of the elementary invariant flow for deducing a first integral, and indirectly state conjectures.

Now we select some ideas of Sabba Ştefănescu in the commentary of the paper [85]. The basic configuration analysed in this paper consists of four infinite rectilinear currents of the same intensity forming two complete equipollent angles in two parallel planes and having their centres on the same vertical Oz (Fig.115). In case of nonplanar electric circuits, the shape of magnetic lines becomes particularly intricate, sometimes apparently chaotic as far as the electric field generating the magnetic field deviates from planarity (e.g. a skewed square circuit, Fig.116).

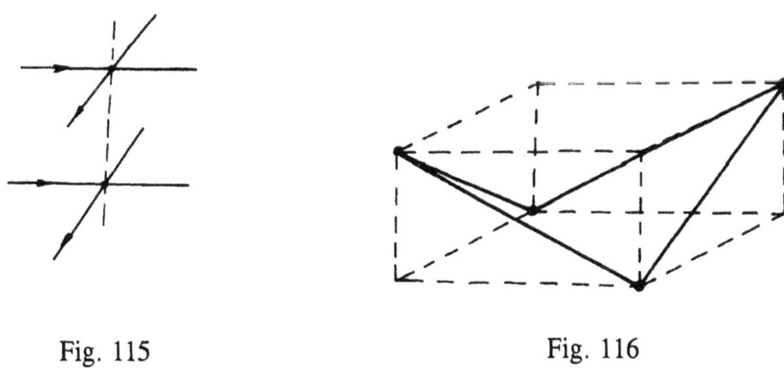

Fig. 115 Fig. 116

From the theoretical point of view, it is very interesting to know whether in the complicated structure of magnetic phase portraits, especially of those due to nonplanar electric circuits, one can detect simpler structural elements. The investigations undertaken in this direction lead to identification of the existence of certain algebraic first integrals for describing magnetic lines. These first integrals determine pencils of algebraic surfaces on which there are wound magnetic lines, generally transcendental ones. The complete determination of magnetic lines may be reduced in these cases to Abelian quadratures and in their turn, these quadratures, under entirely special conditions, are reducible to elliptical integrals and even to elementary transcendental ones.

The Sabba Ştefănescu Conjecture. *The differential system describing the lines of a magnetic field generated by a configuration of piecewise rectilinear electric circuits admits an algebraic first integral.*

Open problem. *Which are the Cartesian implicit equations and the shape of the magnetic lines around $n > 2$ equal rectilinear currents placed arbitrarily in space?*

The commentary of Sabba Ştefănescu made in paper [86] contains also many interesting ideas. First he mentions that some controversies in the Romanian technical world are due to the wrong idea that magnetic lines around filiform electric circuits are always closed. Also, the existence of open magnetic lines was almost unanimously ascribed to the fact that the system of two equal infinite rectilinear currents cannot constitute by any means a closed circuit. This objection is fully grounded. But, if it is admitted that the two currents are closed at infinity through filiform rectilinear junctions, one may prove that these junctions determine, within large finite distance, a negligible magnetic field, and consequently, this part of the field cannot modify the quasi-helicoidal form of the magnetic lines [76]. Other examples of open magnetic lines [74, [75], [80], [85], [86] raised similar objections. The careful investigation of these problems led Sabba Ştefănescu to the conclusion that the closedness (nonclosedness) of the magnetic lines is due not to the continuity (discontinuity) of the generating electric field or circuits but to the fact that the circuits are (are not) planar. Given the complexity of the differential system governing the magnetic lines, the mathematical proof of this assertion appears as difficult and till now has not been approached.

The basic configuration exploited in the paper [86] is an electric circuit of skew square type (obtained by connecting in series four diagonals of the faces of an upright prism whose basis is a square), and it has surely open magnetic lines of helicoidal type (Fig.116). During the decrease of each angle toward zero, the magnetic lines remain open, of infinite length, but their turns become progressively closer. The paper [5] of S.Bobbio shows that confinement of thermonuclear plasma requires stationary and quasi-stationary magnetic fields,and consequently the ideas of Sabba Ştefănescu are very modern and topical.Also, S.Bobbio mentions the **Grad Conjecture** (confirmed by all numerical experiments performed recently): *without symmetry, the existence of a rational magnetic surface, immersed in a set of irrational surface, is not possible* (see [5] p.138). This conjecture is strongly related to the Sabba Ştefănescu conjecture (see also, [69], [71]-[77], [88]).

Between 1985 and 1986, the ideas of Sabba Ştefănescu were taken over and were used by Alexandru Timotin and his student Liviu Milea at the Politehnica University of Bucharest.

Starting from 1987, the ideas of Sabba Ştefănescu [63]-[88] were developed by our research team in a series of papers [49]- [51], [89], [98], [99], [104], [120]-[130], [132], [133], [135], etc.

10.3. MAGNETIC DYNAMICS AROUND FILIFORM ELECTRIC CIRCUITS OF RIGHT ANGLE TYPE

This theory is contained in details in [49], [51], [89], [98], [99], [120]-[130].

10.3.1. Magnetic flows and magnetic surfaces

Let $H = (H_x, H_y, H_z)$ be a C^∞ stationary magnetic field, i.e., an irrotational and solenoidal vector field, defined on an open set D in R^3. The relations $\text{rot}H = 0$, $\text{div}H = 0$ imply $\Delta H = 0 = (\Delta H_x, \Delta H_y, \Delta H_z)$ and therefore H is a harmonic vector field.

Zeros of H are constant field lines (points). These are called the *equilibrium points* of the differential system (1) or of the magnetic field H.

Let $\varphi : D_1 \subset D \to R$ be the potential of H, i.e., $H = \text{grad}\varphi$ on $D_1 \subset D$. The field lines of H contain the gradient lines of φ.

A maximal magnetic line $\alpha_{(x,y,z)} : I(x,y,z) \to D \subset R^3$ at $(x,y,z) \in D$ is defined on an open interval $I(x,y,z) = (t_-(x,y,z), t_+(x,y,z))$ containing 0 in R. The flow

$$T: \mathcal{D}(H) \to D,\ T_t(x,y,z) = \alpha_{(x,y,z)}(t),$$

where

$$\mathcal{D}(\boldsymbol{H}) = \{(t; x, y, z) \in R \times D | t_-(x,y,z) < t < t_+(x,y,z)\}$$

is a map of class C^∞ defined on the open subset $\mathcal{D}(\boldsymbol{H})$ of $R \times D$. This flow preserves the volume because $\operatorname{div} H = 0$.

Let $f: D \to R$, $f = \frac{1}{2}(H_x^2 + H_y^2 + H_z^2)$ be the energy of the magnetic field H, leaving aside the multiplicative factor μ [130]. The energy f cannot be upper bounded, since the functions H_x, H_y, H_z are unbounded as harmonic functions on an open set D.

Let $\alpha : I \to D$, $\alpha(t) = (x(t), y(t), z(t))$ be a magnetic line. The motion of a particle along the magnetic line α is included in the motion described by the conservative differential system with three degrees of freedom associated to the potential $V = -f$, i.e.,

$$\frac{d^2x}{dt^2} = \frac{\partial f}{\partial x}, \quad \frac{d^2y}{dt^2} = \frac{\partial f}{\partial y}, \quad \frac{d^2z}{dt^2} = \frac{\partial f}{\partial z}.$$

Denoting

$$\frac{dx}{dt} = -u, \quad \frac{dy}{dt} = -v, \quad \frac{dz}{dt} = -w$$

the conservative system is transformed into the phase space $R^6 = \{(x,y,z,u,v,w)\}$ in a Hamiltonian system,

$$\frac{dx}{dt} = -u, \quad \frac{dy}{dt} = -v, \quad \frac{dz}{dt} = -w$$

$$\frac{du}{dt} = -\frac{\partial f}{\partial x}, \quad \frac{dv}{dt} = -\frac{\partial f}{\partial y}, \quad \frac{dw}{dt} = -\frac{\partial f}{\partial z}$$

with the *Hamiltonian (mechanical energy)*

$$\mathcal{H}(x,y,z,u,v,w) = \frac{1}{2}(u^2 + v^2 + w^2) - f(x,y,z).$$

Denote by (,) the scalar product on R^3. Differentiating along a field line of the magnetic field H and replacing $\frac{dx}{dt}$ by H_x, etc, we find the prolongations

$$\begin{aligned} \frac{d^2x}{dt^2} &= \left(\frac{\partial \boldsymbol{H}}{\partial x}, \boldsymbol{H}\right) = \frac{\partial f}{\partial x} \\ \frac{d^2y}{dt^2} &= \left(\frac{\partial \boldsymbol{H}}{\partial y}, \boldsymbol{H}\right) = \frac{\partial f}{\partial y} \\ \frac{d^2z}{dt^2} &= \left(\frac{\partial \boldsymbol{H}}{\partial z}, \boldsymbol{H}\right) = \frac{\partial f}{\partial z}; \end{aligned} \tag{3}$$

$$\begin{aligned} \frac{d^3x}{dt^3} &= \left(\frac{\partial^2 \boldsymbol{H}}{\partial x^2}, \boldsymbol{H}\right) + \left(\frac{\partial \boldsymbol{H}}{\partial x}, \frac{\partial \boldsymbol{H}}{\partial x}\right) = \frac{\partial^2 f}{\partial x^2} H_x + \frac{\partial^2 f}{\partial x \partial y} H_y + \frac{\partial^2 f}{\partial x \partial z} H_z = L \\ \frac{d^3y}{dt^3} &= \left(\frac{\partial^2 \boldsymbol{H}}{\partial y^2}, \boldsymbol{H}\right) + \left(\frac{\partial \boldsymbol{H}}{\partial y}, \frac{\partial \boldsymbol{H}}{\partial y}\right) = \frac{\partial^2 f}{\partial x \partial y} H_x + \frac{\partial^2 f}{\partial y^2} H_y + \frac{\partial^2 f}{\partial z \partial y} H_z = M \end{aligned} \tag{4}$$

$$\frac{d^3 z}{dt^3} = \left(\frac{\partial^2 \boldsymbol{H}}{\partial z^2}, \boldsymbol{H}\right) + \left(\frac{\partial \boldsymbol{H}}{\partial z}, \frac{\partial \boldsymbol{H}}{\partial z}\right) = \frac{\partial^2 f}{\partial x \partial z} H_x + \frac{\partial^2 f}{\partial y \partial z} H_y + \frac{\partial^2 f}{\partial z^2} H_z = N.$$

So the following statement is true.

Theorem. *Let* $\boldsymbol{H}$ *be a magnetic field of class* C^∞ *and* $\alpha : I \to D$, $\alpha(t) = (x(t), y(t), z(t))$ *be a nonconstant field line of* $\boldsymbol{H}$.

1) α *is a straight line iff the vector fields* $\boldsymbol{H} \circ \alpha$ *and* $\operatorname{grad} f \circ \alpha$ *are collinear.*

2) α *is a plane curve iff the vector fields* $\boldsymbol{H} \circ \alpha$, $\operatorname{grad} f \circ \alpha$ *and* $(L, M, N) \circ \alpha$ *are coplanar.*

Proof. 1) α is a straight line iff its curvature is identically zero, i.e., $\alpha' \times \alpha'' = 0$.

2) α is a plane curve iff its torsion is identically zero, i.e., $(\alpha' \times \alpha'', \alpha''') = 0$.

Let $\varphi : D_1 \to R$ be the local potential of $\boldsymbol{H}$. We find

$$H_x \frac{\partial f}{\partial x} + H_y \frac{\partial f}{\partial y} + H_z \frac{\partial f}{\partial z} = \operatorname{Hess} \varphi (\boldsymbol{H}, \boldsymbol{H}) \tag{5}$$

and hence the energy f is a solution of a magnetic differential equation. It follows that generally the magnetic lines are transversal to the surfaces $\Sigma_c : f(x,y,z) = c$. If a magnetic line α is included in Σ_c, then it is a geodesic of Σ_c because the acceleration $\alpha'' = \operatorname{grad} f \circ \alpha$ is normal to Σ_c.

The restrictions of the functions L, M, N to D_1 can be written in the form

$$L = \frac{\partial}{\partial x} \operatorname{Hess} \varphi(\boldsymbol{H}, \boldsymbol{H}) - \left(\frac{\partial \boldsymbol{H}}{\partial x}, \nabla f\right)$$

$$M = \frac{\partial}{\partial y} \operatorname{Hess} \varphi(\boldsymbol{H}, \boldsymbol{H}) - \left(\frac{\partial \boldsymbol{H}}{\partial y}, \nabla f\right)$$

$$N = \frac{\partial}{\partial z} \operatorname{Hess} \varphi(\boldsymbol{H}, \boldsymbol{H}) - \left(\frac{\partial \boldsymbol{H}}{\partial z}, \nabla f\right).$$

Theorem. *1) If the magnetic field* H *has a closed field line*

$$\alpha : [t_1, t_2] \to D, \ \alpha(t) = (x(t), y(t), z(t)),$$

then

$$\oint_\alpha \frac{\operatorname{Hess} \varphi (\boldsymbol{H}, \boldsymbol{H})}{\sqrt{2f}} \circ \alpha \, ds = 0,$$

where

$$ds = \sqrt{2f} \circ \alpha \, dt.$$

2) Suppose that $\boldsymbol{H}$ *has closed field surfaces and denote by* V *the domain between two closed magnetic surfaces. Then*

$$\int_V \text{Hess}\,\varphi\,(\boldsymbol{H},\boldsymbol{H})\,dv = 0.$$

Proof. One uses the relation (5).

1) By hypotheses, $t_1 < t_2$ and $\alpha(t_1) = \alpha(t_2)$. The restriction to α of the left member of the relation (5) can be written as $\frac{d}{dt} f \circ \alpha$ and therefore

$$\oint_\alpha \frac{\text{Hess}\,\varphi\,(\boldsymbol{H},\boldsymbol{H})}{\sqrt{2f}} \circ \alpha\, ds = \int_{t_1}^{t_2} \frac{d}{dt} f \circ \alpha\, dt = f(\alpha(t))\Big|_{t_1}^{t_2} = 0.$$

2) Since $\text{div}\,\boldsymbol{H} = 0$, the left member of the relation (5) can be written as $\text{div}(\boldsymbol{H}f)$. By the Gauss theorem, the integral on V transforms into an integral on ∂V, and the normal versor field of the boundary ∂V (union of magnetic surfaces) is orthogonal to $\boldsymbol{H}$. Hence

$$\int_V \text{div}(\boldsymbol{H}f)\,dv = \int_{\partial V} (\boldsymbol{H}f, n)\,d\sigma = 0.$$

Corollary. *If* $\boldsymbol{H}$ *admits closed field lines or closed field surfaces, then there exists at least one point* $(x_0, y_0, z_0) \in D_1$ *at which* $\text{Hess}\,\varphi\,(\boldsymbol{H},\boldsymbol{H})(x_0, y_0, z_0) = 0$.

Remark. Since φ is a harmonic function, i.e., $\Delta\varphi = 0$, the Hessian $d^2\varphi$ cannot be definite. As a result, the surfaces of constant potential $S_c : \varphi(x,y,z) = c$ cannot be orientable and compact or convex. These surfaces are surely unbounded.

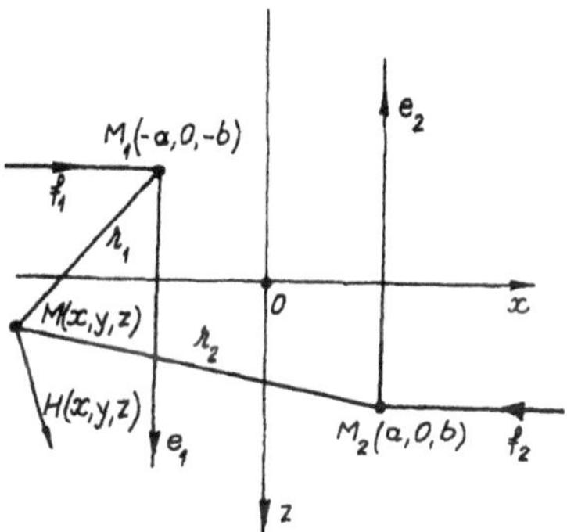

Fig. 117

10.3.2. Magnetic lines around two coplanar filiform electric circuits of right angle type with currents of opposite sense

The configuration of Fig.117 and the Biot-Savart-Laplace law permit computation of the magnetic field $\boldsymbol{H} = (H_x, H_y, H_z)$,

$$H_x = \frac{-y}{r_1(r_1 - z - b)} + \frac{y}{r_2(r_2 + z - b)}$$

$$H_y = \frac{x+a}{r_1(r_1 - z - b)} - \frac{z+b}{r_1(r_1 + x + a)} - \frac{x-a}{r_2(r_2 + z - b)} + \frac{z-b}{r_2(r_2 - x + a)}$$

$$H_z = \frac{y}{r_1(r_1 + x + a)} - \frac{y}{r_2(r_2 - x + a)},$$

where

$$r_1^2 = (x+a)^2 + y^2 + (z+b)^2, \; r_2^2 = (x-a)^2 + y^2 + (z-b)^2.$$

The domain of definition of this vector field is

$$D = R^3 - (e_1 \cup f_1 \cup e_2 \cup f_2),$$

where

$$f_1 : x \le -a, \; y = 0, \; z = -b; \; e_1 : x = -a, \; y = 0, \; z \ge -b$$

$$f_2 : x \ge a, \; y = 0, \; z = b; \; e_2 : x = a, \; y = 0, \; z \le b.$$

We remark that the functions H_x, H_y, H_z are bounded with respect to y for fixed x, z. For example,

$$H_x \le \frac{1}{r_1 - z - b} + \frac{1}{r_2 + z - b}$$

$$H_y \le \frac{1}{r_1 - z - b} + \frac{1}{r_1 + x + a} + \frac{1}{r_2 + z - b} + \frac{1}{r_2 - x + a}$$

$$H_z \le \frac{1}{r_1 + x + a} + \frac{1}{r_2 - x + a},$$

$$r_1^2 = (x+a)^2 + (z+b)^2, \; r_2^2 = (x-a)^2 + (z-b)^2.$$

Suppose that the parameters a and b do not vanish simultaneously.

Theorem. *1) If $a \le 0$, $b > 0$, then the set of equilibrium points of H is the ellipse of equations*

$$y = 0, \; r_1 + r_2 = 2(b-a)$$

without the points $(a, 0, -b)$ and $(-a, 0, b)$.

2) If $ab > 0$ and $a \ne b$, then the set of equilibrium points of H consists of two points

$$\left(0; \frac{\pm\sqrt{2ab(a^2+b^2)}}{b-a}; 0\right).$$

3) In the other cases the set of equilibrium points is void.

Theorem. *1) The field line through (x_0, y_0, z_0) is congruent to the field line through $(x_0, -y_0, z_0)$.*

2) The field line through (x_0, y_0, z_0) is congruent to the field line through $(-x_0, y_0, -z_0)$.

Proof. 1) The symmetry with respect to the plane xOy is

$$x' = x, \; y' = -y, \; z' = z.$$

One deduces that the differential system (1) is changed into

$$\frac{dx'}{dt} = -H_{x'}, \quad \frac{dy'}{dt} = -H_{y'}, \quad \frac{dz'}{dt} = -H_{z'}.$$

Considering (1), (3), (4), the field line through (x_0, y_0, z_0) is congruent to the field line through $(x_0, -y_0, z_0)$, having the same speed, same curvature and the same absolute value of torsion.

2) Analogously, the symmetry with respect to Oy being $x' = -x$, $y' = y$, $z' = -z$, the differential system (1) is changed into

$$\frac{dx'}{dt} = H_{x'}, \quad \frac{dy'}{dt} = H_{y'}, \quad \frac{dz'}{dt} = H_{z'}.$$

The formulas (1), (3), (4), show that the field line through (x_0, y_0, z_0) has the same speed, same curvature and the same torsion as the field line through $(-x_0, y_0, -z_0)$.

The preceding theorems show that the nonconstant field lines can be fixed by initial conditions of the type

$$x(0) = x_0, \; y(0) = 0, \; z(0) = z_0$$

or of the type

$$x(0) = 0, \; y(0) = y_0, \; z(0) = 0,$$

under the condition that these are not zeros of H. Since

$$H_x(x_0, 0, z_0) = 0, \; H_y(x_0, 0, z_0) \neq 0, \; H_z(x_0, 0, z_0) = 0$$

$$H_x(0, y_0, 0) = 0, \; H_y(0, y_0, 0) \neq 0, \; H_z(0, y_0, 0) = 0,$$

the nonconstant magnetic lines that intersect the plane xOy are perpendicular to it, and the nonconstant magnetic lines which meet Oy are included in this axis.

Theorem. *The nonconstant field line through* $x(0) = x_0$, $y(0) = y_0$, $z(0) = z_0$ *is symmetrical with respect to the plane* xOz.

Proof. Let $(x(t), y(t), z(t))$, $t \in (-\varepsilon, \varepsilon)$ be the solution of the Cauchy problem

$$\frac{dx}{dt} = H_x(x(t), y(t), z(t))$$

$$\frac{dy}{dt} = H_y(x(t), y(t), z(t))$$

$$\frac{dz}{dt} = H_z(x(t), y(t), z(t)), \; x(0) = x_0, \; y(0) = y_0, \; z(0) = z_0.$$

Changing t into $-t$ we find

$$\frac{dx}{dt} = -H_x(x(-t), y(-t), z(-t)) - H_x(x(-t), \; y(-t), z(-t))$$

$$\frac{dx}{dt} = H_y(x(-t),\ -y(-t),\ z(-t))$$

$$\frac{dz}{dt} = H_z(x(-t),\ -y(-t),\ z(-t))$$

$$x(0) = x_0,\ y(0) = y_0,\ z(0) = z_0.$$

By the existence and uniqueness theorem applied to this Cauchy problem we find

$$x(-t) = x(t),\ -y(-t) = y(t),\ z(-t) = z(t)$$

and hence the curve $\alpha : (-\varepsilon, \varepsilon) \to D$, $\alpha(t) = (x(t), y(t), z(t))$ is symmetrical with respect to the plane xOz.

Corollary. *The field lines of* $\boldsymbol{H}$, *which do not admit zeros of* $\boldsymbol{H}$ *as limit points, are closed curves either around the wire* $e_1 \cup f_1$ *or around the wire* $e_2 \cup f_2$.

Proof. Consequence of the "right-hand rule" and of the symmetry with respect to the plane xOz.

Theorem. *Let* $(x_0, 0, z_0)$ *be a point that is not a zero of* $\boldsymbol{H}$.

1) The curvature at $(x_0, 0, z_0)$ *of the magnetic line through* $(x_0, 0, z_0)$ *is zero iff* $x_0 = z_0 = 0$.

2) The torsion at $(x_0, 0, z_0) \neq (0,0,0)$ *of the magnetic line through* $(x_0, 0, z_0)$ *is zero. The osculating plane at such a point is parallel to* Oy.

There exist points on the field line through $(x_0, 0, z_0) \neq (0,0,0)$ *at which the torsion is not zero.*

Proof. Let

$$r_1^2 = (x+a)^2 + (z+b)^2,\ r_2^2 = (x-a)^2 + (z-b)^2.$$

It turns out that

$$H_x(x,0,z) = 0,\ H_z(x,0,z) = 0$$

$$H_y(x,0,z) = \frac{2(r_1 + r_2 + 2a - 2b)}{[r_1 + x + a - (z+b)][r_2 + (z-b) - (x-a)]};$$

$$\frac{\partial f}{\partial x}(x,0,z) = \frac{\partial H_y}{\partial x} H_y(x,0,z) = \left(\frac{1}{r_2(r_2 + z - b)} - \frac{1}{r_1(r_1 - z - b)}\right) H_y(x,0,z)$$

$$\frac{\partial f}{\partial y}(x,0,z) = \frac{\partial H_y}{\partial y} H_y(x,0,z) = 0$$

$$\frac{\partial f}{\partial z}(x,0,z) = \frac{\partial H_y}{\partial z} H_y(x,0,z) = \left(\frac{1}{r_1(r_1 + x + a)} - \frac{1}{r_2(r_2 - x + a)}\right) H_y(x,0,z);$$

$$L(x,0,z) = \frac{\partial^2 f}{\partial x \partial y} H_y(x,0,z) = 0$$

$$M(x,0,z) = \frac{\partial^2 f}{\partial y^2} H_y(x,0,z) = \left(\frac{1}{r_2(r_2+z-b)} - \frac{1}{r_1(r_1-z-b)} \right)^2$$

$$+ \left(\frac{1}{r_1(r_1+x+a)} - \frac{1}{r_2(r_2-x+a)} \right)^2 + \frac{\partial^2 H_y}{\partial y^2} H_y(x,0,z)$$

$$N(x,0,z) = \frac{\partial^2 f}{\partial y \partial z} H_y(x,0,z) = 0.$$

1) Taking into account the formula

$$k = \frac{\|\alpha' \times \alpha''\|}{\|\alpha'\|^3}$$

and the relations (1), (3) we infer

$$k(0) = 0 \Leftrightarrow \frac{\partial f}{\partial x}(x_0, 0, z_0) = 0, \ \frac{\partial f}{\partial z}(x_0, 0, z_0) = 0 \Leftrightarrow \ x_0 = z_0 = 0.$$

2) Analogously,

$$\tau = \frac{(\alpha' \times \alpha'', \alpha''')}{\|\alpha' \times \alpha''\|^2}$$

and the formulas (1), (3), (4) lead to $\tau(0) = 0$.

The equation of the specified osculating plane is

$$(x - x_0) \frac{\partial f}{\partial z}(x_0, 0, z_0) - (z - z_0) \frac{\partial f}{\partial x}(x_0, 0, z_0) = 0.$$

The last assertion devolves from the torsion formula and from the formulas (1), (3), (4).

Corollaries. *1) The magnetic field H admits field lines that are not plane curves.*

2) If there exist plane magnetic lines, then these curves are contained in the planes passing by Oy.

Proof. 2) The orbits through the points $(x_0, y_0, z_0), (x_0, -y_0, z_0)$ are congruent to the orbit through the points $(-x_0, y_0, -z_0), (-x_0, -y_0, -z_0)$. These four points are in a plane passing by Oy. If there exists a plane orbit, i.e., one included in its osculating plane, then necessarily the osculating plane passes by Oy.

We suspect that the only plane orbits are those in the next

Theorem (Fig.118). *1) If $b < a$, then the axis Oy is a nonconstant field line.*

2) If $b > a$, $ab > 0$, then the axis Oy is composed from two equilibrium points E_1, E_2 and from three nonconstant field lines, and the circle

$$C:\begin{cases} x^2+y^2+z^2=2ab(a^2+b^2)(b-a)^{-2} \\ ax+bz=0 \end{cases}$$

is constituted from two equilibrium points E_1, E_2 *and two nonconstant field lines (semicircles).*

3) If $b>a,\ ab<0,\ (\Leftrightarrow a<0, b>0)$, *then the axis* Oy' *is a nonconstant field line.*

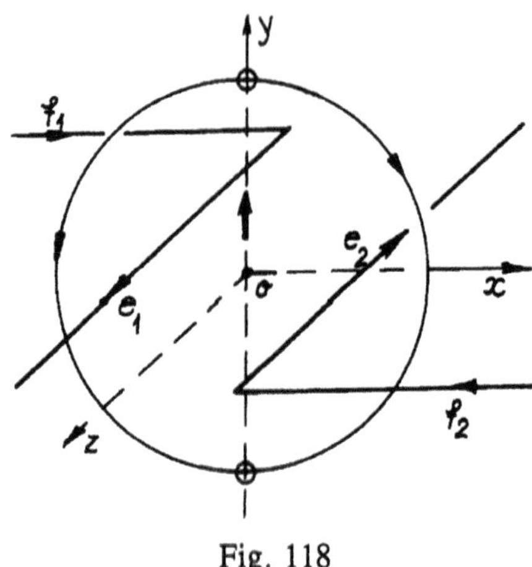

Fig. 118

10.3.3. Magnetic lines around two coplanar filiform electric circuits of right angle type with currents of same sense

The configuration of Fig.119 and the Biot-Savart-Laplace law produce the magnetic field $\boldsymbol{H}=(H_x, H_y, H_z)$,

$$H_x=-\frac{y}{r_1(r_1-z-b)}-\frac{y}{r_2(r_2+z-b)}$$

$$H_y=\frac{x+a}{r_1(r_1-z-b)}-\frac{z+b}{r_1(r_1+x+a)}+\frac{x-a}{r_2(r_2+z-b)}-\frac{z-b}{r_2(r_2-x+a)}$$

$$H_z=\frac{y}{r_1(r_1+x+a)}+\frac{y}{r_2(r_2-x+a)},$$

where

$$r_1^2=(x+a)^2+y^2+(z+b)^2,\ r_2^2=(x-a)^2+y^2+(z-b)^2.$$

The domain of the vector field $\boldsymbol{H}$ is the set D described in the preceding paragraph.

One observes that H_x, H_y, H_z are bounded with respect to y for fixed x, z since

$$H_x \leq \frac{1}{r_1 - z - b} + \frac{1}{r_2 + z - b}$$

$$H_y \leq \frac{1}{r_1 - z - b} + \frac{1}{r_1 + x + a} + \frac{1}{r_2 + z - b} + \frac{1}{r_2 - x + a}$$

$$H_z \leq \frac{1}{r_1 + x + a} + \frac{1}{r_2 - x + a},$$

where

$$r_1^2 = (x+a)^2 + (z+b)^2, \ r_2^2 = (x-a)^2 + (z-b)^2.$$

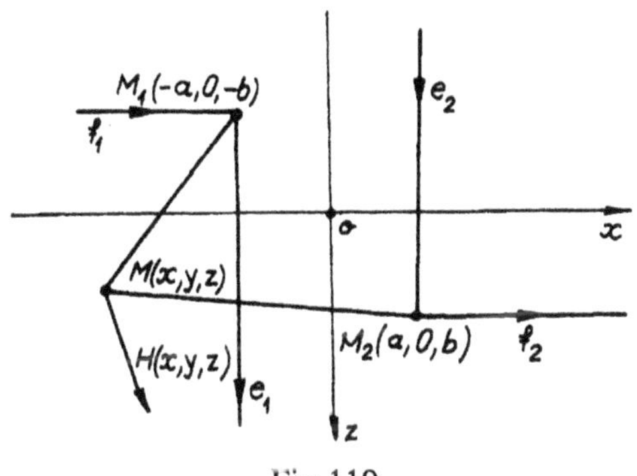

Fig 119

Suppose that the parameters a and b do not vanish simultaneously.

Theorem. *The set of equilibrium points of* H *is the curve*

$$\Gamma : y = 0, \ r_1 - r_2 = 2(x - z).$$

Theorem. *1) The field line through* (x_0, y_0, z_0) *is congruent to the field line through* $(x_0, -y_0, z_0)$.

2) The field line through (x_0, y_0, z_0) *is congruent to the field line through* $(-x_0, y_0, -z_0)$.

Proof. 1) The symmetry $x' = x, \ y' = -y, \ z' = z$ changes the differential system (1) into the differential system

$$\frac{dx'}{dt} = -H_{x'}, \ \frac{dy'}{dt} = -H_{y'}, \ \frac{dz'}{dt} = -H_{z'}.$$

So the field lines through (x_0, y_0, z_0) and $(x_0, -y_0, z_0)$ respectively are congruent.

The preceding theorems suggest that nonconstant field lines can be fixed by initial conditions of the type

$$x(0) = x_0, \ y(0) = 0, \ z(0) = z_0$$

or of the type

$$x(0) = 0, \ y(0) = y_0, \ z(0) = 0,$$

excluding the zeros of H. Since

$$H_x(x_0, 0, z_0) = 0, \ H_y(x_0, 0, z_0) \neq 0, \ H_z(x_0, 0, z_0) = 0;$$

$$H_x(0, y_0, 0) \neq 0, \ H_y(0, y_0, 0) = 0, \ H_z(0, y_0, 0) \neq 0,$$

the nonconstant magnetic lines that come across the plane xOz are perpendicular to this plane, and the nonconstant magnetic lines which meet Oy are perpendicular to this axis.

Theorem. *The nonconstant field line through* $x(0) = x_0, \ y(0) = y_0, \ z(0) = z_0$ *is symmetrical with respect to the plane* xOz.

Corollary. *The field lines of* $\boldsymbol{H}$, *which do not admit zeros of* $\boldsymbol{H}$ *as limit points, are closed curves either around the wire* $e_1 \cup f_1$, *around the wire* $e_2 \cup f_2$, *or around both of them.*

Theorem. *Let* $(x_0, 0, z_0)$ *be a point that is not a zero of* H.

1) The curvature at $(x_0, 0, z_0)$ *of the magnetic line through* $(x_0, 0, z_0)$ *is strictly positive.*

2) The torsion at $(x_0, 0, z_0)$ *of the magnetic line through* $(x_0, 0, z_0)$ *is zero. The osculating plane at such a point is parallel to the axis* Oy.

There exist points on the field line through $(x_0, 0, z_0)$ *at which the torsion is not zero.*

Proof. Let $r_1^2 = (x+a)^2 + (z+b)^2, \ r_2^2 = (x-a)^2 + (z-b)^2$. We find

$$H_x(x,0,z) = 0, \ H_z(x,0,z) = 0$$

$$H_y(x,0,z) = \frac{2(r_2 - r_1 + 2z - 2x)}{[r_1 + x + a - (z+b)][r_2 + (z-b) - (x-a)]};$$

$$\frac{\partial f}{\partial x}(x,0,z) = \frac{\partial H_y}{\partial x} H_y(x,0,z) = -\left(\frac{1}{r_1(r_1 - z - b)} + \frac{1}{r_2(r_2 + z - b)} \right) H_y(x,0,z)$$

$$\frac{\partial f}{\partial y}(x,0,z) = \frac{\partial H_y}{\partial y} H_y(x,0,z) = 0$$

$$\frac{\partial f}{\partial z}(x,0,z) = \frac{\partial H_y}{\partial z} H_y(x,0,z) = \left(\frac{1}{r_1(r_1 + x + a)} + \frac{1}{r_2(r_2 - x + a)} \right) H_y(x,0,z);$$

$$L(x,0,z) = \frac{\partial^2 f}{\partial x \partial y} H_y(x,0,z) = 0$$

$$M(x,0,z) = \frac{\partial^2 f}{\partial y^2} H_y(x,0,z) = \left(\frac{1}{r_1(r_1 - z - b)} + \frac{1}{r_2(r_2 + z - b)} \right)^2 +$$

$$+\left(\frac{1}{r_1(r_1+x+a)}+\frac{1}{r_2(r_2-x+a)}\right)^2+\frac{\partial^2 H_y}{\partial y^2}H_y(x,0,z)$$

$$N(x,0,z)=\frac{\partial^2 f}{\partial y\partial z}H_y(x,0,z).$$

1) One observes that $H\circ\alpha$ and $\mathrm{grad}f\circ\alpha$ cannot be collinear.

2) The formulas (1), (3), (4) lead to $\tau(0)=0$. The equation of the specified osculating plane is

$$(x-x_0)\frac{\partial f}{\partial z}(x_0,0,z_0)-(z-z_0)\frac{\partial f}{\partial x}(x_0,0,z_0)=0.$$

Obviously, there exist points at which the vectors $H\circ\alpha$, $\mathrm{grad}f\circ\alpha$, $(L,M,N)\circ\alpha$ are not coplanar.

Theorem. *If* $a+b=0$, *then there exist at least two points of the type* $(0,y,0)$, $y\neq 0$, *at which the curvature of the magnetic line through such a point is zero.*

Proof. On the axis Oy we have $r_1=r_2=\sqrt{a^2+y^2+b^2}$. For $y\neq 0$ we find

$$H_x(0,y,0)\neq 0,\ H_y(0,y,0)=0,\ H_z(0,y,0)\neq 0,$$

$$\frac{\partial f}{\partial x}(0,y,0)=0$$

$$\frac{\partial f}{\partial y}(0,y,0)=\left(H_x\frac{\partial H_x}{\partial y}+H_z\frac{\partial H_z}{\partial y}\right)(0,y,0)$$

$$=-\frac{2y}{r_1(r_1-b)}\left(\frac{-2}{r_1(r_1-b)}+\frac{2y^2(2r_1-b)}{r_1^3(r_1-b)^2}\right)+\frac{2y}{r_1(r_1+a)}\left(\frac{2}{r_1(r_1+a)}-\frac{2y^2(2r_1+a)}{r_1^3(r_1+a)^2}\right)$$

$$\frac{\partial f}{\partial z}(0,y,0)=0.$$

If $a+b\neq 0$, then the equations

$$\frac{\partial H_x}{\partial y}(0,y,0)=0,\quad \frac{\partial H_z}{\partial y}(0,y,0)=0,$$

with the unknown r_1, have no common solutions. If $a+b=0$, then these equations have a common solution $r_1\geq\sqrt{a^2+b^2}$ and therefore the solutions $\pm y_1$ with respect to y. At the points $(0,\pm y_1,0)$, the curvature is zero, since these are critical points of f.

The existence of plane magnetic lines is still an open problem.

10.3.4. Stationary magnetic field with heteroclinic structure

Let $\boldsymbol{H}=(H_1, H_2, H_3)$ be a stationary magnetic field, i.e., a C^∞ irrotational ($\mathrm{rot}\,\boldsymbol{H}=0$) and solenoidal ($\mathrm{div}\,\boldsymbol{H}=0$) vector field, defined on an open set D in R^3.

Theorem. *Let $p=(x_0^1, x_0^2, x_0^3)$ be an equilibrium point of the magnetic dynamical system. If p is an isolated equilibrium point of the linear approximation around p, then it is a hyperbolic equilibrium point of the magnetic dynamical system.*

Proof. The matrix

$$L=(L_{ij}),\quad L_{ij}=\frac{\partial H_i}{\partial x^j}(p),\quad i,j=1,2,3,$$

of the linear approximation

$$\frac{dx^i}{dt}=\frac{\partial H_i}{\partial x^j}(p)(x^j-x_0^j)$$

is symmetric since $\mathrm{rot}\,\boldsymbol{H}=0$. Therefore its proper values are real numbers. This matrix is nonsingular since $p=(x_0^1, x_0^2, x_0^3)$ is an isolated equilibrium point, and it is indefinite because its trace is zero as a consequence of $\mathrm{div}\,\boldsymbol{H}=0$.

Consequently, the linear approximation has three nonzero real proper values $\lambda_1, \lambda_2, \lambda_3$, two of them having the same sign, and the third having opposite sign. Assuming, $\lambda_1, \lambda_2<0$, $\lambda_3>0$, the space $T_{x_0}R^3$ decomposes as a direct sum

$$T_pR^3=E^s\oplus E^u,$$

where E^s is the stable manifold (plane) and E^u is the unstable manifold (straight line) for the linear approximation.

Taking into account the Stable Manifold Theorem for equilibrium of finite-dimensional vector fields we obtain

Theorem. *Let p be a hyperbolic equilibrium point and $T_t(x)$ be the flow of the magnetic dynamical system. Let $L: T_pR^3\to T_pR^3$ be the linearization of $\boldsymbol{H}$ at p. Assume that $T_pR^3=E^s\oplus E^u$, with the spectrum of $L|_{E^s}$ consisting of two numbers in $(-\infty,0)$ and the spectrum of $L|_{E^u}$ consisting of one number in $(0,\infty)$. Then there exists a C^∞ magnetic surface W^s, and C^∞ magnetic line W^u passing through p, with tangent spaces E^s and E^u respectively, and*

$$W^s=\{x\in D\,|\,T_t(x)\to p \text{ as } t\to\infty\},$$

$$W^u=\{x\in D\,|\,T_t(x)\to p \text{ as } t\to-\infty\}.$$

If $T_t(x)$ is complete, i.e., the parameter t refers to the whole real line, then W^s, W^u are one-to-one immersions of Euclidean spaces into D.

W^s is called *the stable manifold of* p *and* W^u is called *the unstable manifold of* p.

Theorem. *Let* p *be a hyperbolic point of the magnetic dynamical system with* $\dim W^s = 2$, $\dim W^u = 1$. *The stable manifold* W^s *(unstable manifold* W^u*) of* p *is a ruled surface (a geodesic) in the Riemann-Jacobi manifold*

$$(D\setminus\{p\},\, g_{ij} = (\mathcal{H}+f)\,\delta_{ij},\ i,j = 1,2,3).$$

Proof. The map $t \to T_t(M)$ is a reparametrized geodesic of the Riemann-Jacobi metric. So W^s, W^u are generated by geodesics of the associated Riemann-Jacobi manifold. The stable manifold is a cone with the vertex p.

Remark. 1) The Gauss curvature of the surface W^s is at most zero because W^s is a (ruled) magnetic surface.

2) For computing stable and unstable manifolds attached to a hyperbolic equilibrium point of a magnetic dynamical system, we can use algorithms for computing geodesics, since they display the geometry of the Riemann-Jacobi manifold in a way that naive computation of trajectories does not.

3) The relation $\lambda_1 + \lambda_2 + \lambda_3 = 0$ is equivalent to $\lambda_i = 2\lambda_i + \lambda_j + \lambda_k$, $i, j, k = 1, 2, 3$, $i \neq j \neq k$, and consequently the proper values of a saddle type equilibrium point of $\boldsymbol{H}$ are resonant of order four.

Suppose that the vector field $\boldsymbol{H}$ exhibits the symmetries of R^3 given by the matrices

$$R = \begin{bmatrix} 1 & 0 & 0 \\ 0 & -1 & 0 \\ 0 & 0 & 1 \end{bmatrix}, \quad S = \begin{bmatrix} -1 & 0 & 0 \\ 0 & 1 & 0 \\ 0 & 0 & -1 \end{bmatrix},$$

in the sense

$$R(D) = D,\ \boldsymbol{H}\circ R = -R\circ \boldsymbol{H},\ S(D) = D,\ \boldsymbol{H}\circ S = S\circ \boldsymbol{H}.$$

Denoting by T_t the flow of $\boldsymbol{H}$, these relations imply

$$T_{-t}\circ R = R\circ T_t,\ T_t\circ S = S\circ T_t.$$

Automatically, if p_+ is an isolated equilibrium point of $\boldsymbol{H}$, then $p_- = R(p_+)$ is also an isolated equilibrium point of $\boldsymbol{H}$, and the field $\boldsymbol{H}$ admits a heteroclinic structure.

Theorem. *Let* $L_\pm = D\boldsymbol{H}(p_\pm)$ *be the linearizations of the vector field* $\boldsymbol{H}$ *around the equilibrium points* $p_\pm$. *Then* λ *is a proper value of* L_+ *iff* $-\lambda$ *is a proper value of* L_-.

Proof. R is an involution of the space, i.e., $R^2 = I$. The relation $\boldsymbol{H} = -R\circ \boldsymbol{H}\circ R$ implies $L_+ = -RL_-R$. Therefore

$$\det(L_+ - \lambda I) = \det(-RL_-R + \lambda(RR)) = \det(-R(L_- + \lambda I)R) = -\det(L_- + \lambda I).$$

Corollary. *The proper subspaces of* L_+, *and* L_- *coincide.*

Theorem. *The stable and unstable magnetic manifolds associated to the equilibrium points* $p_\pm$ *of the magnetic field* $\boldsymbol{H}$ *are related by*

$$R(W^u(p_+)) = W^s(p_-),\ R(W^s(p_+)) = W^u(p_-).$$

Let us now explain the heteroclinic structure of the magnetic fields produced by two coplanar filiform electric circuits of right angle type, with currents of opposite sense. As was shown by our research team, the results are true for a family of pairs of angles.

10.3.5. Heteroclinic structure of magnetic field produced by two coplanar filiform electric circuits of angle type

For simplicity we study the dynamics of the stationary magnetic field produced by the formula of Biot-Savart-Laplace around two coplanar filiform electric circuits of right angle type, with currents of opposite senses. As was shown by the research team Constantin Udrişte, Aneta Udrişte, Vladimir Bălan, Emilia Petrişor, Mihai Postolache, the results are true for pairs of a family of angles and give the first example of an elementary magnetic field having a heteroclinic behaviour. Our vector field $\boldsymbol{H}$ has the components (Fig.117)

$$H_x = \frac{-y}{r_1(r_1 - x - b)} + \frac{y}{r_2(r_2 + z - b)}$$

$$H_y = \frac{x+a}{r_1(r_1 - z - b)} - \frac{z+b}{r_2(r_2 + x + a)} - \frac{x-a}{r_2(r_2 + z + b)} + \frac{z-b}{r_2(r_2 - x + a)}$$

$$H_z = \frac{y}{r_1(r_1 + x + a)} - \frac{y}{r_2(r_2 - x + a)},$$

where

$$r_1^2 = (x+a)^2 + y^2 + (z+b)^2,\ r_2^2 = (x-a)^2 + y^2 + (z-b)^2.$$

The domain of definition of the vector field $\boldsymbol{H}$ is

$$D = R^3 - \{e_1 \cup f_1 \cup e_2 \cup f_2\},$$

where

$$f_1 : x \le -a,\ y = 0,\ z = -b;\ e_1 : x = -a,\ y = 0,\ z \ge -b$$

$$f_2 : x \ge a,\ y = 0,\ z = b;\ e_2 : x = a,\ y = 0,\ z \le b.$$

The study of such a magnetic field was suggested by the geophysycist Sabba Ştefănescu.

If $ab > 0$ and $a \ne b$, then the set of equilibrium points of $\boldsymbol{H}$ consists of two points (see 10.3.2)

$$p_\pm = \left(0,\ \pm\frac{\sqrt{2ab(a^2+b^2)}}{b-a},\ 0\right).$$

To establish the type of isolated equilibrium points $p_\pm$, we investigate the spectrum of the linearizations of the vector field $\boldsymbol{H}$ around these points. For p_+, we find that the

Jacobian matrix L_+ has the form

$$\begin{bmatrix} L_{11} & 0 & L_{13} \\ 0 & L_{22} & 0 \\ L_{13} & 0 & L_{33} \end{bmatrix}$$

and the proper values of L_+ are

$$\lambda_1 = \frac{L_{11}a^2 - L_{33}b^2}{a^2 - b^2} < 0,\ \lambda_2 = L_{22} < 0,\ \lambda_3 = \frac{L_{33}a^2 - L_{11}b^2}{a^2 - b^2} > 0.$$

The orthogonal proper vectors of L_+ are $v_1(a,0,b)$, $v_2(0,1,0)$, $v_3(-b,0,a)$.

Denote by $S_\lambda(p_+)$, $S_{-\lambda}(p_-)$ the proper subspaces of L_+, respectively L_- corresponding to the proper values λ, respectively $-\lambda$; $v \in S_\lambda(p_+)$ means $L_+(v) = \lambda v$ or equivalently, $L_-(R(v)) = -\lambda R(v)$. But $R(S_\lambda(p_+)) = S_\lambda(p_+)$, therefore $S_\lambda(p_+) = S_{-\lambda}(p_-)$.

The subspace $bx - az = 0$, generated by the proper vectors $v_1(a,0,b)$, $v(0,1,0)$ is the stable subspace for L_+, and unstable subspace for L_-. The stable - unstable plane $bx - az = 0$ is tangent to $W^s(p_+)$ at p_+ and to $W^u(p_-)$ at p_-.

If $b > a$, $ab > 0$, then the axis Oy is composed from two equilibrium points $p_\pm$ and from three nonconstant maximal field lines, and the circle

$$C: ax + bz = 0,\ x^2 + y^2 + z^2 = 2ab(a^2 + b^2)(b - a)^{-2}$$

is constituted from two equilibrium points $p_\pm$ and two nonconstant maximal field lines (semicircles).

This result shows the existence of heteroclinic orbits in the dynamics of our magnetic field. In order to identify the invariant submanifold containing each heteroclinic semicircle of the circle C, we observe that tangent lines to the circle at equilibrium points $p_\pm$ have common direction given by $(-b,0,a)$. Because the vector $v_3(-b,0,a)$ generates the unstable subspace associated to L_+, respectively the stable subspace associated to L_-, we deduced that $C\setminus\{p_-\}$, respectively $C\setminus\{p_+\}$ is $W^u(p_+)$ respectively $W^u(p_-)$. Therefore the circle C is an 1-dimensional heteroclinic submanifold.

Let us comment on the geometry and relative position of the 2-dimensional invariant manifolds associated to the equilibrium points p_+ and p_-.

Note that the subspace $\mathrm{Fix}(S): x = 0,\ z = 0$ is a proper subspace for $L_\pm$, and simultaneously it is flow-invariant. The two equilibrium points belong to it.

So far we have found that the semiline $L_1 = \{(x,y,z) \in R^3 \mid x = 0, z = 0, y \geq y(p_+)\}$ and the interval $L_2 = \{(x,y,z) \in R^3 \mid x = 0, z = 0, y(p_+) \leq y < y(p_-)\}$ of $\mathrm{Fix}(S)$ lie on the stable manifold associated to the point p_+. Moreover the points of $L_2 \setminus \{p_+\}$ have heteroclinic orbits. Hence the two dimensional manifolds $W^s(p_+)$, $W^u(p_-)$ intersect along $L_2 \setminus \{p_+\}$. Because of the preceding results the intersection cannot be transversal. Therefore, excepting the unbounded orbits $L_1 \subset W^s(p_+)$ and $R(L_1) \subset W^u(p_-)$, the orbits lying in 2-dimensional invariant submanifolds are heteroclinic orbits.

Hence, associated to the saddle equilibrium points $p_\pm$ of the vector field $\boldsymbol{H}$, we have a heteroclinic structure consisting of a heteroclinic circle and parts of the 2-dimensional manifolds of the $p_\pm$.

10.4. ENERGY OF MAGNETIC FIELD GENERATED BY FILIFORM ELECTRIC CIRCUITS OF RIGHT ANGLE TYPE

Let $\boldsymbol{H} = (H_x, H_y, H_z)$ *be a stationary magnetic field and* $f = \frac{1}{2}(H_x^2 + H_y^2 + H_z^2)$ *its energy. Section 10.4.1 recalls that critical points of* f *may be minimum points or saddle points only, and points out again that the motion of a certain particle along a magnetic line belongs to the motion in some field of forces generated by the potential* $-f$.

Sections 10.4.2 and 10.4.3 search for the critical points of the energies associated to magnetic fields generated by the currents passing through a coplanar pair of wires of right angle type [121]. These points are important for geophysical and physical theories of plasma.

10.4.1. Energy of a magnetic vector field

Let $\boldsymbol{H} = (H_x, H_y, H_z)$ be a magnetic field that satisfies $\operatorname{div} \boldsymbol{H} = 0$, $\operatorname{rot} \boldsymbol{H} = 0$ on an open set of R^3. Leaving aside the multiplicative factor μ, the function

$$f = \frac{1}{2}(H_x^2 + H_y^2 + H_z^2)$$

is called the *energy* of $\boldsymbol{H}$, while the functions

$$\frac{1}{2}H_x^2,\ \frac{1}{2}H_y^2,\ \frac{1}{2}H_z^2$$

are called *partial energies*. Critical points of f are important for stability theory and controlled thermonuclear fusion research.

Theorem. *1) Critical points of* f *can be minimum points or saddle points only.*

2) Critical points of the partial energies can be minimum points or saddle points only.

Proof. The relations $\operatorname{div}\boldsymbol{H} = 0$, $\operatorname{rot}\boldsymbol{H} = 0$ imply $\Delta \boldsymbol{H} = 0$ and thus $\Delta H_x = 0$, $\Delta H_y = 0$, $\Delta H_z = 0$, where Δ denotes the Laplacian. Thus, $\boldsymbol{H}$ and H_x, H_y, H_z are harmonic functions.

1) It follows that $\Delta f = \|\nabla H_x\|^2 + \|\nabla H_y\|^2 + \|\nabla H_z\|^2 \geq 0$, i.e., f is a subharmonic function. Consequently, the critical points of f cannot be maximum points.

2) By analogy, the partial energies are subharmonic functions

$$\left(\Delta\ \frac{1}{2}H_x^2 = \|\nabla H_x\|^2\ ,\ etc\right).$$

Those critical points of partial energies that are not zeros of these energies are saddle points.

Critical points of f are the solutions of the algebraic system

$$\frac{\partial f}{\partial x} = H_x \frac{\partial H_x}{\partial x} + H_y \frac{\partial H_y}{\partial x} + H_z \frac{\partial H_z}{\partial x} = 0$$

$$\frac{\partial f}{\partial y} = H_x \frac{\partial H_x}{\partial y} + H_y \frac{\partial H_y}{\partial y} + H_z \frac{\partial H_z}{\partial y} = 0 \tag{6}$$

$$\frac{\partial f}{\partial z} = H_x \frac{\partial H_x}{\partial z} + H_y \frac{\partial H_y}{\partial z} + H_z \frac{\partial H_z}{\partial z} = 0.$$

Obviously, every zero of $\boldsymbol{H}$ is a critical point of f. At such a point, (6) does not provide any limitations on the derivatives of the components of $\boldsymbol{H}$. However, if the critical point is not a zero of $\boldsymbol{H}$, then (6) gives us some additional relationships among the first derivatives of components of $\boldsymbol{H}$. Critical points of the functions H_x, H_y, H_z are critical points of saddle type, since these are harmonic functions on an open set. The points (x_0, y_0, z_0), that simultaneously are critical points of H_x, H_y, H_z, are also critical points of the energy f and the relationship

$$d^2 f = (dH_x)^2 + (dH_y)^2 + (dH_z)^2 + H_x d^2 H_x + H_y d^2 H_y + H_z d^2 H_z$$

yields $\Delta f(x_0, y_0, z_0) = 0$.

Any field line of $\boldsymbol{H}$ is a solution of a conservative differential system with three degrees of freedom and with potential $-f$. The motion of a particle along a magnetic line is included in the motion of a particle in a field of forces produced by the potential $-f$. Critical points of the energy f appear as points at which the acceleration of the particle is zero.

For plasma traps it is of interest to consider the regions of critical (eventually minimum) energy f with nonvanishing intensity $\sqrt{2f}$.

10.4.2. Critical points of the energy of a magnetic field generated by currents of opposite sense through two coplanar wires of right angle type

We consider the magnetic field $\boldsymbol{H} = (H_x, H_y, H_z)$ of components (Fig.117)

$$H_x = \frac{-y}{r_1(r_1 - z - b)} + \frac{y}{r_2(r_2 + z - b)}$$

$$H_y = \frac{x+a}{r_1(r_1 - z - b)} - \frac{z+b}{r_1(r_1 + x + a)} - \frac{x-a}{r_2(r_2 + z - b)} + \frac{z-b}{r_2(r_2 - x + a)}$$

$$H_z = \frac{y}{r_1(r_1 + x + a)} - \frac{y}{r_2(r_2 - x + a)},$$

where

$$r_1^2 = (x+a)^2 + y^2 + (z+b)^2, \quad r_2^2 = (x-a)^2 + y^2 + (z-b)^2.$$

The domain of definition of this field is

$$D = R^3 \setminus \{e_1 \cup f_1 \cup e_2 \cup f_2\},$$

where

$$f_1 : x \le -a,\ y = 0,\ z = -b; \quad e_1 : x = -a,\ y = 0,\ z \ge -b;$$

$$f_2 : x \ge a,\ y = 0,\ z = b; \quad e_2 : x = a,\ y = 0,\ z \le b.$$

Obviously, $\boldsymbol{H}$ is an irrotational and solenoidal (and thus harmonic) vector field. We assume that a and b do not vanish simultaneously.

Theorem. *The plane xOz is the single set of critical points of the partial energies $\frac{1}{2}H_x^2$, $\frac{1}{2}H_z^2$. This plane is included in the set of all zeros of these functions.*

Proof. The critical points of the function $\frac{1}{2}H_x^2$ are the solutions of the system

$$H_x \frac{\partial H_x}{\partial x} = 0,\ H_x \frac{\partial H_x}{\partial y} = 0,\ H_x \frac{\partial H_x}{\partial z} = 0.$$

Therefore any zero of H_x is also a critical point of $\frac{1}{2}H_x^2$. Let us find the critical points of the function H_x, that is, the solutions of the system

$$\frac{\partial H_x}{\partial x} = \frac{y(x+a)(2r_1 - z - b)}{r_1^3 (r_1 - z - b)^2} - \frac{y(x-a)(2r_2 + z - b)}{r_2^3 (r_2 + z - b)^2} = 0$$

$$\frac{\partial H_x}{\partial y} = \frac{-1}{r_1(r_1 - z - b)} + \frac{y^2(2r_1 - z - b)}{r_1^3 (r_1 - z - b)^2} + \frac{1}{r_2(r_2 + z - b)} - \frac{y^2(2r_2 + z - b)}{r_2^3(r_2 + z - b)^2} = 0$$

$$\frac{\partial H_x}{\partial z} = -\frac{y}{r_1^3} - \frac{y}{r_2^3} = 0.$$

It is seen that the points of the curve

$$\Gamma_1 : y = 0,\ r_1(z+b) + r_2(z-b) = 4ax + 4bz,$$

with

$$r_1^2 = (x+a)^2 + (z+b)^2,\ r_2^2 = (x-a)^2 + (z-b)^2,$$

are critical points of H_x only. These are also zeros of H_x. Since H_x is a harmonic function, its critical points are of the saddle type only. It follows that the partial energy $\frac{1}{2}H_x^2$ has no other local minimum than the global minimum zero.

By analogy, it follows that the critical points of the harmonic function H_z are located on the curve,

$$\Gamma_2 : y = 0,\ r_1(x+a) + r_2(x-a) = -4ax - 4bz,$$

where

$$r_1^2 = (x+a)^2 + (z+b)^2,\ r_2^2 = (x-a)^2 + (z-b)^2.$$

Because $H_z|_{\Gamma_2} = 0$, it follows that the partial energy $\frac{1}{2}H_z^2$ has no nonzero local minima.

By calculation we find

$$H_y(x,0,z) = \frac{2}{r_1 + (x+a) - (z+b)} + \frac{2}{r_2 + (z-b) - (x-a)} =$$

$$= \frac{2(r_1 + r_2 + 2a - 2b)}{[r_1 + (x+a) - (z+b)][r_2 + (z-b) - (x-a)]}.$$

Theorem. *1) If* $a < b,\ ab < 0$ *or* $a = b$ *or* $b < a$, *then* $(0,0,0)$ *is the single critical point of the partial energy* $\frac{1}{2}H_y^2$ *situated on the* y*-axis.*

2) If $a < b,\ ab > 0$, *then* $\frac{1}{2}H_y^2$ *has three critical points*

$$(0, -y_1, 0),\ (0,0,0),\ (0, y_1, 0),\ y_1 \neq 0.$$

Proof. The critical points (saddle points) of the harmonic function H_y are solutions of the system

$$\frac{\partial H_y}{\partial x} = \frac{\partial H_x}{\partial y} = 0$$

$$\frac{\partial H_y}{\partial y} = -\frac{(x+a)y(2r_1 - z - b)}{r_1^3(r_1 - z - b)^2} + \frac{(z+b)y(2r_1 + x + a)}{r_1^3(r_1 + x + z)^2}$$

$$+ \frac{(x+a)y(2r_2 + z - b)}{r_2^3(r_2 + z - b)^2} - \frac{(z-b)y(2r_2 - x + a)}{r_2^3(r_2 - x + a)^2} = 0$$

$$\frac{\partial H_y}{\partial z} = \frac{\partial H_z}{\partial y} = \frac{1}{r_1(r_1 + x + a)} - \frac{y^2(2r_1 + x + a)}{r_1^3(r_1 + x + a)^2}$$

$$- \frac{1}{r_2(r_2 - x + a)} + \frac{y^2(2r_2 - x + a)}{r_2^3(r_2 - z + a)^2} = 0.$$

Because $\Gamma_1 \cap \Gamma_2 = \{(0,0,0)\}$, the origin is the only critical point located in the xOy plane. This critical point is not a zero of H. The first and the last equations are identically verified by the points $(0, y, 0)$. Therefore, it remains to solve the equation

$$\frac{\partial H_y}{\partial y}(0,y,0) = \frac{2y}{r_1^3}\left[\frac{b(2r_1 + a)}{(r_1 + a)^2} - \frac{a(2r_1 - b)}{(r_1 - b)^2}\right] = 0, \tag{7}$$

where

$$r_1 = \sqrt{a^2 + y^2 + b^2} \geq \sqrt{a^2 + b^2},\ r_1 \neq -a,\ r_1 \neq b.$$

The equation (7) admits $y = 0$ as a solution, therefore $(0,0,0)$ is a critical point of H_y.

If $a < 0,\ b > 0 (\Leftrightarrow a < b, ab < 0)$ or $a = b$, then the equation (7) admits $y = 0$ as a solution and $(0, 0, 0)$ is the single critical point of H_y. For the converse, we employ the equation extended to the whole real axis

$$\varphi(r_1) = b(2r_1 + a)(r_1 - b)^2 - a(2r_1 - b)(r_1 + a)^2 = 0,$$

that is

$$\varphi(r_1) = 2r_1^3(b-a) + 2r_1^2(ab - 2a^2 - 2b^2)$$
$$+ 2r_1(b-a)(a^2+b^2) + ab(a^2+b^2) = 0.$$

If $a \neq b$, then the signs of the numbers

$$b - a,\quad \varphi(0) = ab(a^2+b^2)$$

$$\varphi(\sqrt{a^2+b^2}) = (a^2+b^2)\,[4\sqrt{a^2+b^2}(b-a) + 3ab - 4a^2 - 4b^2],$$

$$\sum_{i=1}^{3} r_{1i}^2 = \frac{2a^4 + 2b^4 + 5a^2b^2}{b-a}$$

can resolve the existence of solutions of the equation (7).

Obviously, $3ab - 4a^2 - 4b^2 < 0$. If $b < a$, then the sum of the squares of the roots is negative and then $\varphi(r_1) = 0$ has a single real solution. The table of signs

r_1	$-\infty$	0	$\sqrt{a^2+b^2}$	$+\infty$
$\varphi(r_1)$	+	±	-	-

shows that this solution does not belong to the straight semiline $(\sqrt{a^2+b^2}, +\infty)$. Then $(0, 0, 0)$ is the single critical point of H_y.

If $b > a,\ ab > 0$, then the table of signs

r_1	$-\infty$	0	$\sqrt{a^2+b^2}$	$+\infty$
$\varphi(r_1)$	-	+	-	+

shows that the equation $\varphi(r_1) = 0$ has a solution on $(\sqrt{a^2+b^2}, \infty)$ to which will correspond two solutions y_1, $-y_1$ with respect to y. Therefore H_y has three critical points $(0,0,0)$, $(0,y_1,0)$, $(0,-y_1,0)$, $y_1 \neq 0$.

Since H_y is a harmonic function, its critical points are saddle points. In general, these points are not zeros of H_y. Indeed,

$$H_x(0,y,0) = 0, \; H_z(0,y,0) = 0$$

$$H_y(0,y,0) = \frac{2}{r_1}\left(\frac{a}{r_1 - b} - \frac{b}{r_1 + a}\right) = \frac{2}{r_1}\frac{(a-b)r_1 + a^2 + b^2}{(r_1 - b)(r_1 + a)},$$

where

$$r_1 = r_2 = \sqrt{a^2 + y^2 + b^2}.$$

If $a > b$, then $H_y(0,y,0) > 0$.

If $a < b$, $ab > 0$, then the equation $H_y(0,y,0) = 0$ has two solutions

$$y_{1,2} = \frac{\pm\sqrt{2ab(a^2 + b^2)}}{b - a},$$

and $H_y(0,y,0)$ is positive between zeros and negative outside them.

If $a < b$, $ab < 0$ $(\Leftrightarrow a < 0, b > 0)$, then $H_y(0,y,0) < 0$.

Corollary. *The partial energy* $\frac{1}{2}H_y^2$ *admits critical points that are not zeros.*

Theorem. *1) The critical values of the energy* f *are at least equal to the critical values of the partial energy* $\frac{1}{2}H_y^2$.

2) The critical point $(0,0,0)$ *is a saddle point of the energy* f *and of the partial energy* $\frac{1}{2}H_y^2$.

Proof. The energy f and the partial energies are invariant with respect to the symmetry upon xOy and to that upon Oy.

1) It is seen that $H_x^2 + H_y^2 + H_z^2 \geq H_y^2$, and the critical points of H_y^2 are critical points of f. The problem of existence of critical points of f, which are different from those of H_y^2, remains open.

2) We find $d^2f(0,0,0) = H_y(0,0,0)\,d^2H_y(0,0,0)$ and $d^2H_y(0,0,0)$ cannot be definite since $\Delta H_y = 0$.

10.4.3. Critical points of the energy of a magnetic field generated by currents of the same sense through two coplanar wires of right angle type

For the configuration of (Fig.119), the Biot-Savart-Laplace law determines the magnetic field $\boldsymbol{H} = (H_x, H_y, H_z)$,

$$H_x = \frac{-y}{r_1(r_1 - z - b)} - \frac{y}{r_2(r_2 + z - b)}$$

$$H_y = \frac{x+a}{r_1(r_1 - z - b)} - \frac{z+b}{r_1(r_1 + z + b)} + \frac{x-a}{r_2(r_2 + x - b)} - \frac{z-b}{r_2(r_2 - x + a)}$$

$$H_z = \frac{y}{r_1(r_1 + x + a)} + \frac{y}{r_2(r_2 - z + a)},$$

where

$$r_1^2 = (x+a)^2 + y^2 + (z+b)^2, \; r_2^2 = (x-a)^2 + y^2 + (z-b)^2.$$

The domain of definition of this field is the same set D as in 10.4.2.

Obviously, $\boldsymbol{H}$ is an irrotational and solenoidal (and thus, harmonic) vector field.

We assume that a and b do not vanish simultaneously.

Theorem. *Let $\boldsymbol{H}$ be the magnetic field defined above. Then the set of all zeros of $\boldsymbol{H}$ is the curve*

$$y = 0, \; r_2 - r_1 = 2(x - z).$$

Theorem. *1) If $a \neq 0$, $b \in \boldsymbol{R}$ or $a = 0$, $b < 0$, then the partial energy $\frac{1}{2}H_x^2$ has critical points of type $(0, -y_1, 0)$, $(0, y_1, 0)$, $y_1 \neq 0$.*

2) If $a = 0$, $b > 0$, then the partial energy $\frac{1}{2}H_x^2$ has no critical points on the y-axis.

3) The plane xOy is a set of critical points of the partial energy $\frac{1}{2}H_x^2$ that coincides with the set of all zeros of this function.

Proof. The critical points of the function $\frac{1}{2}H_x^2$ are solutions of the system

$$H_x \frac{\partial H_x}{\partial x} = 0, \; H_x \frac{\partial H_x}{\partial y} = 0, \; H_x \frac{\partial H_x}{\partial z} = 0.$$

Therefore the zeros of H_x are critical points of $\frac{1}{2}H_x^2$. Since

$$\frac{\partial H_x}{\partial x} = \frac{y(x+a)(2r_1 - z - b)}{r_1^3(r_1 - z - b)^2} + \frac{y(x-a)(2r_2 + z - b)}{r_2^3(r_2 + z - b)^2}$$

$$\frac{\partial H_x}{\partial y} = -\frac{1}{r_1(r_1 - z - b)} + \frac{y^2(2r_1 - z - b)}{r_1^3(r_1 - z - b)^2} - \frac{1}{r_2(r_2 + z - b)} + \frac{y^2(2r_2 + z - b)}{r_2^3(r_2 + z - b)^2}$$

$$\frac{\partial H_x}{\partial z} = -\frac{y}{r_1^3} + \frac{y}{r_2^3},$$

it follows that the harmonic function H_x has no critical points in the plane $xOz: y = 0$, where $H_x(x, 0, z) = 0$, but H_x may have some critical points that lie on the y-*axis*: $x = 0$, $z = 0$, with $y \neq 0$, where $H_x(0, y, 0) = \dfrac{-2y}{r_1(r_1 - b)}$.

Indeed,

$$\frac{\partial H_x}{\partial x}(0, y, 0) = 0, \quad \frac{\partial H_x}{\partial z}(0, y, 0) = 0$$

and it remains to discuss the equation

$$\frac{\partial H_x}{\partial y}(0, y, 0) = -\frac{2}{r_1(r_1 - b)} + \frac{2y^2(2r_1 - b)}{r_1^3(r_1 - b)^2} = 0, \tag{8}$$

where

$$r_1 - \sqrt{a^2 + y^2 + b^2} \geq \sqrt{a^2 + b^2},\ r_1 \neq b.$$

This equation may be extended by

$$\psi(r_1) = r_1^3 - 2r_1(a^2 + b^2) + b(a^2 + b^2) = 0.$$

We assume that the function ψ is extended to the whole real axis and we calculate

$$\psi(-\sqrt{a^2 + b^2}) = (a^2 + b^2)(b + \sqrt{a^2 + b^2}) \geq 0,$$

$$\psi(\sqrt{a^2 + b^2}) = (a^2 + b^2)(b - \sqrt{a^2 + b^2}) \leq 0.$$

Let $a \neq 0$. The table of signs

r_1	$-\infty$	$-\sqrt{a^2 + b^2}$	$\sqrt{a^2 + b^2}$	∞
$\psi(r_1)$	$-$	$+$	$-$	$+$

shows that the equation (8) has a single solution with respect to r_1 and then it has two solutions y_1, $-y_1$ with respect to y.

Let $a = 0$. The solutions of the equation $\psi(r_1) = 0$ are b and $\dfrac{-b \pm b\sqrt{5}}{2}$. If $b > 0$, then the equation (8) has no solution. If $b < 0$, then the equation (8) has the solution

$r_1 = \dfrac{-b(1+\sqrt{5})}{2}$, and then it has two solutions $y_1, -y_1$, with respect to y. Since H_x is a harmonic function on an open set, its critical points are saddle points.

Theorem. *1) If* $a \in R,\ b \neq 0$ *or* $a > 0,\ b = 0$, *then the partial energy* $\frac{1}{2}H_z^2$ *has critical points of the type* $(0, y_1, 0),\ (0, -y_1, 0),\ y_1 \neq 0$.

2) If $a < 0,\ b = 0$, *then the partial energy* $\frac{1}{2}H_z^2$ *has no critical points on the* y*-axis.*

3) The plane xOy *is a set of critical points of the partial energy* $\frac{1}{2}H_z^2$ *that coincides with the set of all zeros of this function.*

Proof. We find

$$\frac{\partial H_z}{\partial x} = \frac{\partial H_x}{\partial z} = -\frac{y}{r_1^3} + \frac{y}{r_2^3}$$

$$\frac{\partial H_z}{\partial y} = \frac{1}{r_1(r_1+x+a)} - \frac{y^2(2r_1+x+a)}{r_1^3(r_1+x+a)^2} + \frac{1}{r_2(r_2-x+a)} - \frac{y^2(2r_2-x+a)}{r_2^3(r_2-x+a)^2}$$

$$\frac{\partial H_z}{\partial z} = -\frac{y(z+b)(2r_1+x+a)}{r_1^3(r_1+x+a)^2} - \frac{y(z-b)(2r_2-x+a)}{r_2^3(r_2-x+a)^2}.$$

Thus, the harmonic function H_z has no critical points that lie on the plane xOz: $y = 0$, where $H_z(x, 0, z) = 0$, but it may have some critical points that lie on the y - *axis*: $x = 0,\ z = 0$, where $H_z(0, y, 0) = \dfrac{2y}{r_1(r_1+a)}$. Since

$$\frac{\partial H_z}{\partial x}(0, y, 0) = 0, \quad \frac{\partial H_z}{\partial z}(0, y, 0) = 0,$$

it remains to discuss the equation

$$\frac{\partial H_z}{\partial y}(0, y, 0) = \frac{2}{r_1(r_1+a)} - \frac{2y^2(2r_1+a)}{r_1^3(r_1+a)^2} = 0, \tag{9}$$

where

$$r_1 = \sqrt{a^2+y^2+b^2} \geq \sqrt{a^2+b^2},\ r_1 \neq -a.$$

This equation may be extended by

$$\chi(r_1) = r_1^3 - 2r_1(a^2+b^2) - a(a^2+b^2) = 0.$$

We calculate

$$\chi(-\sqrt{a^2+b^2}) = (a^2+b^2)(\sqrt{a^2+b^2} - a) \geq 0$$

$$\chi(\sqrt{a^2+b^2}) = -(a^2+b^2)(\sqrt{a^2+b^2}+a) \le 0.$$

For $b \neq 0$, we find the table of signs

r_1	$-\infty$	$-\sqrt{a^2+b^2}$	$\sqrt{a^2+b^2}$	∞
$\chi(r_1)$	$-$	$+$	$-$	$+$

that shows that the equation (9) has a single solution with respect to r_1, and then it has two solutions y_1, $-y_1$, with respect to y.

Let $b = 0$. The solutions of the equation $\chi(r_1) = 0$ are $-a$, $\dfrac{a \pm a\sqrt{5}}{2}$. If $a > 0$, then the equation (9) has the solution $r_1 = \dfrac{a(1+\sqrt{5})}{2}$, and then it has two solutions y_1, $-y_1$, with respect to y. If $a > 0$, then (9) has no solution.

All critical points of H_z are saddle points of H_z.

Theorem. *Critical points of the partial energy* $\frac{1}{2}H_y^2$ *are zeros of it, only.*

Proof. We consider the harmonic function H_y with the partial derivatives

$$\frac{\partial H_y}{\partial x} = \frac{\partial H_x}{\partial y} = -\frac{1}{r_1(r_1-z-b)} + \frac{y^2(2r_1-z-b)}{r_1^3(r_1-z-b)^2}$$

$$-\frac{1}{r_2(r_2+z-b)} + \frac{y^2(2r_2+z-b)}{r_2^3(r_2+z-b)^2},$$

$$\frac{\partial H_y}{\partial y} = -\frac{(x+a)y(2r_1-z-b)}{r_1^3(r_1-z-b)^2} + \frac{(z+b)y(2r_1+x+a)}{r_1^3(r_1+x+a)^2}$$

$$-\frac{(x-a)y(2r_2+z-b)}{r_2^3(r_2+z-b)^2} + \frac{(z-b)y(2r_2-x+a)}{r_2^3(r_2-x+a)^2},$$

$$\frac{\partial H_y}{\partial z} = \frac{\partial H_z}{\partial y} = \frac{1}{r_1(r_1+x+a)} - \frac{y^2(2r_1+x+a)}{r_1^3(r_1+x+a)^2} +$$

$$+\frac{1}{r_2(r_2-x+a)}-\frac{y^2(2r_2-x+a)}{r_2^3(r_2-x+a)^2}.$$

We get

$$\frac{\partial H_y}{\partial x}(x,0,z)<0,\ \frac{\partial H_y}{\partial y}(x,0,z)=0,\ \frac{\partial H_y}{\partial z}(x,0,y)>0$$

and, respectively,

$$H_y(0,y,0)=0$$

$$\frac{\partial H_y}{\partial x}(0,y,0)=\frac{\partial H_x}{\partial y}(0,y,0)=-\frac{2}{r_1(r_1-b)}+\frac{2y^2(2r_1-b)}{r_1^3(r_1-b)^2},\quad \frac{\partial H_y}{\partial y}(0,y,0)=0,$$

$$\frac{\partial H_y}{\partial z}(0,y,0)=\frac{\partial H_z}{\partial y}(0,y,0)=\frac{2}{r_1(r_1+a)}-\frac{2y^2(2r_1+a)}{r_1^3(r_1+a)^2},$$

where

$$r_1=\sqrt{a^2+y^2+b^2},\ r_1\neq -a,b.$$

If $a+b\neq 0$, then the equations have no common roots. If $a+b=0$, then these equations have a common root $r_1\geq\sqrt{a^2+b^2}$, and then H_y admits two critical points of type $(0,-y_1,0)$, $(0,y_1,0)$, $y_1\neq 0$, but these are zeros of H_y.

Theorem. *The critical values of the energy f are at least equal to the critical values of the function* $\frac{1}{2}H_x^2+\frac{1}{2}H_z^2$.

Proof. The energy f and the partial energies are invariant with respect to the symmetry upon the plane xOy and that upon the y-*axis*. Also, $H_x^2+H_y^2+H_z^2\geq H_x^2+H_z^2$.

10.5. ELECTROMAGNETIC DYNAMICAL SYSTEMS AS HAMILTONIAN SYSTEMS [130]

Section 10.5.1 transcribes the Lorentz-Udriste world-force law in the Hamiltonian language using suitable symplectic forms and Hamiltonians.

Section 10.5.2 presents the classical theory of motion of a particle in an electromagnetic field, to show that this is different from the geometric electromagnetic dynamics discovered by us.

Section 10.5.3 studies the field lines of vector fields that appear in Maxwell's equations. Original mathematical constructions show that the equations of motion of a particle in an electric field or in a magnetic field are Hamiltonian equations, with respect to certain symplectic forms and Hamiltonians.

Section 10.5.4 analyses the electromagnetic dynamical systems appearing in the relativistic model.

10.5.1. Hamiltonian formulation of the Biot-Savart-Laplace dynamical systems

Now we want to explain the dynamics induced by the Biot-Savart-Laplace vector field in the language of exterior forms and Hamiltonian theory.

Let M be a manifold and Ω a 2-form on M. The pair (M, Ω) is called a *symplectic manifold* if Ω satisfies

1) $d\Omega = 0$ (i.e., Ω is closed),
2) Ω is nondegenerate.

Let (M, Ω) be a symplectic manifold and let $\varphi \in \mathcal{F}(M)$. Let X_φ be the unique vector field on M satisfying

$$\Omega_p(X_\varphi(p), v) = d\varphi(p) \cdot v, \ \forall\, v \in T_p M.$$

We call X_φ the *Hamiltonian vector field of* φ. Hamiltonian equations are the differential equations on M given by

$$\dot{p} = X_\varphi(p).$$

Let T_s be the flow of the Hamiltonian equations, i.e., $T_s(p)$ is a field line of X_φ starting at p. Then the energy φ is conserved, i.e., $\varphi \circ T_s = \varphi$.

Theorem. *The equations of motion of a particle moving in a Biot-Savart-Laplace magnetic field are Hamiltonian, with respect to the energy*

$$\mathcal{H} = \frac{1}{2}\delta_{ij}\dot{x}^i\dot{x}^j - f(x^1, x^2, x^3).$$

1) If the particle belongs to $\mathrm{int}(R^3 \setminus D)$, *then the symplectic form is*

$$\Omega = \delta_{ij}\, dx^i \wedge d\dot{x}^j,$$

where "." stands for the derivative with respect to s.

2) If the particle belongs to D, then the symplectic form is

$$\Omega = \delta_{ij}\, dx^i \wedge d\dot{x}^j + J,$$

where the current density J *is viewed as a closed 2-form*

$$J = J_1 dx^2 \wedge dx^3 + J_2 dx^3 \wedge dx^1 + J_3 dx^1 \wedge dx^2$$

with which we associate the solenoidal vector field

$$J = J_1 i_1 + J_2 i_2 + J_3 i_3 .$$

Proof. Let

$$\Omega = \begin{cases} \delta_{ij}\, dx^i \wedge d\dot{x}^j + J & \text{on } D \times R^3 \\ \delta_{ij}\, dx^i \wedge d\dot{x}^j & \text{on } (\text{ext}\overline{D}) \times R^3 . \end{cases}$$

Denote

$$X_{\mathcal{H}} = (u^1, u^2, u^3, \dot{u}^1, \dot{u}^2, \dot{u}^3)$$

and we focus on the case $D \times R^3$. The condition

$$i_{X_{\mathcal{H}}} \Omega = d\mathcal{H}$$

which defines $X_{\mathcal{H}}$, is written

$$u^1 d\dot{x}^1 - \dot{u}^1 dx^1 + u^2 d\dot{x}^2 - \dot{u}^2 dx^2 + u^3 d\dot{x}^3 - \dot{u}^3 dx^3$$

$$+ J_1 u^2 dx^3 - J_1 u^3 dx^2 + J_2 u^3 dx^1 - J_2 u^1 dx^3 + J_3 u^1 dx^2 - J_3 u^2 dx^1$$

$$= \dot{x}^1 d\dot{x}^1 + \dot{x}^2 d\dot{x}^2 + \dot{x}^3 d\dot{x}^3 - \left(\frac{\partial f}{\partial x_1} dx^1 + \frac{\partial f}{\partial x_2} dx^2 + \frac{\partial f}{\partial x_3} dx^3 \right) .$$

By identification we find

$$u^1 = \dot{x}^1 ,\ u^2 = \dot{x}^2 ,\ u^3 = \dot{x}^3$$

$$\dot{u}^1 = \frac{\partial f}{\partial x^1} + J_2 u^3 - J_3 u^2$$

$$\dot{u}^2 = \frac{\partial f}{\partial x^2} + J_3 u^1 - J_1 u^3$$

$$\dot{u}^3 = \frac{\partial f}{\partial x^3} + J_1 u^2 - J_2 u^1 ,$$

i.e.,

$$\ddot{x}^1 = \frac{\partial f}{\partial x^1} + J_2 \dot{x}^3 - J_3 \dot{x}^2$$

$$\ddot{x}^2 = \frac{\partial f}{\partial x^2} + J_3 \dot{x}^1 - J_1 \dot{x}^3$$

$$\ddot{x}^3 = \frac{\partial f}{\partial x^3} + J_1 \dot{x}^2 - J_2 \dot{x}^1$$

which is the same as the system analysed in 10.1.2.

Obviously $\operatorname{div} X_{\mathcal{H}} = 0$ and hence the flow generated by $X_{\mathcal{H}}$ preserves the volume.

10.5.2. Classical equations of motion for a charged particle in a stationary electromagnetic field

To avoid some misunderstandings we recall some well-known facts. Let

$$B = B_1 dx^2 \wedge dx^3 + B_2 dx^3 \wedge dx^1 + B_3 dx^1 \wedge dx^2$$

be a closed two-form on R^3 and

$$\boldsymbol{B} = B_1 \boldsymbol{i}_1 + B_2 \boldsymbol{i}_2 + B_3 \boldsymbol{i}_3$$

the associated divergence-free vector field. The connection between the magnetic induction $\boldsymbol{B}$ and the magnetic vector field $\boldsymbol{H}$ is $\boldsymbol{B} = \mu_0 \boldsymbol{H}$. Thinking of $\boldsymbol{B}$ as a magnetic field and taking the electromagnetic field on R^3 given by the electric field $\boldsymbol{E}$ and the magnetic field $\boldsymbol{B}$, the equations of motion, for a particle with charge e and mass m in the electromagnetic field, are given by the Lorentz force law $m \dfrac{dv}{dt} = \dfrac{e}{c}(\boldsymbol{E} + v \times \boldsymbol{B})$, where $v = \dot{x}^1 \boldsymbol{i}_1 + \dot{x}^2 \boldsymbol{i}_2 + \dot{x}^3 \boldsymbol{i}_3$ is the field of velocities, and the dot "." denotes the derivative with respect to t. Since $\operatorname{rot}\boldsymbol{E} = 0$ $(\partial_t \boldsymbol{B} = 0)$ we can write (locally) $\boldsymbol{E} = \operatorname{grad}\varphi$.

On $R^3 \times R^3$, i.e., on $(x^1, x^2, x^3, \dot{x}^1, \dot{x}^2, \dot{x}^3)$-space, we consider the symplectic form

$$\Omega_B = m\,\delta_{ij}\,dx^i \wedge d\dot{x}^j - \frac{e}{c} B$$

and the Hamiltonian (total energy)

$$\mathcal{H} = \frac{m}{2}\,\delta_{ij}\,\dot{x}^i \dot{x}^j + \frac{e}{c}\,\varphi(x)\,.$$

Denoting

$$X_{\mathcal{H}}(u^1, u^2, u^3) = (u^1, u^2, u^3, \dot{u}^1, \dot{u}^2, \dot{u}^3)$$

the condition of defining $X_{\mathcal{H}}$, i.e.,

$$i_{X_{\mathcal{H}}} \Omega_B = d\mathcal{H}$$

becomes

$$m(u^1 d\dot{x}^1 - \dot{u}^1 dx^1 + u^2 d\dot{x}^2 - \dot{u}^2 dx^2 + u^3 d\dot{x}^3 - \dot{u}^3 dx^3)$$

$$= m(\dot{x}^1 d\dot{x}^1 + \dot{x}^2 d\dot{x}^2 + \dot{x}^3 d\dot{x}^3) + \frac{e}{c}\left(\frac{\partial\varphi}{\partial x^1}dx^1 + \frac{\partial\varphi}{\partial x^2}dx^2 + \frac{\partial\varphi}{\partial x^3}dx^3\right).$$

Consequently

$$u^1 = \dot{x}^1,\ u^2 = \dot{x}^2,\ u^3 = \dot{x}^3$$

$$m\dot{u}^1 = \frac{e}{c}(E_1 + B_3 u^2 - B_2 u^3),\ m\dot{u}^2 = \frac{e}{c}(E_2 + B_1 u^3 - B_3 u^1),\ m\dot{u}^3 = \frac{e}{c}(E_3 + B_2 u^1 - B_1 u^2)$$

or

$$m\ddot{x}^1 = \frac{e}{c}(E_1 + B_3\dot{x}^2 - B_2\dot{x}^3),\ m\ddot{x}^2 = \frac{e}{c}(E_2 + B_1\dot{x}^3 - B_3\dot{x}^1),\ m\dot{x}^3 = \frac{e}{c}(E_3 + B_2\dot{x}^1 - B_1\dot{x}^2)$$

which are the same as the classical Lorentz equations. Thus the equations of motion for a charged particle in an electromagnetic field are Hamiltonian, with energy equal to the total energy $\mathcal{H}$ and with the symplectic form Ω_B.

10.5.3. Electromagnetic dynamical systems

The mathematical ingredients of electromagnetism are: $\boldsymbol{E}$ = *the electric vector field (electric intensity)*, $\boldsymbol{H}$ = *the magnetic vector field (magnetizing force)*, $\boldsymbol{B}$ = *the magnetic induction*, $\boldsymbol{D}$ = *the electric displacement (electric induction)*, $\boldsymbol{J}$ = *the electric current density (conduction density)*, ρ = *the electric charge density*, t = *the time*, ∂_t = *the time derivative operator*, μ = *the scalar permeability*, ε = *the permitivity*. These satisfy the Maxwell equations $\operatorname{div}\boldsymbol{D} = \rho$, $\operatorname{rot}\boldsymbol{H} = \boldsymbol{J} + \partial_t\boldsymbol{D}$, $\operatorname{div}\boldsymbol{B} = 0$, $\operatorname{rot}\boldsymbol{E} = -\partial_t\boldsymbol{B}$, the associated constitutive equations relating the fields being $\boldsymbol{B} = \mu\boldsymbol{H}$, $\boldsymbol{D} = \varepsilon\boldsymbol{E}$, for linear homogeneous isotropic media $U \subset R^3$.

Let $\boldsymbol{E} = \boldsymbol{E}(x,t)$, $\boldsymbol{E} = E_1 i_1 + E_2 i_2 + E_3 i_3$ be the electric vector field on the domain $U \times R$. The electric line α which starts at the moment $s = 0$ from the point (x_0^1, x_0^2, x_0^3) is the oriented curve $\alpha : (-\varepsilon, \varepsilon) \to U$, $\alpha(s) = (x^1(s), x^2(s), x^3(s))$, a solution of the Cauchy problem

$$\frac{dx^i}{ds} = E_i,\ x^i(0) = x_0^i,\ i = 1, 2, 3.$$

The set of all images of maximal electric lines is called the *phase portrait* of the electric field $\boldsymbol{E}$. The parameter t can produce bifurcations in the flow generated by $\boldsymbol{E}(x,t)$.

Let

$$f : U \to R, \quad f = \frac{1}{2}(E_1^2 + E_2^2 + E_3^2)$$

be the energy of $\boldsymbol{E}$, leaving aside the multiplicative factor ε.

Theorem. *Every electric line is the trajectory of a nonpotential dynamical system with three degrees of freedom for which the energy*

$$\mathcal{H} = \frac{1}{2}\delta_{ij}\dot{x}^i\dot{x}^j - f(x^1, x^2, x^3)$$

is conserved.

Proof. Differentiating $\frac{dx^i}{ds} = E_i$ along a solution α, using $\mathrm{rot}\boldsymbol{E} = -\partial_t \boldsymbol{B}$, and replacing $\frac{dx^i}{ds}$ only in terms that allows to recover ∇f, we find the prolongation

$$\frac{d^2x^i}{ds^2} = \frac{\partial f}{\partial x^i} + \left(\frac{\partial E_i}{\partial x^j} - \frac{\partial E_j}{\partial x^i}\right)\frac{dx^j}{ds}$$

or otherwise written

$$\frac{d^2x^1}{ds^2} = \frac{\partial f}{\partial x^1} + \partial_t B_3 \frac{dx^2}{ds} - \partial_t B_2 \frac{dx^3}{ds}$$

$$\frac{d^2x^2}{ds^2} = \frac{\partial f}{\partial x^2} + \partial_t B_1 \frac{dx^3}{ds} - \partial_t B_3 \frac{dx^1}{ds}$$

$$\frac{d^2x^3}{ds^2} = \frac{\partial f}{\partial x^3} + \partial_t B_2 \frac{dx^1}{ds} - \partial_t B_1 \frac{dx^2}{ds}.$$

Multiplying by $\frac{dx^i}{ds}$ and summing, we find $\frac{d}{ds}\mathcal{H} = 0$.

The vector field $\frac{d\alpha}{ds} \times \partial_t \boldsymbol{B}$ does not produce a dissipation of energy along the electric line α, since it is orthogonal to α.

Theorem. *The equations of motion of a particle moving in an electric field* $\mathbf{E}$ *are Hamiltonian, with respect to the energy*

$$\mathcal{H} = \frac{1}{2}\delta_{ij}\dot{x}^i\dot{x}^j - f(x^1, x^2, x^3),$$

and the symplectic form

$$\Omega = \delta_{ij}\, dx^i \wedge d\dot{x}^j - \partial_t B,$$

where the magnetic induction $\mathbf{B}$ *is viewed as a closed 2-form*

$$B = B_1\, dx^2 \wedge dx^3 + B_2\, dx^3 \wedge dx^1 + B_3\, dx^1 \wedge dx^2$$

associated to the solenoidal vector field

$$\mathbf{B} = B_1 \mathbf{i}_1 + B_2 \mathbf{i}_2 + B_3 \mathbf{i}_3.$$

Remarks. 1) Another prolongation on U of the kinematic system of order one

$$\frac{dx^i}{ds} = E_i, \quad i = 1, 2, 3,$$

is the nonconservative dynamical system of order two

$$\frac{d^2x^i}{ds^2} = \frac{\partial f}{\partial x^i} + E_j\partial_t B_k - E_k\partial_t B_j, \quad i, j, k = \text{ permutation of the set } \{1, 2, 3\}.$$

2) The flow generated by $X_{\mathcal{H}}$ conserves the volume.

3) For the magnetic lines (the field lines of $\mathbf{H}$) one obtains similar results. The difference is that the symplectic form contains the closed 2-form $J + \partial_t D$ associated to the solenoidal vector field $\mathbf{J} + \partial_t \mathbf{D}$.

Open problems. 1) Find the properties for the field lines of the Poynting vector field

$$\mathbf{S} = \mathbf{E} \times \mathbf{H}.$$

2) Study the electromagnetic geometric dynamics defined by a vector field in the distribution generated by the vector fields **E** and **H**.

10.5.4. Electromagnetic dynamical systems in the relativistic model

Let M be a connected 4-dimensional differentiable manifold and g a Lorentz metric on M. The pair (M, g) is called a *Lorentz manifold.*

Definition. A *spacetime* (M, g, ∇) is a connected 4-dimensional, oriented, and time-oriented Lorentz manifold (M, g) together with its Levi-Civita connection ∇.

Let F be the electromagnetic field as a 2-form on M. We denote by $(M, \mathcal{M}, F)$ a relativistic model and by J the charge-current density of the matter model $\mathcal{M}$.

Definition. $(M, \mathcal{M}, F)$ or (M, F, J) satisfies the *Maxwell equations* if:

1) F is closed, i.e., $dF = 0$;

2) $\operatorname{div} \hat{F} = J$, where $\hat{F}$ is the $(1,1)$ tensor field physically equivalent to F via the Lorentz metric g.

As a consequence of 1), locally, there exists a 1-form η such that $F = d\eta$. We denote by ξ the vector field physically equivalent to η via the Lorentz metric g.

Obviously, J is a solenoidal vector field, i.e.,

$$\operatorname{div} J = \operatorname{div} \operatorname{div} \hat{F} = 0.$$

Usually, the authors study the influence of spacetime M and of the matter model $\mathcal{M}$ on the electromagnetic field F.

Let F_{ij} be the components of F. Then $dF = 0$ is equivalent to

$$F_{ij|k} + F_{jk|i} + F_{ki|j} = 0$$

and

$$\operatorname{div} \hat{F} = J$$

is equivalent to

$$F^{j}{}_{i|j} = -J_i .$$

If M and J are given ab initio, and the influence of F on M and on $\mathcal{M}$ is neglected, then the Maxwell equations become conditions detecting F. Here, we use the Maxwell equations to obtain information about the dynamical systems generated by η and J.

Examples. 1) *Constant magnetic field.* Set $E = 0$, and let $F = 2B\,dx^3 \wedge dx^1$ be an electromagnetic field on the Minkowski space (R^4, g); B is a scalar field on R^4, and the electric field E in covariant constant (parallel, inertial) reference frame ∂_4 is everywhere zero. The condition $dF = 0$ is equivalent to $\partial_4 B = 0 = \partial_2 B$. The condition $\operatorname{div} \hat{F} = 0$ (zero source J) gives $\partial_3 B = 0 = \partial_1 B$. Consequently $B = \text{constant}$

2) *Waves.* Let (R^4, g) be a Minkowski space. Near the origin of 3-space are some electric charges that move back and forth in the ∂_1 direction of 3-space. An electromagnetic field is generated. In the observation region ("wave zone"), this field can be described by the 2-form

$$F = 2(f \circ \phi)\, d\phi \wedge dx^1,$$

where $f: R \to R$ is C^∞, and $\phi = (x^3 - x^4): R^4 \to R$. The set $(R^4, F, 0)$ obeys the Maxwell equations,

$$dF = f' \circ \phi \, d\phi \wedge d\phi \wedge dx^1 = 0$$

$$\hat{F} = 2(f \circ \phi)(\partial_3 + \partial_4) \wedge \partial_1$$

$$\operatorname{div} \hat{F} = \partial_1 (f \circ \phi) - (\partial_3 + \partial_4)(f \circ \phi) = 0.$$

F is called a *plane, linearly polarized electromagnetic wave* on Minkowski space.

The *stress-energy tensor* T of an electromagnetic field F on M is a (0,2)-tensor field on M of components

$$T_{ij} = F_{im} F_j^{\ m} - \frac{1}{4} g_{ij} F^{mn} F_{mn}.$$

Theorem. *Let $\hat{T}$ be the (0,2)-tensor field physically equivalent to T via the Lorentz metric g.*

1) $\hat{T}$ is symmetric and $\operatorname{trace} \hat{T} = 0$.

2) $\hat{T}(\omega, \omega) \geq 0$ for every causal 1-form ω.

3) If (M, F, J) obey the Maxwell equations, then $\operatorname{div} \hat{T} = -\hat{F}J$.

Using the components F_{ij} of F, the condition $\operatorname{div} \hat{T} = -\hat{F}J$ is equivalent to $T^{ij}|j = -F^i_{\ m} J^m$.

Remark. The stress-energy tensor T unifies and replaces the classical energy density $\frac{1}{2}(\varepsilon \|E\|^2 + \mu \|B\|^2)$, Poynting vector $S = E \times B$ and Maxwell stress tensor

$$t^{\alpha\beta} = -(\epsilon E^\alpha E^\beta + \mu H^\alpha H^\beta - \frac{1}{2} \delta^{\alpha\beta} (\epsilon \|E\|^2 + \mu \|H\|^2)).$$

We consider the vector field ξ of components ξ^i, $i = 1, 2, 3, 4$, physically equivalent to the 1-form η via the Lorentz metric g. The energy associated to ξ is $f: M \to R$, $f = \frac{1}{2} g(\xi, \xi)$. Obviously

$$f = \frac{1}{2} g_{ij} \xi^i \xi^j = \frac{1}{2} g^{ij} \eta_i \eta_j.$$

The field line α of ξ which starts from the point $(x_0^1, x_0^2, x_0^3, x_0^4)$ at the moment $s = 0$ is the oriented curve $\alpha: (-\varepsilon, \varepsilon) \to M$, $\alpha(s) = (x^1(s), x^2(s), x^3(s), x^4(s))$ that satisfies the Cauchy problem

$$\frac{dx^i}{ds} = \xi^i,\ x^i(0) = x_0^i,\ i = 1, 2, 3, 4.$$

Since ξ is an irrotational vector field the following theorem is true.

Theorem. *Every field line of ξ is a trajectory of a potential dynamical system with four degrees of freedom associated to the potential $V = -f$.*

We can obtain automatically a new version of the Lorentz law determined by ξ.

Now we consider the vector field J of components J^i, $i = 1, 2, 3, 4$. The energy associated to J is $\varphi : M \to R$, $\varphi = \frac{1}{2} g(J, J)$, and the field line of J which starts from the point $(x_0^1, x_0^2, x_0^3, x_0^4)$ at the moment $s = 0$ is the oriented curve $\alpha : (-\varepsilon, \varepsilon) \to M$, $\alpha(s) = (x^1(s), x^2(s), x^3(s), x^4(s))$ that satisfies the Cauchy problem

$$\frac{dx^i}{ds} = J^i,\ x^i(0) = x_0^i,\ i = 1, 2, 3, 4.$$

We can obtain easily the prolongation of this kinematic system to a conservative dynamical system of order two and therefore a new Lorentz law. The flow generated by J conserves the volume because J is a solenoidal vector field.

Suppose that J has no zero on M. Then $J = \|J\| J_0$, $\|J_0\| = 1$, and the restriction of the energy φ to a field line $\alpha(s)$, $s \in I$ of J_0 (s being here the curvilinear abscissa) is well determined by the restriction of $\operatorname{div} J_0$ to that line. Indeed, denoting $l = \|J\| \circ \alpha$, $m = \operatorname{div} J_0$ and taking into account that

$$0 = \operatorname{div} J = D_{J_0} \|J\| + \|J\| \operatorname{div} J_0,$$

we find

$$\frac{dl}{ds} = -lm.$$

Consequently

$$l(s) = l_0 \exp\left(-\int_{s_0}^{s} m(t)\,dt\right),\ l(s_0) = l_0.$$

If m is nowhere zero, the field line α cannot be closed (a field line of J_0 is a reparametrization of a field line of J).

11. BIFURCATIONS IN THE MECHANICS OF HYPOELASTIC GRANULAR MATERIALS

By Lucia Drăguşin

This chapter analyses the behavior of a hypoelastic material obtained by the combination of two granular hypoelastic materials, each of which retains a memory of its initial stress state and of its stress work, depending on its stress history. The modification of behavior under small variations of the material parameters is described by using elements of bifurcation theory.

The constitutive equation of the new material is deduced by means of the constitutive equations of the components. Consequently, the mechanical properties of the components strongly interact, producing domains of stability and unstability for the new material, as well as surfaces on which the strain-stress system is not invertible. In the axial symmetric case, starting from the volumetric stress power and from the total stress power, we find three bifurcation relations between the constitutive parameters. Using the same components, but varying proportions, we also obtain materials with different mechanical behavior. Therefore, to realise new materials, suitable for practical use, we need to choose properly the components, their relative proportions, and the forming process. Of course, from the point of view of mathematical modelling, the choice of the components means the choice of constitutive equations, the proportion of components fixes the stability domain for the new granular material, and the forming process is conditioned by dependence of the stability domain of the new material on the initial stress states of the component materials.

11.1. CONSTITUTIVE EQUATIONS

The constitutive equation of a hypoelastic material (using Truesdell's definition [1]) can be regarded as a linear mapping from the vector space of the deformation rates (D_{11}, D_{22}, D_{33}, D_{12}, D_{23}, D_{13}) into the vector space of Jaumann-Noll stress rates ($\mathring{T}_{11}, \mathring{T}_{22}, \mathring{T}_{33}, \mathring{T}_{12}, \mathring{T}_{23}, \mathring{T}_{13}$).

The material to be analysed has a constitutive equation deduced from the constitutive equations established in [2], [3] for the granular materials.

For the hypoelastic material of a second degree and for the hypoelastic material of a third degree we select the forms

$$\dot{\mathbf{T}}_I = (\alpha_0 x - \frac{\alpha_{15}}{9}x^2 + \frac{\alpha_{15}}{6}y)I_D\mathbf{I} + (-3\alpha_0 x + \frac{\alpha_{13}}{9}x^2 - \frac{\alpha_{15}}{6}y)\mathbf{D} + \alpha_7 x I_D \mathbf{T}' + (\alpha_7 + \frac{\alpha_{13}}{3} + \frac{\alpha_{15}}{9})x\,\mathrm{tr}(\mathbf{T}'\mathbf{D})\mathbf{I} -$$

$$- \frac{\alpha_{15}}{3}x(\mathbf{TD}+\mathbf{DT}) - \frac{\alpha_{15}}{3}I_D\mathbf{T}^2 + \alpha_{13}\mathrm{tr}(\mathbf{TD})\mathbf{T} - \frac{\alpha_{15}}{3}\mathrm{tr}(\mathbf{T}^2\mathbf{D})\mathbf{I} + \frac{\alpha_{15}}{2}(\mathbf{T}^2\mathbf{D}+\mathbf{DT}^2) \quad (1)$$

$$\overset{\circ}{\mathbf{T}}_{II} = (\beta_0 x^3 + \beta_1 xy - \frac{\beta_5}{3}z)I_D\mathbf{I} + (\beta_3 x^3 + \beta_4 xy + \beta_5 z)\mathbf{D} + \beta_6 x^2 I_D\mathbf{T} + (\beta_8 x^2 + \beta_9 y)\mathrm{tr}(\mathbf{TD})\mathbf{I}$$

$$+ (-\frac{\beta_{15}}{3}x^2 + \frac{\beta_{11}}{2}y)(\mathbf{TD}+\mathbf{DT}) + \beta_{12}xI_D\mathbf{T}^2 + \beta_{13}x\,\mathrm{tr}(\mathbf{TD})\mathbf{T} + \beta_{14}x\,\mathrm{tr}(\mathbf{T}^2\mathbf{D})\mathbf{I} \quad (2)$$

$$+ \frac{\beta_{15}}{2}x(\mathbf{T}^2\mathbf{D}+\mathbf{DT}^2) - \beta_5\mathrm{tr}(\mathbf{TD})\mathbf{T}^2 - \beta_{11}\mathrm{tr}(\mathbf{T}^2\mathbf{D})\mathbf{T},$$

where $\mathbf{I}$ is the *unit tensor*, $\mathbf{T}$ is *Cauchy's stress tensor* (defined by means of the internal normal), $\overset{\circ}{\mathbf{T}} = \dot{\mathbf{T}} + \mathbf{WT} - \mathbf{TW}$ is the *Jaumann-Noll stress rate tensor*, $\mathbf{W}$ is the *spin tensor*, $\mathbf{D} = \frac{1}{2}(\mathbf{L}+\mathbf{L}^T)$ is the *deformation rate tensor* ($\mathbf{L} = -\,\mathrm{grad}\,\mathbf{v}$ being the spatial gradient of velocity), $I_D = \mathrm{tr}\mathbf{D}$, $x = \mathrm{tr}\mathbf{T}$, $y = \mathrm{tr}(\mathbf{T}^*)^2$, $z = \mathrm{tr}(\mathbf{T}^*)^3$, $\mathbf{T}^* = \mathbf{T} - \frac{1}{3}x\mathbf{I}$ and

$$\beta_0 = -\frac{1}{81}(27\beta_3 - 3\beta_5 + 27\beta_8 + 2\beta_{11} + 3\beta_{13} - 2\beta_{15}),$$

$$\beta_1 = -\frac{1}{18}(3\beta_5 + 27\beta_8 + 2\beta_{11} + 3\beta_{13} - 11\beta_{15}),$$

$$\beta_4 = \frac{1}{6}(\beta_5 + 27\beta_8 + 2\beta_{11} + 3\beta_{13} - 9\beta_{15}), \quad \beta_6 = -\beta_{12} = -\frac{1}{3}(\beta_5 - \beta_{15}), \quad \beta_9 = \frac{1}{3}(\beta_5 - \beta_{11}),$$

$$\beta_{14} = \frac{1}{3}(\beta_{11} - \beta_{15}).$$

The superimposed dot means the *material time derivative*. It is assumed that there are two functions φ_1, φ_2 such that $\dot{\varphi}_1 = \frac{x}{3}(I_D)_I$, $\dot{\varphi}_2 = \frac{x}{3}(I_D)_{II}$, and two functions ψ_1, ψ_2 such that $\dot{\psi}_1 = = \mathrm{tr}(\mathbf{TD})_I$, $\dot{\psi}_2 = \mathrm{tr}(\mathbf{TD})_{II}$. For such materials, the stress work w_1, w_2 related to the initial configuration having the initial volume V_o, would depend on stress history

$\mathbf{T} = \mathbf{T}(\tau)$, $\tau \in [t_o, t]$

$$w_I(\mathbf{T}(\cdot))(t) = \int_{V_0}\Big(\int_{t_0}^{t}\big(\frac{\rho_0}{\rho}\big)_I\mathrm{tr}(\mathbf{TD})_I\,d\tau\Big)\,dv_0, \quad w_{II}(\mathbf{T}(\cdot))(t) = \int_{V_0}\Big(\int_{t_0}^{t}\big(\frac{\rho_0}{\rho}\big)_{II}\mathrm{tr}(\mathbf{TD})_{II}\,d\tau\Big)\,dv_0.$$

From equations (1) and (2) we get $(I_D)_I$, $\mathrm{tr}(\mathbf{TD})_I$, $\mathrm{tr}(\mathbf{T}^2\mathbf{D})_I$, respectively $(I_D)_{II}$, $\mathrm{tr}(\mathbf{TD})_{II}$, $\mathrm{tr}(\mathbf{T}^2\mathbf{D})_{II}$ as functions of x, y, z, $\dot{x}$, $\dot{y}$, $\dot{z}$.

If the total mass of new material is denoted by m and the constituent masses by m_1, m_2, then between them is the relation $m = m_1 + m_2$. If we consider the mass density of new material $\rho = m/v$, and the apparent mass densities of constituent materials $\rho_1 = m_1/v$, $\rho_2 = m_2/v$, v being the total volume of new material, then

$$\rho = \rho_1 + \rho_2, \quad \frac{\dot{\rho}}{\rho} = \frac{\dot{\rho}_1}{\rho_1}\cdot\frac{\rho_1}{\rho} + \frac{\dot{\rho}_2}{\rho_2}\cdot\frac{\rho_2}{\rho} \quad \text{or} \quad \frac{\dot{\rho}}{\rho} = \frac{\dot{\rho}_1}{\rho_1}\cdot\frac{m_1}{m} + \frac{\dot{\rho}_2}{\rho_2}\cdot\frac{m_2}{m}.$$

From the *equation of continuity* $\frac{\dot{\rho}}{\rho} = -\operatorname{div}\mathbf{v}$, we have $I_{\mathrm{D}} = \frac{\dot{\rho}}{\rho}$, $(I_{\mathrm{D}})_{\mathrm{I}} = \frac{\dot{\rho}_1}{\rho_1}$, $(I_{\mathrm{D}})_{\mathrm{II}} = \frac{\dot{\rho}_2}{\rho_2}$. We obtain the constitutive equation of new hypoelastic granular material taking

$$I_{\mathrm{D}} = \frac{m_1}{m}\left[(I_{\mathrm{D}})_{\mathrm{I}} + \frac{m_2}{m_1}(I_{\mathrm{D}})_{\mathrm{II}}\right],$$

$$\operatorname{tr}(\mathbf{TD}) = \frac{m_1}{m}\left[\operatorname{tr}(\mathbf{TD})_{\mathrm{I}} + \frac{m_2}{m_1}\operatorname{tr}(\mathbf{TD})_{\mathrm{II}}\right],$$

$$\operatorname{tr}(\mathbf{T}^2\mathbf{D}) = \frac{m_1}{m}\left[\operatorname{tr}(\mathbf{T}^2\mathbf{D})_{\mathrm{I}} + \frac{m_2}{m_1}\operatorname{tr}(\mathbf{T}^2\mathbf{D})_{\mathrm{II}}\right],$$

where $\frac{m_2}{m_1}$ indicates the share of constituent materials.

Replacing $(I_{\mathrm{D}})_{\mathrm{I}}$, $(I_{\mathrm{D}})_{\mathrm{II}}$, $\operatorname{tr}(\mathbf{TD})_{\mathrm{I}}$, $\operatorname{tr}(\mathbf{TD})_{\mathrm{II}}$, $\operatorname{tr}(\mathbf{T}^2\mathbf{D})_{\mathrm{I}}$, $\operatorname{tr}(\mathbf{T}^2\mathbf{D})_{\mathrm{II}}$ with their expressions deduced from constitutive equations (1), (2), we find

$$I_{\mathrm{D}} = 3\frac{m_1}{m}\cdot\frac{1}{(3\alpha_7 - \alpha_{15})(1+\mu)x^5(2\alpha x - y)}\Big\{[\mu x^3 y + x^3(2\alpha x - y) + 3\beta(2x^2 - 3\gamma y)(2\alpha x - y)]\dot{x}$$
$$- x[\mu x^3 - 3\beta\gamma(2\alpha x - y)]\dot{y}\Big\},$$

$$\operatorname{tr}(\mathbf{TD}) = \frac{m_1}{m}\cdot\frac{1}{(3\alpha_7 - \alpha_{15})(1+\mu)x^4(2\alpha x - y)}\Big\{[-x^3 y + x^3(2\alpha x - y) + 3\beta(2x^2 - 9\lambda y)(2\alpha x - y)]\dot{x}$$
$$+ x[x^3 + 9\beta\lambda(2\alpha x - y)]\dot{y}\Big\}, \tag{3}$$

$$\operatorname{tr}(\mathbf{T}^2\mathbf{D}) = \frac{m_1}{m}\cdot\frac{1}{6\alpha(3\alpha_7 - \alpha_{15})(1+\mu)x^5(2\alpha x - y)[2x^3 + 2\delta xy - 3(9\lambda + 2\delta)z]}\Big\{\Big[2\alpha x^3[2x^3$$
$$+ 2\delta xy - 3(9\lambda + 2\delta)z][2\alpha x^3 + 6\alpha xy \; (3 + \mu)x^2 y - 3(1+\mu)xz - 3(1-\mu)y^2] + 3\alpha\beta(2\alpha x - y)[8x^7$$
$$+ 4(3\gamma + 2\delta - 18\lambda + 6)x^5 y + 12(\gamma\delta + 2\delta - 6\lambda\delta - 3\gamma)x^3 y^2 + 27(2\lambda\delta - 2\gamma\delta + 9\lambda^2 - 3\lambda\gamma)xy^3$$
$$+ 12(3\gamma - 2\delta - 18\lambda)x^4 z + 18(6\lambda\delta - 9\lambda\gamma + 54\lambda^2 - 18\lambda - 4\delta)x^2 yz + 54\gamma(9\lambda + 2\delta)y^2 z]\Big]\dot{x}$$
$$+ \Big[x^3[2x^3 + 2\delta xy - 3(9\lambda + 2\delta)z][2\alpha(2+\mu)x^2 - 6\alpha\mu y + 3(1+\mu)z] + 3\alpha\beta(2\alpha x - y)[4(6\lambda - \gamma)x^5$$
$$+ 4(6\lambda\delta - \gamma\delta + 3\gamma)x^3 y + 9(2\delta\gamma - 2\delta\lambda - 9\lambda^2 + 3\gamma)xy^2 - 18\gamma(9\lambda + 2\delta)yz + 18\lambda(3\gamma - 18\lambda - 2\delta)x^2 z]\Big]x\dot{y} +$$

$$+ 2(2\alpha x - y)\Big[(1+\mu)[2x^3 + 2\delta xy - 3(9\lambda + 2\delta)z] + 12\alpha\beta(3\lambda - \gamma)x\Big]x^4\dot{z}\Big\},\ \text{where}$$

$$\alpha = -\frac{3\alpha_0}{3\alpha_7 - \alpha_{15}} > 0,\ \mu = \frac{9\alpha_7 + 6\alpha_{13} - \alpha_{15}}{3(3\alpha_7 - \alpha_{15})} < 0,\ \gamma = 3\frac{\beta_5 - 9\beta_8 - 3\beta_{13} + 2\beta_{15}}{9\beta_3 - \beta_{15}} > 0,$$

$$\lambda = -\frac{3\beta_5 + 27\beta_8 + 2\beta_{11} + 3\beta_{13} - 8\beta_{15}}{3(9\beta_3 - \beta_{15})} > 0,\ \delta = 3\frac{\beta_5 + 27\beta_8 + 4\beta_{11} + 3\beta_{13} - 8\beta_{15}}{2(9\beta_3 - \beta_{15})} < 0,$$

$$\beta = \frac{m_2}{m_1}\cdot\frac{3(1+\mu)(3\alpha_7 - \alpha_{15})}{2(3\lambda - \gamma)(9\beta_3 - \beta_{15})} < 0,$$

and $1 + 2\mu > 0,\ 3\alpha_7 - \alpha_{15} \neq 0,\ \ 9\beta_3 - \beta_{15} \neq 0,\ 3\lambda - \gamma \neq 0.$

The preceding functions are defined on the domain

$$\mathcal{D} = \{\mathbf{T}\in\mathbb{R}^6 \mid x \neq 0,\ 2\alpha x - y \neq 0,\ 2x^3 + 2\delta xy - 3(9\lambda + 2\delta)z \neq 0\}.$$

11.2. THE AXIAL SYMMETRIC CASE

We shall study the axial symmetric case

$$\mathbf{T} = \begin{bmatrix} T_1 & 0 & 0 \\ 0 & T_1 & 0 \\ 0 & 0 & T_3 \end{bmatrix}, \qquad \mathbf{D} = \begin{bmatrix} D_1 & 0 & 0 \\ 0 & D_1 & 0 \\ 0 & 0 & D_3 \end{bmatrix}.$$

If $p = \frac{1}{3}(2T_1 + T_3),\ q = T_3 - T_1,$ then $x = 3p,\ y = \frac{2}{3}q^2,\ z = \frac{2}{9}q^3,$

$$\mathrm{tr}(\mathbf{T}^2\mathbf{D}) = -\frac{1}{9}(9p^2 + 3pq - 2q^2)I_{\mathbf{D}} + \frac{1}{3}(6p + q)\mathrm{tr}(\mathbf{TD}).$$

Since the granular materials interact strongly under compression, we shall consider the domain

$$\mathcal{D}_+ = \{(p,q) \mid 9\alpha p - q^2 > 0,\ 81p^3 + 6\delta pq^2 - (9\lambda + 2\delta)q^3 > 0\} \subset \mathcal{D}.$$

The system (3) becomes

$$I_{\mathbf{D}} = \frac{m_1}{m}\frac{3\{9\mu p^3q^2 + [9p^2(p+2\beta) - 2\beta\gamma q^2](9\alpha p - q^2)\}\dot{p} - 2pq[27\mu p^3 - 2\beta\gamma(9\alpha p - q^2)]\dot{q}}{27(1+\mu)(3\alpha_7 - \alpha_{15})p^5(9\alpha p - q^2)}, \tag{4}$$

$$\mathrm{tr}(\mathbf{TD}) = \frac{m_1}{m}\frac{3\{-3p^3q^2 + [3p^2(p+2\beta) - 2\beta\lambda q^2](9\alpha p - q^2)\}\dot{p} + 2pq[9p^3 + 2\beta\lambda(9\alpha p - q^2)]\dot{q}}{9(1+\mu)(3\alpha_7 - \alpha_{15})p^4(9\alpha p - q^2)}.$$

From the system (4), we can find $\dot{p}$, $\dot{q}$ as functions of p, q, D_1, D_3, respectively T_1, T_3, D_1, D_3, if in addition the condition

$$q\left\{9p(p+2\beta)[3(1+\mu)p^2+2\alpha\beta(3\lambda-\gamma)]-2\beta q^2\{[3\lambda(1+2\mu)+\gamma]p+2\beta(3\lambda-\gamma)\}\right\}\neq 0$$

is satisfied.

11.2.1. Bifurcations for the differential equation $I_D = 0$

The differential equation $I_D = 0$ was studied in [4], using bifurcation theory (see [7], [8], [9]). From $(4)_1$, the equation $3pI_D = 0$ may be written

$$[F_2(p,q,\beta,\mu)\dot{p} - F_1(p,q,\beta,\mu)\dot{q}]\Big/N(p,q,\mu) = 0, \tag{5}$$

where

$$F_1(p,q,\beta,\mu) = 2pq[27\mu p^3 - 2\beta\gamma(9\alpha p - q^2)],$$

$$F_2(p,q,\beta,\mu) = [27\mu p^3 - 2\beta\gamma(9\alpha p - q^2)]q^2 + (9\alpha p - q^2)(27p^3 + 54\beta p^2 - 4\beta\gamma q^2),$$

$$N(p,q,\mu) = [9m(1+\mu)(3\alpha_7 - \alpha_{15})\big/m_1]p^4(9\alpha p - q^2).$$

The singular points of differential equation (5) are the points where the theorem of existence and uniqueness of the initial-value problems solution cannot be applied. They are equilibrium points for the differential system

$$\begin{cases} \dfrac{dp}{dt} = F_1(p,q,\beta,\mu)\Big/N(p,q,\mu) \\ \dfrac{dq}{dt} = F_2(p,q,\beta,\mu)\Big/N(p,q,\mu), \end{cases} \tag{6}$$

namely they are the solutions of the algebraic system

$$\begin{cases} F_1(p,q,\beta,\mu) = 0 \\ F_2(p,q,\beta,\mu) = 0. \end{cases} \tag{7}$$

In $\mathcal{D}_+$ the system (7) is equivalent to

$$\begin{cases} q[27\mu p^3 - 2\beta\gamma(9\alpha p - q^2)] = 0 \\ 27p^3 + 54\beta p^2 - 4\beta\gamma q^2 = 0. \end{cases}$$

First we have the solution $(-2\beta, 0)$, and at most four solutions deduced from the system

$$\begin{cases} 3(1+2\mu)p^2 + 6\beta p - 4\alpha\beta\gamma = 0 \\ q^2 = \dfrac{27}{4\beta\gamma}p^2(p+2\beta). \end{cases} \tag{8}$$

If $\frac{\alpha\gamma}{6\mu} < \beta < -\frac{4\alpha\gamma}{3}(1+2\mu)$, $-\frac{1}{4} < \mu < 0$, then the system (8) has the solutions (p_1,q_1), $(p_1,-q_1)$, (p_2,q_2), $(p_2,-q_2)$, where

$$p_1 = \frac{-3\beta - \sqrt{3\beta[3\beta + 4\alpha\gamma(1+2\mu)]}}{3(1+2\mu)}, \quad p_2 = \frac{-3\beta + \sqrt{3\beta[3\beta + 4\alpha\gamma(1+2\mu)]}}{3(1+2\mu)},$$

$$q_1 = \frac{3p_1}{2}\sqrt{\frac{3(p_1+2\beta)}{\beta\gamma}}, \quad q_2 = \frac{3p_2}{2}\sqrt{\frac{3(p_2+2\beta)}{\beta\gamma}}.$$

Consequently on $\mathcal{D}_+$ we have:

(i) if $\frac{\alpha\gamma}{6\mu} < \beta < -\frac{4\alpha\gamma}{3}(1+2\mu)$, $-\frac{1}{4} < \mu < 0$, there are five singular points

$$(-2\beta,0),\ (p_1,\pm q_1),\ (p_2,\pm q_2);$$

(ii) if $\beta = \frac{\alpha\gamma}{6\mu}$, $-\frac{1}{4} < \mu < 0$, there are three singular points

$$(-2\beta,0),\ \left(\frac{2\alpha\gamma}{3(1+2\mu)},\ \pm\frac{\alpha}{1+2\mu}\sqrt{\frac{6\gamma(1+4\mu)}{1+2\mu}}\right);$$

(iii) if $\beta = \frac{\alpha\gamma}{6\mu}$, $-\frac{1}{2} \le \mu \le -\frac{1}{4}$, there is only one singular point $(-2\beta,0)$;

(iv) if $\beta < \frac{\alpha\gamma}{6\mu}$, $-\frac{1}{2} < \mu < 0$, there are three singular points $(-2\beta,0)$, $(p_1,\pm q_1)$;

(v) if $\beta < -\frac{\alpha\gamma}{3}$, $\mu = -\frac{1}{2}$, there are three singular points

$$(-2\beta,0),\ \left(\frac{2}{3}\alpha\gamma,\ \pm\alpha\sqrt{\frac{2\gamma}{\beta}(3\beta+\alpha\gamma)}\right);$$

(vi) if $\beta = -\frac{4\alpha\gamma}{3}(1+2\mu)$, $-\frac{1}{4} < \mu < 0$, there are three singular points

$$(-2\beta,0),\ \left(\frac{4}{3}\alpha\gamma,\ \pm 2\alpha\sqrt{\frac{3\gamma(1+4\mu)}{1+2\mu}}\right);$$

(vii) if $\frac{\alpha\gamma}{6\mu} < \beta < 0$, $-\frac{1}{2} < \mu < -\frac{1}{4}$ or $-\frac{4\alpha\gamma}{3}(1+2\mu) < \beta < 0$, $-\frac{1}{4} \le \mu < 0$, there is only one singular point $(-2\beta,0)$.

Fig.120 shows those seven zones with the number of the singular points in each zone (in Arabic numbers) in the (β, μ)-plane.

Let (p_s,q_s) be a singular point of the equation (5). The solution $p(t) = p_s$, $q(t) = q_s$ is an equilibrium solution for the differential system (6). In the variables $u_1 = p - p_s$, $u_2 = q - q_s$, this differential system becomes

$$\begin{cases} \dfrac{du_1}{dt} = dF_1(u_1,u_2) + \dfrac{1}{2!}d^2F_1(u_1,u_2) + \dfrac{1}{3!}d^3F_1(u_1,u_2) + \dfrac{1}{4!}d^4F_1(u_1,u_2) + \dfrac{1}{5!}d^5F_1(u_1,u_2) \\ \dfrac{du_2}{dt} = dF_2(u_1,u_2) + \dfrac{1}{2!}d^2F_2(u_1,u_2) + \dfrac{1}{3!}d^3F_2(u_1,u_2) + \dfrac{1}{4!}d^4F_2(u_1,u_2) + \dfrac{1}{5!}d^5F_2(u_1,u_2), \end{cases}$$

where the differentials of the functions F_1, F_2 have been calculated in (p_s,q_s,β,μ).

Let us study the stability of the equilibrium solution $u_1(t) = 0$, $u_2(t) = 0$ of the linearized system

$$\begin{cases} \dfrac{du_1}{dt} = u_1\left(\dfrac{\partial F_1}{\partial p}\right)_{(p_s,q_s,\beta,\mu)} + u_2\left(\dfrac{\partial F_1}{\partial q}\right)_{(p_s,q_s,\beta,\mu)} \\ \dfrac{du_2}{dt} = u_1\left(\dfrac{\partial F_2}{\partial p}\right)_{(p_s,q_s,\beta,\mu)} + u_2\left(\dfrac{\partial F_2}{\partial q}\right)_{(p_s,q_s,\beta,\mu)} \end{cases}.$$

If $(p_s,q_s) = (-2\beta,0)$, the matrix attached to the system,

$$J_{(-2\beta,0,\beta,\mu)} = \begin{bmatrix} \dfrac{\partial F_1}{\partial p} & \dfrac{\partial F_1}{\partial q} \\ \dfrac{\partial F_2}{\partial p} & \dfrac{\partial F_2}{\partial q} \end{bmatrix}_{(-2\beta,0,\beta,\mu)} = \begin{bmatrix} 0 & -144\beta^3(\alpha\gamma - 6\beta\mu) \\ -1944\alpha\beta^3 & 0 \end{bmatrix},$$

has the eigenvalues $\nu_{1,2} = \pm 216\beta^3\sqrt{6\alpha(\alpha\gamma - 6\beta\mu)}$.

If $\alpha\gamma - 6\beta\mu > 0$, the solution $p(t) = -2\beta$, $q(t) = 0$ of the nonlinear system (6) is unstable. If $\alpha\gamma - 6\beta\mu = 0$, we have two zero eigenvalues $\nu_{1,2} = 0$. If $\alpha\gamma - 6\beta\mu < 0$, we have two purely imaginary eigenvalues. In the last two cases, the stability of the equilibrium solution of the nonlinear system (6) cannot be deduced from the stability of the equilibrium solution for the linearized system.

According to [6,7,8] the bifurcation of the solution appears when at least one eigenvalue of the linearized system is null, i.e., when $\det J_{(-2\beta,0,\beta,\mu)} = 0$.

It follows that the bifurcation relation for the equilibrium solution $p(t) = -2\beta$, $q(t) = 0$ has the form $\alpha\gamma - 6\beta\mu = 0$.

We replace now (p_s,q_s) by (p_1,q_1) or $(p_1,-q_1)$ or (p_2,q_2) or $(p_2,-q_2)$. The matrix

$$J_{(p_s,q_s,\beta,\mu)} = \begin{bmatrix} 12\beta\gamma q_s(6\alpha p_s - q_s^2) & 8\beta\gamma p_s q_s^2 \\ -9[54\alpha\beta p_s^2 + (\frac{27}{2}p_s^2 + 21\beta p_s - 16\alpha\beta\gamma)q_s^2] & -12\beta\gamma q_s(6\alpha p_s - q_s^2) \end{bmatrix}$$

has the eigenvalues $\nu_{1,2} = \pm\, 12\beta q_s\sqrt{\gamma p_s(9\alpha p_s - q_s^2)(4\alpha\gamma - 3p_s)}$.

If $p_s < \frac{4}{3}\alpha\gamma$, the solution of the nonlinear system (6) $p(t) = p_s$, $q(t) = q_s$ is unstable. If $p_s \geq \frac{4}{3}\alpha\gamma$, the stability of the equilibrium solution of the nonlinear system (6) cannot be deduced from the study of the stability for the linearized system. On condition that $p_s = \frac{4}{3}\alpha\gamma$ should satisfy equation $(8)_1$, we obtain the bifurcation relation $4\alpha\gamma(1+2\mu) + 3\beta = 0$. For $\beta = -\frac{4\alpha\gamma}{3}(1+2\mu)$, there are two equilibrium solutions $p(t) = \frac{4}{3}\alpha\gamma$, $q(t) = 2\alpha\sqrt{\frac{3\gamma(1+4\mu)}{1+2\mu}}$ and $p(t) = \frac{4}{3}\alpha\gamma$, $q(t) = -2\alpha\sqrt{\frac{3\gamma(1+4\mu)}{1+2\mu}}$, while the matrix $\mathbf{J}_{\left(\frac{4}{3}\alpha\gamma,\, \pm 2\alpha\sqrt{\frac{3\gamma(1+4\mu)}{1+2\mu}},\, -\frac{4}{3}\alpha\gamma(1+2\mu),\, \mu\right)}$ has the eigenvalues $\nu_{1,2} = 0$.

It follows that:

(i) if $\frac{\alpha\gamma}{6\mu} < \beta < -\frac{4\alpha\gamma}{3}(1+2\mu)$, $-\frac{1}{4} < \mu < 0$ ($4\alpha\gamma - 3p_1 > 0$ $4\alpha\gamma - 3p_2 < 0$), the equilibrium solutions of the nonlinear system (6) $p(t) = p_1$, $q(t) = \pm q_1$; $p(t) = -2\beta$, $q(t) = 0$ are unstable [$(p_1, \pm q_1)$, $(-2\beta, 0)$ are saddle points], while the equilibrium solutions $p(t) = p_2$, $q(t) = \pm q_2$ are stable;

(ii) if $\beta = \frac{\alpha\gamma}{6\mu}$, $-\frac{1}{4} < \mu < 0$ ($4\alpha\gamma - 3p_1 > 0$), the equilibrium solutions of the nonlinear system (6), $p(t) = p_1$, $q(t) = \pm q_1$, are unstable [$(p_1, \pm q_1)$ are saddle points], while the solution $p(t) = -2\beta$, $q(t) = 0$ bifurcates;

(iii) if $\beta = \frac{\alpha\gamma}{6\mu}$, $-\frac{1}{2} \leq \mu \leq -\frac{1}{4}$, the equilibrium solution $p(t) = -2\beta$, $q(t) = 0$ bifurcates;

(iv) if $\beta < \frac{\alpha\gamma}{6\mu}$, $-\frac{1}{2} < \mu < 0$ ($4\alpha\gamma - 3p_1 > 0$), the equilibrium solutions of the nonlinear system (6), $p(t) = p_1$, $q(t) = \pm q_1$, are unstable [$(p_1, \pm q_1)$ are saddle points], while the solution $p(t) = -2\beta$, $q(t) = 0$ is stable;

(v) if $\beta < -\frac{\alpha\gamma}{3}$, $\mu = -\frac{1}{2}$, the solutions $p(t) = \frac{2}{3}\alpha\gamma$, $q(t) = \pm\alpha\sqrt{\frac{2\gamma}{\beta}(3\beta + \alpha\gamma)}$ are unstable [$\left(\frac{2}{3}\alpha\gamma, \pm\alpha\sqrt{\frac{2\gamma}{\beta}(3\beta + \alpha\gamma)}\right)$ are saddle points], while the solution $p(t) = -2\beta$, $q(t) = 0$ is stable;

(vi) if $\beta = -\frac{4\alpha\gamma}{3}(1+2\mu)$, $-\frac{1}{4} < \mu < 0$, the solution $p(t) = -2\beta$, $q(t) = 0$ is unstable

$[(-2\beta, 0)$ is a saddle point], while the solutions $p(t) = \frac{4}{3}\alpha\gamma$, $q(t) = \pm 2\alpha\sqrt{\frac{3\gamma(1+4\mu)}{1+2\mu}}$ bifurcate;

(vii) if $\frac{\alpha\gamma}{6\mu} < \beta < 0$, $-\frac{1}{2} < \mu < -\frac{1}{4}$ or $-\frac{4\alpha\gamma}{3}(1+2\mu) < \beta < 0$, $-\frac{1}{4} \le \mu < 0$, the solution $p(t) = -2\beta$, $q(t) = 0$ is unstable $[(-2\beta, 0)$ is a saddle point].

11.2.2. Bifurcations for the differential equation tr(TD) = 0

The differential equation tr(**TD**) = 0 was studied in [5]. From $(4)_2$ the equation tr(**TD**)=0 may be written

$$[G_2(p,q,\beta,\lambda)\dot{p} - G_1(p,q,\beta,\lambda)\dot{q}]\big/N(p,q,\mu) = 0, \tag{9}$$

where

$$G_1(p,q,\beta,\lambda) = -2pq[9p^3 + 2\beta\lambda(9\alpha p - q^2)]$$
$$G_2(p,q,\beta,\lambda) = 3\{-3p^3q^2 + [3p^2(p+2\beta) - 2\beta\lambda q^2](9\alpha p - q^2)\}.$$

The singular points of the differential equation (9) are the equilibrium points for the differential system

$$\begin{cases} \dfrac{dp}{dt} = G_1(p,q,\beta,\lambda)\big/N(p,q,\mu) \\ \dfrac{dq}{dt} = G_2(p,q,\beta,\lambda)\big/N(p,q,\mu), \end{cases} \tag{10}$$

namely they satisfy the algebraic system

$$\begin{cases} G_1(p,q,\beta,\lambda) = 0 \\ G_2(p,q,\beta,\lambda) = 0. \end{cases} \tag{11}$$

In $\mathcal{D}_+$, the system (11) has a solution $(-2\beta, 0)$, and at most four solutions deduced from the system

$$\begin{cases} p^2 - 2\beta p + 4\alpha\beta\lambda - 0 \\ q^2 = \dfrac{9}{4\beta\lambda}p^2(p+2\beta). \end{cases}$$

It results that

(i) if $\beta < -\frac{\alpha\lambda}{2}$, there are three singular points $(-2\beta, 0)$, $(p_3, \pm q_3)$ in $\mathcal{D}_+$, where

$$p_3 = \beta + \sqrt{\beta(\beta - 4\alpha\lambda)}, \; q_3 = 6\alpha\sqrt{\frac{\beta\lambda(2\beta + \alpha\lambda)}{\beta(2\beta - 5\alpha\lambda) + (\alpha\lambda - 2\beta)\sqrt{\beta(\beta - 4\alpha\lambda)}}};$$

(ii) if $-\frac{\alpha\lambda}{2} \le \beta < 0$, there is only one singular point $(-2\beta, 0)$ in $\mathcal{D}_+$.

We study now the stability of the equilibrium solution $u_1(t) = p(t) - p_s = 0$, $u_2(t) = q(t) - q_s = 0$ of linearized system

$$\begin{cases} \dfrac{du_1}{dt} = u_1\left(\dfrac{\partial G_1}{\partial p}\right)_{(p_s, q_s, \beta, \lambda)} + u_2\left(\dfrac{\partial G_1}{\partial q}\right)_{(p_s, q_s, \beta, \lambda)} \\ \dfrac{du_2}{dt} = u_1\left(\dfrac{\partial G_2}{\partial p}\right)_{(p_s, q_s, \beta, \lambda)} + u_2\left(\dfrac{\partial G_2}{\partial q}\right)_{(p_s, q_s, \beta, \lambda)} \end{cases},$$

where (p_s, q_s) is an equilibrium point.

If $(p_s, q_s) = (-2\beta, 0)$, the matrix attached to the preceding differential system

$$\mathbf{J}_{(-2\beta, 0, \beta, \lambda)} = \begin{bmatrix} \dfrac{\partial G_1}{\partial p} & \dfrac{\partial G_1}{\partial q} \\ \dfrac{\partial G_2}{\partial p} & \dfrac{\partial G_2}{\partial q} \end{bmatrix}_{(-2\beta, 0, \beta, \lambda)} = \begin{bmatrix} 0 & -144\beta^3(2\beta + \alpha\lambda) \\ -648\alpha\beta^3 & 0 \end{bmatrix}$$

has the eigenvalues $\nu_{1,2} = \pm 216\beta^3\sqrt{2\alpha(2\beta + \alpha\lambda)}$.

If $2\beta + \alpha\lambda > 0$, the solution $p(t) = -2\beta$, $q(t) = 0$ of the nonlinear system (10) is unstable.

If $2\beta + \alpha\lambda \le 0$, the stability of the equilibrium solution of the nonlinear system (10) cannot be deduced from the stability of the equilibrium solution for the linearized system.

Consequently the bifurcation relation for the equilibrium solution $p(t) = -2\beta$, $q(t) = 0$ has the form $2\beta + \alpha\lambda = 0$.

If $2\beta + \alpha\lambda < 0$ and we replace (p_s, q_s) by $(p_3, \pm q_3)$, the matrix

$$\mathbf{J}_{(p_s, q_s, \beta, \lambda)} = \begin{bmatrix} -9p_s^2 q_s(5p_s + 2\beta) & 18p_s^3(p_s + 2\beta) \\ -\dfrac{81}{4\lambda}p_s^3[31p_s - 2(17\alpha\lambda - \beta)] & 9p_s^2 q_s(5p_s + 2\beta) \end{bmatrix}$$

has the eigenvalues $\nu_{1,2} = \pm 27p_s^3\sqrt{\frac{2}{\lambda}(p_s + 2\beta)(p_s - 4\alpha\lambda)}$.

It follows that

(i) if $2\beta + \alpha\lambda < 0$, the equilibrium solutions $p(t) = p_3$, $q(t) = \pm q_3$ of the nonlinear system (10) are unstable, while the equilibrium solution $p(t) = -2\beta$, $q(t) = 0$ is stable;

(ii) if $2\beta + \alpha\lambda > 0$, the equilibrium solution $p(t) = -2\beta$, $q(t) = 0$ of the nonlinear system (10) is unstable.

(iii) if $2\beta + \alpha\lambda = 0$, the equilibrium solution $p(t) = -2\beta$, $q(t) = 0$ bifurcates.

Fig.121 shows those two zones with the number of the singular points in each zone (in Arabic numbers) in the (λ, β)-plane.

Therefore, for the equation $I_D = 0$, the bifurcation relations between the constitutive parameters are

$$\beta = \alpha\gamma/(6\mu) \text{ and } \beta = -4\alpha\gamma(1+2\mu)/3.$$

For the equation $\mathrm{tr}(\mathbf{TD}) = 0$ the bifurcation relation is $\beta = -\alpha\lambda/2$.

We note that

a) the system (4) cannot be inverted at all singular points (p_s, q_s);

b) we have $p_s \leq -2\beta$, for all singular points (p_s, q_s).

Note 1: From (8), it follows that the bifurcation diagrams $p = p(\beta)$ have the equations

$$p = -2\beta, \quad p_{1,2} = \frac{-3\beta \pm \sqrt{3\beta[3\beta + 4\alpha\gamma(1+2\mu)]}}{3(1+2\mu)}. \tag{12}$$

They are plotted in Fig.122 for $\alpha = 1$, $\gamma = 3/4$. We consider: $\mu = -1/3$ in Fig.122a, $\mu = -1/4$ in Fig.122b, $\mu = -1/8$ in Fig.122c.

From (11) the bifurcation diagrams $p = p(\beta)$ have the equations

$$p = -2\beta, \quad p = \beta + \sqrt{\beta(\beta - 4\alpha\lambda)}. \tag{13}$$

These diagrams are plotted in Fig.122d for $\alpha = 1$, $\lambda = 1$.

11.2.3. The accessible stress path for a granular new material

Definition 1: A set $\mathcal{S}$ is a *stability domain of the granular new material* if

$$\mathcal{S} = \{(p,q)\,|\,9\alpha p - q^2 > 0,\ 81p^3 + 6\delta pq^2 - (9\lambda + 2\delta)q^3 > 0,\ p > -2\beta\},$$

when $3\alpha_7 - \alpha_{15} > 0$, and

$$\mathcal{S} = \{(p,q)\,|\,9\alpha p - q^2 > 0,\ 81p^3 + 6\delta pq^2 - (9\lambda + 2\delta)q^3 > 0,\ p < -2\beta\},$$

when $3\alpha_7 - \alpha_{15} < 0$.

Definition 2: A stress path $\mathcal{L}$ is an *accessible path for a granular new material* if its beginning point pertains to a stability domain $\mathcal{S}$ and at each of its points the stress-deformation rate system (4) can be inverted, namely:

$$\mathcal{L} \subset \mathcal{S} \cap \{(p,q)\,|\,9p(p+2\beta)[3(1+\mu)p^2 + 2\alpha\beta(3\lambda-\gamma)] \\ -2\beta q^2[3\lambda(1+2\mu)p + \gamma p + 2\beta(3\lambda-\gamma)] \neq 0\}.$$

Definition 3: A stress path $p = p(q)$ located on $\mathcal{D}_+$ and starting from (p_0, q_0) is

- a *compressible loading path*, if $\dot{p} > 0$, $\dot{w} > 0$, $w(p,q) > w(p_0, q_0)$;

- a *loading path with the volume increase*, if $\dot{p} < 0$, $\dot{w} > 0$, $w(p,q) > w(p_0, q_0)$ (a loading path with dilation);

- a *neutral change path*, if $\dot{w} = 0$;

- an *unloading path*, if $\dot{w} < 0$, $w(p,q) > w(p_0,q_0)$.

The derivatives $\dot{\rho}$ and $\dot{w}$ have the same sign as $\dot{\varphi}$ respectively $\dot{\psi}$ because $\dot{\varphi} = p\dot{\rho}/\rho$, $\dot{\psi} = \rho\dot{w}/\rho_0$.

Note 2: The relations

$$9\alpha p - q^2 = 0,\ 81p^3 + 6\delta pq^2 - (9\lambda + 2\delta)q^3 = 0 \tag{14}$$

can be considered as *failure conditions*.

The relation $p = -2\beta$ can be considered as a *stability condition*.

The relation

$$q\left\{9p(p+2\beta)[3(1+\mu)p^2+2\alpha\beta(3\lambda-\gamma)]-2\beta q^2\{[3\lambda(1+2\mu)+\gamma]p+2\beta(3\lambda-\gamma)\}\right\} = 0 \tag{15}$$

can be considered as an *accessibility condition* for the new material.

Note 3: If the body has plastic behaviour, in the constitutive equation for unloading, different coefficients from those used at loading can be taken even if the stress path is the same but runs in a different direction. There are the same failure, stability and accessibility conditions in loading and unloading if we take the same parameters α, μ, γ, λ, δ, β, but the parameter $(3\alpha_7 - \alpha_{15})$ will be different.

In relation (15), fixing the constituent materials means fixing the constitutive parameters α, μ, γ, λ, δ.

Note 4: We shall study the shape of the accessibility condition (15) as a function of β (the new material parameter).

For different values of parameters we shall obtain the following cases:

I. $3\lambda - \gamma < 0$, $\beta < 0$.

II. $\begin{cases}3\lambda-\gamma>0,\\ 3\lambda\mu+\gamma>0,\end{cases}$

1) $\beta < \dfrac{\alpha[3\lambda(1+2\mu)+\gamma]^2}{6(1+\mu)(\gamma-3\lambda)}$

2) $\beta = \dfrac{\alpha[3\lambda(1+2\mu)+\gamma]^2}{6(1+\mu)(\gamma-3\lambda)}$

3) $\dfrac{\alpha[3\lambda(1+2\mu)+\gamma]^2}{6(1+\mu)(\gamma-3\lambda)} < \beta < \dfrac{\alpha(\gamma-3\lambda)}{6(1+\mu)}$

4) $\beta = \dfrac{\alpha(\gamma-3\lambda)}{6(1+\mu)}$

5) $\dfrac{\alpha(\gamma-3\lambda)}{6(1+\mu)} < \beta < 0$

III $\begin{cases}3\lambda-\gamma>0,\\ 3\lambda\mu+\gamma=0,\end{cases}$

1) $\beta < \dfrac{\alpha(\gamma-3\lambda)}{6(1+\mu)}$

2) $\beta = \dfrac{\alpha(\gamma-3\lambda)}{6(1+\mu)}\ \left(= \dfrac{\alpha\gamma}{6\mu} = -\dfrac{\alpha\lambda}{2}\right)$

(bifurcation relation for $I_D = 0$ and for tr(**TD**) $= 0$)

3) $\dfrac{\alpha(\gamma-3\lambda)}{6(1+\mu)} < \beta < 0$

IV $\begin{cases} 3\lambda-\gamma > 0, \\ 3\lambda\mu+\gamma < 0, \end{cases}$

1) $\beta < \dfrac{\alpha(\gamma-3\lambda)}{6(1+\mu)}$

2) $\beta = \dfrac{\alpha(\gamma-3\lambda)}{6(1+\mu)}$

3) $\dfrac{\alpha(\gamma-3\lambda)}{6(1+\mu)} < \beta < \dfrac{\alpha[3\lambda(1+2\mu)+\gamma]^2}{6(1+\mu)(\gamma-3\lambda)}$

4) $\beta = \dfrac{\alpha[3\lambda(1+2\mu)+\gamma]^2}{6(1+\mu)(\gamma-3\lambda)}$

5) $\dfrac{\alpha[3\lambda(1+2\mu)+\gamma]^2}{6(1+\mu)(\gamma-3\lambda)} < \beta < 0$

These cases of the accessibility condition (15) are plotted in Fig.123.
We are using the notations:

$$a = -\frac{2\beta(3\lambda-\gamma)}{3\lambda(1+2\mu)+\gamma}, \quad b = \sqrt{\frac{-2\alpha\beta(3\lambda-\gamma)}{3(1+\mu)}}.$$

Note 5: Let $\dot{\varphi} = pI_D$ be the volume stress power. From $(4)_1$, the solution of the Pfaff equation $\dot{\varphi} = pI_D$ passing through the point (p_o, q_o, φ_o) has the form

$$\frac{m}{m_1}\frac{(1+\mu)}{(-\mu)}(3\alpha_7-\alpha_{15})(\varphi-\varphi_o) = \frac{\mu-1}{\mu}\ln\frac{p}{p_o} + \ln\frac{9\alpha p_o - q_o^2}{9\alpha p - q^2} + \frac{2\beta}{\mu p}\left(1-\frac{\gamma q^2}{27p^2}\right) - \frac{2\beta}{\mu p_o}\left(1-\frac{\gamma q_o^2}{27p_o^2}\right). \tag{16}$$

Let $\dot{\psi}$ = tr(**TD**) be the total stress power. From $(4)_2$, the solution of the Pfaff equation $\dot{\psi}$ = tr(**TD**) passing through the point (p_o, q_o, ψ_o) has the form

$$\frac{m}{m_1}(1+\mu)(3\alpha_7-\alpha_{15})(\psi-\psi_o) = \ln\frac{p^2(9\alpha p_o - q_o^2)}{p_o(9\alpha p - q^2)} - \frac{2\beta}{p}\left(1-\frac{\lambda q^2}{9p^2}\right) + \frac{2\beta}{p_o}\left(1-\frac{\lambda q_o^2}{9p_o^2}\right). \tag{17}$$

Note 6: Since the stress power is tr(**TD**) = tr(**T*D**)$+pI_D$, where **T*** = **T**$-\frac{1}{3}I_T$**I** we have some information about the deviatoric stress power tr(**T*D**).

11.2.4. The physical significance of the accessibility condition

To find the significance of the accessibility condition (15), we will study three loading (see [6]).

I. Let us consider the stress path

$$T_1(t) = T_2(t) = T_3(t) = p(t). \tag{18}$$

Since, here, $q = 0$, from (4) we have

$$\frac{\dot{\rho}}{\rho} = \frac{m_1}{m}\cdot\frac{(p+2\beta)\dot{p}}{(1+\mu)(3\alpha_7-\alpha_{15})p^3}$$

$$\mathrm{tr}(\mathbf{TD}) = \frac{m_1}{m}\cdot\frac{(p+2\beta)\dot{p}}{(1+\mu)(3\alpha_7-\alpha_{15})p^2}.$$

Integrating, we obtain

$$\frac{\rho}{\rho_i}(p) = \exp\left[\frac{m_1}{m(1+\mu)(3\alpha_7-\alpha_{15})}\left(\frac{p_i+\beta}{p_i^2}-\frac{p+\beta}{p^2}\right)\right],$$

$$w(p)-w_i = \int_{p_i}^{p}\frac{\rho_i}{\rho}\mathrm{tr}(\mathbf{TD})dp$$

$$= \exp\left[-\frac{m_1}{m(1+\mu)(3\alpha_7-\alpha_{15})}\left(\frac{p_i+\beta}{p_i^2}+\frac{1}{4\beta}\right)\right]\sum_{n=0}^{\infty}\frac{\ln\frac{p}{p_i}+\sum_{k=1}^{2n+1}\frac{(2\beta)^k}{k}C_{2n+1}^k\left(\frac{1}{p_i^k}-\frac{1}{p^k}\right)}{n!(4\beta)^n[m(1+\mu)(3\alpha_7-\alpha_{15})/m_1]^{n+1}},$$

where $\rho_i = \rho(p_i)$, $w_i = w(p_i)$ are the initial mass density, respectively the initial stress work.

The mass density is represented in Fig.124a, for $3\alpha_7-\alpha_{15}>0$ and in Fig.124b, for $3\alpha_7-\alpha_{15}<0$.

If $3\alpha_7-\alpha_{15} > 0$, we say that the material is *uncompacted* for $p_i < -2\beta$, it is *normal compacted* for $p_i = -2\beta$ and it is *supercompacted* for $p_i > -2\beta$. The stress work w decreases for $p < -2\beta$ and increases for $p > -2\beta$.

If $3\alpha_7-\alpha_{15} <0$ and $p_i < -2\beta$, we say that the material has a *dilation* for $p > -2\beta$. The stress work increases for $p < -2\beta$ and decreases for $p > -2\beta$.

II. We shall study the particular case: $\alpha = \lambda = 1$, $\gamma = 3/4$, $\mu = -1/4$, $\delta = -9/8$, when $3\lambda - \gamma > 0$, $3\lambda\mu + \gamma = 0$ (case III). We consider $m(3\alpha_7 - \alpha_{15})/m_1 = 4/3$ and $(p_o,q_o,\varphi_o) = (p_o,q_o,\psi_o) = (-2\beta,0,1)$.

Figs.125a, 125b represent the surfaces $\varphi = \varphi(p,q)$ and $\psi = \psi(p,q)$ (see (16), (17)) for $\alpha = \lambda = 1$, $\gamma = 3/4$, $\mu = -1/4$, $\beta = -1$ and $(p,q)\in[1,4]\times[-2.9,2.9]$.

The contour curves for (16), (17) were plotted in Figs.126a, 126b if $\beta = -1$, in Figs.127a, 127b if $\beta = -1/2$ and in Figs.128a, 128b if $\beta = -0.3$.
See too ([4], Fig.5) and ([5], Fig.5) for Figs.126a, 126b, ([4], Fig.3) and ([5], Fig.4) for Figs.127a, 127b and ([5], Fig.3) for Fig.128b.

In Figs.126a,126b we have $\mathcal{L}\subset\mathcal{S} = \{(p,q)\mid q^2<9p,\ q<2p,\ p>2\}$. For $\varphi=\varphi(p,q)$ the saddle points are $(2-\sqrt{2},\ \pm3(2-\sqrt{2})\sqrt[4]{2})\notin\mathcal{S}$ (see **11.2.1.**iv), and for $\psi = \psi(p,q)$ the saddle points are $(\sqrt{5}-1,\ \pm3\sqrt{2}(3-\sqrt{5})/2)\notin\mathcal{S}$ (see **11.2.2.**i.). In Figs.127a, 127b we have $\mathcal{L}\subset\mathcal{S} = \{(p,q)\mid q^2 < 9p,\ q<2p,\ p>1\}$, and in Figs.128a, 128b we have

$$\mathcal{L}\subset\{(p,q)\mid q^2<9p,\ q<2p,\ p>0.6\}\cap\{(p,q)\mid q^2\neq3p(3-5p^2)\}.$$

The accessibility condition (15) becomes

$$(\Gamma_a):\ q(p+2\beta)[9p(p^2+2\beta)-2\beta q^2]=0. \tag{19}$$

From (4), on the line $(\Gamma_a)_1$: $p=-2\beta$, the curves $\varphi=$ const. and $\psi=$ const. have the same tangent of slope

$$\left.\frac{dq}{dp}\right|_{p=-2\beta}=-3q\frac{q^2+18\beta+12\beta^2}{4\beta(q^2+18\beta+36\beta^2)}.$$

On the line $q=0$, and on the curve $(\Gamma_a)_2$: $9p(p^2+2\beta)=2\beta q^2$ there are the extremal points for the functions $p=p(q)$ implicitly defined by the equations of the contour curves.

We assume that for the stress path (16), the material with the initial mass density $\rho_i=\rho(p_i)$, $p_i\geq-2\beta$ was compacted until the mass density reached the value $\rho_1=\rho(p_1)$, $p_1\geq p_i$. From (16), for $(p_0,q_0)=(p_1,0)$ and $\varphi_1=\varphi(p_1,0)$, we get

$$\varphi-\varphi_1=\frac{1}{4}\ln\frac{9p^5}{9p-q^2}-\frac{2\beta}{p}+\frac{2\beta}{p_1}-\ln p_1+\frac{\beta q^2}{18p^3}. \tag{20}$$

In the first part of loading (18) the value $\psi_1=\psi(p_1,0)$ is reached. From (17), we obtain

$$\psi-\psi_1=\ln\frac{9p^2}{9p-q^2}-\frac{2\beta}{p}+\frac{2\beta}{p_1}-\ln p_1+\frac{2\beta q^2}{9p^3}. \tag{21}$$

Let $(p_1,0)$ be, $-2\beta=0.6<p_1<p_a=\sqrt{3/5}$, $(p_a,0)\in(\Gamma_a)_2$.
We consider the stress path (20), $(\Gamma_1)_\varphi$: $\varphi(p,q)=\varphi_1$, $\varphi_1=1.04$ (see the double line in Fig.129). The curves $(\Gamma_1)_\varphi$ and $(\Gamma_1)_\psi$: $\psi(p,q)=\psi_1$, $\psi_1=1.01$ are tangent to each other at the point $P(p_1,0)$. When q increases on the stress path $(\Gamma_1)_\varphi$, having the start point P, the work w decreases ($\dot{w}=\frac{\rho_1}{\rho}\dot{\psi}<0$) until the curves $(\Gamma_1)_\varphi$ and $\psi(p,q)=\psi_2<\psi_1$ become tangent at the intersection point with the accessibility curve $(\Gamma_a)_2$. This may indicate that the stress work has been used to rearrange the material grains. After that, when q increases, the work w increases until the curve $(\Gamma_1)_\varphi$ intersects the accessibility line $(\Gamma_a)_1$: $p=0.6$.

Let $(p_2,0)$ be, $p_2>p_a>-2\beta=0.6$.

We consider the stress path $(\Gamma_2)_\varphi$: $\varphi(p,q)=\varphi_2$, $\varphi_2=\varphi(p_2,0)=1.2$. The curves $(\Gamma_2)_\varphi$ and $(\Gamma_2)_\psi$: $\psi(p,q)=\psi_3$, $\psi_3=\psi(p_2,0)=1.05$ are tangent to each other at $Q(p_2,0)$. When p decreases on the stress path $(\Gamma_2)_\varphi$, having the start point Q, the work w increases ($\dot{w}=\frac{\rho_2}{\rho}\dot{\psi}>0$) until the curves $(\Gamma_2)_\varphi$ and $\psi(p,q)=\psi_4$, $\psi_4>\psi_3$ become tangent to each other. The point at which those two curves are tangent is found on the accessibility line $(\Gamma_a)_1$: $p=0.6$. If p decreases, the curve $(\Gamma_2)_\varphi$ intersects again the curve $(\Gamma_2)_\psi$, therefore the work w decreases ($\dot{w}=\frac{\rho_2}{\rho}\dot{\psi}<0$) and the failure appears.

The curve (19) and the contour curves for the surfaces (20), (21) are represented in

Fig.129 for $\beta = -0.3$, $\varphi_1 = \varphi(p_1,0) = 1.04$, $\varphi_2 = \varphi(p_2,0) = 1.2$, $\psi(p,q) = k$, k=0.98; 1; 1.01; 1.05; 1.07; 1.1; 1.2.

We note that, for an incompressible material (when ρ = const.), there is only the stress path $\varphi(p,q)$ = const.

III. We shall consider axis-symmetric compression. The stress path

$$T_1(t) = T_2(t) = p_0 > p_i$$

is characterized by the relation $p = q/3 + p_0$. From (4) we obtain

$$\frac{\dot{\rho}}{\rho} = \frac{m_1}{m}\cdot\frac{3\dot{q}}{(1+\mu)(3\alpha_7-\alpha_{15})(q+3p_0)^5(-q^2+3\alpha q+9\alpha p_0)}\Big\{-\mu q(q+6p_0)(q+3p_0)^3$$
$$+(-q^2+3\alpha q+9\alpha p_0)[(q+3p_0)^2(q+3p_0+6\beta)-2\beta\gamma q(q-6p_0)]\Big\} \tag{22}$$

$$\mathrm{tr}(\mathbf{TD}) = \frac{m_1}{m}\cdot\frac{\dot{q}}{(1+\mu)(3\alpha_7-\alpha_{15})(q+3p_0)^4(-q^2+3\alpha q+9\alpha p_0)}\Big\{q(q+6p_0)(q+3p_0)^3$$
$$+(-q^2+3\alpha q+9\alpha p_0)[(q+3p_0)^2(q+3p_0+6\beta)-6\beta\lambda q(q-6p_0)]\Big\}. \tag{23}$$

Since $\mathrm{tr}(\mathbf{TD}) = pI_{\mathbf{D}} + q\dot{\varepsilon}$, where $\dot{\varepsilon} = \frac{2}{3}(D_3 - D_1)$, from (4) it follows that

$$\dot{\varepsilon} = \frac{m_1}{m}\cdot\frac{1}{27(1+\mu)(3\alpha_7-\alpha_{15})p^4(9\alpha p-q^2)}\Big\{3[-9(1+\mu)p^3q+2\beta(\gamma-3\lambda)q(9\alpha p-q^2)]\dot{p}$$
$$+2p[27(1+\mu)p^3-2\beta(\gamma-3\lambda)(9\alpha p-q^2)]\dot{q}\Big\}.$$

For the stress path $p = q/3 + p_0$ we obtain

$$\dot{\varepsilon} = \frac{m_1}{m}\cdot\frac{(1+\mu)(q+6p_0)(q+3p_0)^3+2\beta(\gamma-3\lambda)(-q^2+3\alpha q+9\alpha p_0)(q-6p_0)}{(1+\mu)(3\alpha_7-\alpha_{15})(q+3p_0)^4(-q^2+3\alpha q+9\alpha p_0)}\dot{q}. \tag{24}$$

We will study the material behavior for particular values of the constitutive parameters and different initial conditions.

For $\alpha=\lambda=1$, $\gamma=3/4$, $\mu=-1/4$, $m(3\alpha_7-\alpha_{15})/m_1 = 4/3$, $\beta=-0.3$, (see Fig.129), the solutions of equations (22), (24), having initial conditions $\rho=\rho_0$, $q_0 = 0$ and $\varepsilon_0 = q_0 = 0$ are plotted in Figs.130a, 130b, when $p_0 = 0.5$ and $p_0 = 0.6$ $(= -2\beta)$.

Remark 1. If $p_0 = 0.5$, from (22), (23), (24) we find

$$\frac{\dot{\rho}}{\rho} = 18\frac{-4q^5+9.2q^4+101.4q^3+110.7q^2+2.7q-16.2}{(3+2q)^5(-q^2+3q+4.5)}\dot{q},$$

$$\dot{\varepsilon} = 3\frac{4q^4 + 22.8q^3 + 124.2q^2 + 62.1q - 56.7}{(3+2q)^4(-q^2+3q+4.5)}\dot{q},$$

$$\mathrm{tr}(\mathbf{TD}) = 6\frac{16q^4 + 112.8q^3 + 86.4q^2 - 27q - 8.1}{(3+2q)^4(-q^2+3q+4.5)}\dot{q}.$$

It follows that q_m=0.3728 is an approximation of the solution of the equation $16q^4 + 112.8q^3 + 86.4q^2 - 27q - 8.1 = 0$, as $\dot{w} = \frac{\rho_0}{\rho}\mathrm{tr}(\mathbf{TD}) < 0$ for $0 < q < q_m$ and $\dot{w} \geq 0$ for $q \geq q_m$.

Here the system (4) is not invertible if

$$q(p - 0.6)[3p(3 - 5p^2) - q^2] = 0 .$$

Intersecting with the stress path $p = (1.5 + q)/3$ we find

$$q = 0.3 \text{ and } 40q^3 + 252q^2 + 54q - 189 = 0. \tag{25}$$

The minimum values $(q_m)_\rho$=0.3256 for the function $\rho = \rho(q)$, $(q_m)_\varepsilon$=0.4572 for $\varepsilon = \varepsilon(q)$, q_m=0.3728 for $w = w(q)$ and the root q_a=0.7294 of the equation $(25)_2$ are in the relation $(q_m)_\rho < q_m < (q_m)_\varepsilon < q_a$. Therefore, for $q > q_a$ the stress work increases.
For $0 < q < q_a$ this may indicate that the stress work has been used to rearrange the material grains.

Remark 2. If $p_0 = 0.6$, we have $\dot{w} \geq 0$ for $q \geq 0$ [see Fig.130c].

Remark 3. Fig.129 shows that an accessible path is a loading path if it has the start point

$$(p_0, q_0) \in \{(p,q)/9p - q^2 > 0,\ 12p^3 - pq^2 - q^3 > 0,\ p > 0.6,\ q > 0,\ 9p(p^2 - 0.6) + 0.6q^2 > 0\}.$$

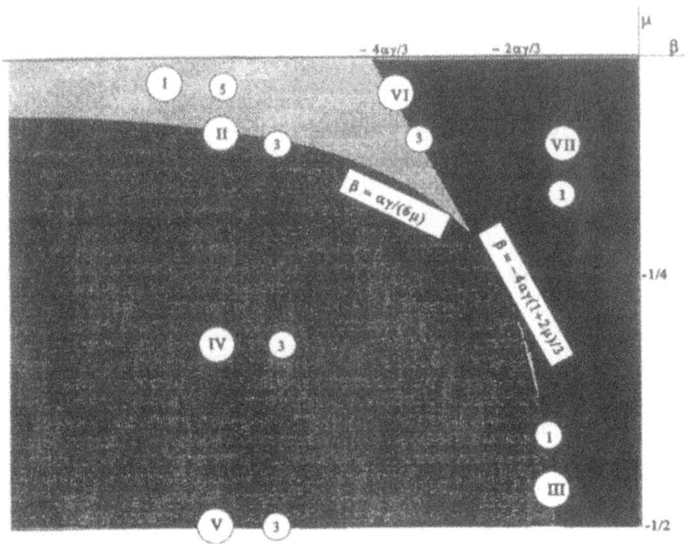

Fig.120. Number of the singular points in the (β,μ) - plane, for the bifurcation relations $\beta=\alpha\gamma/(6\mu)$ and $\beta=-4\alpha\gamma(1+2\mu)/3$.

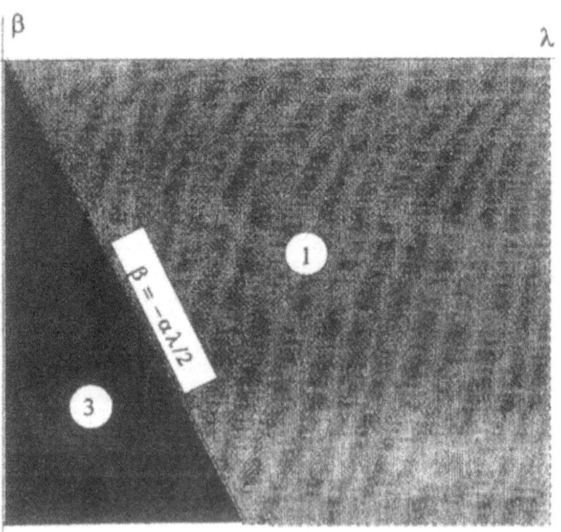

Fig.121. Number of singular points in the (λ,β) - plane, for the bifurcation relation $\beta=-\alpha\lambda/2$.

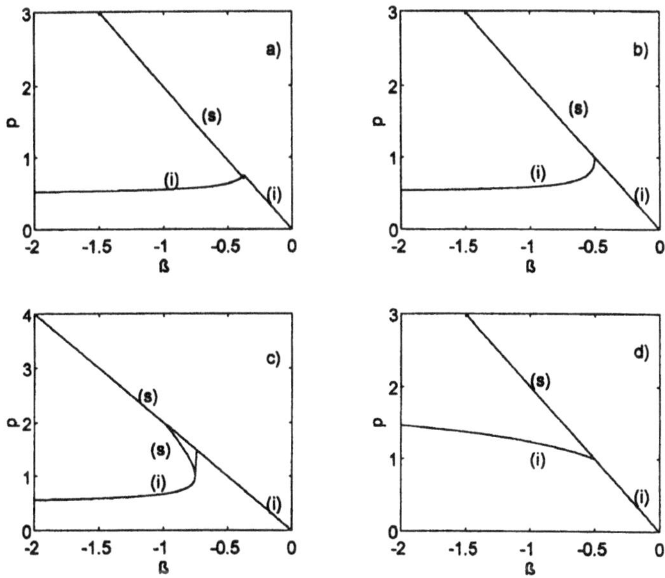

Fig. 122 a, b, c, d. Bifurcation diagrams (12), (13) ((i) - instability, (s) - stability).

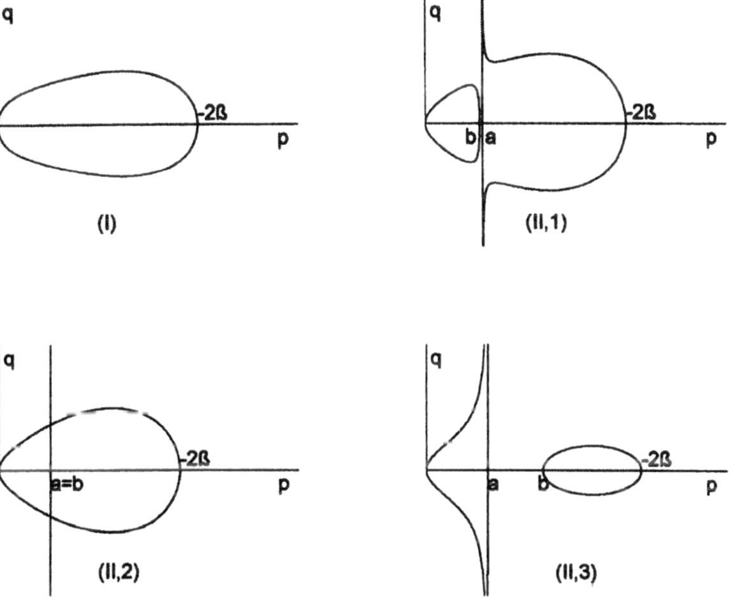

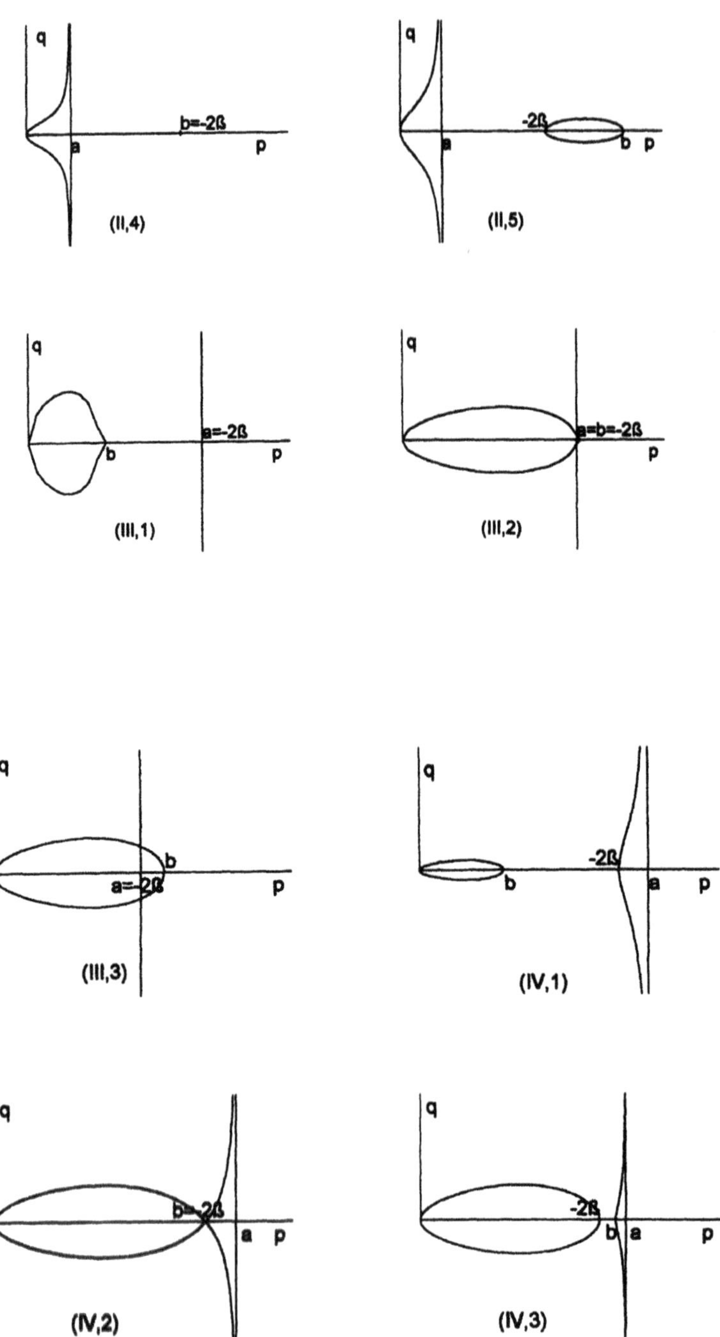
q
b=-2ß
a
p
(II,4)
q
-2ß
a
b p
(II,5)
q
a=-2ß
b
p
(III,1)
q
a=b=-2ß
p
(III,2)
q
b
a=-2ß
p
(III,3)
q
-2ß
b
a p
(IV,1)
q
b=-2ß
a p
(IV,2)
q
-2ß
b a
p
(IV,3)

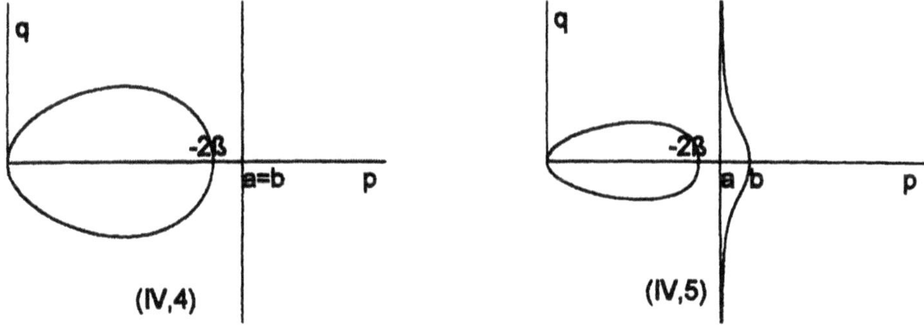

Fig. 123. The accessibility curves (15).

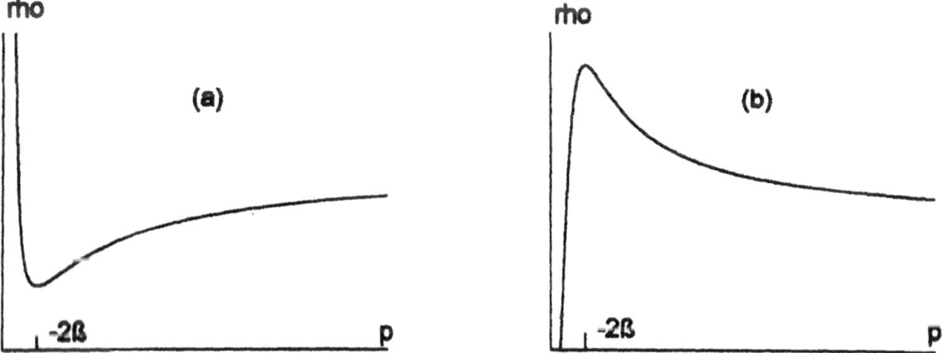

Fig. 124 a,b. Mass density ρ as a function of pressure p.

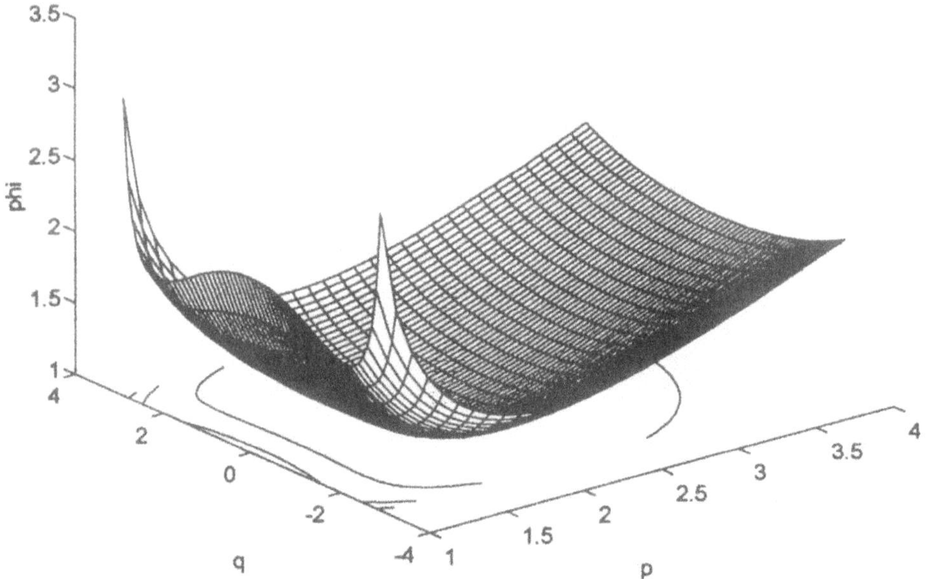

Fig. 125 a. Surface $\varphi = \varphi(p,q)$, if $\alpha = \lambda = 1$, $\gamma = 3/4$, $\mu = -1/4$, $\beta = -1$ and $(p,q) \in [1,4] \times [-2.9, 2.9]$.

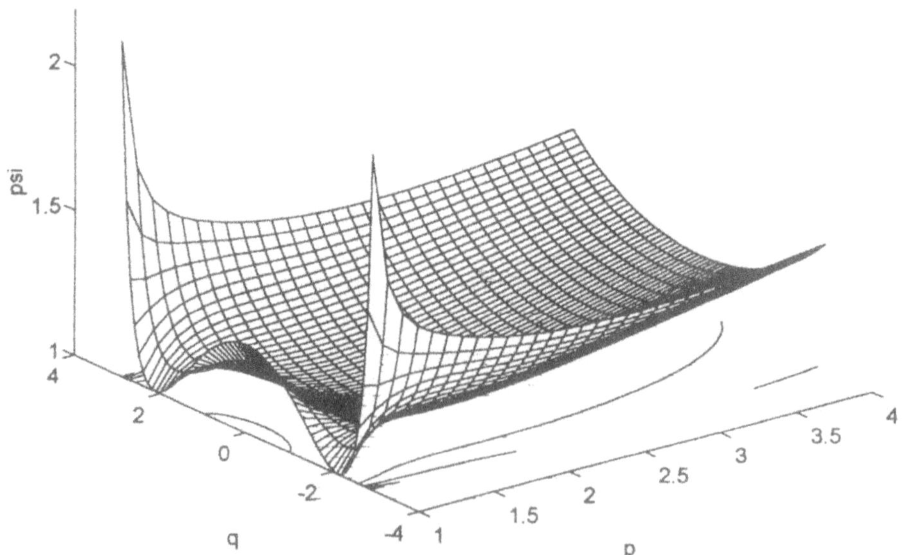

Fig. 125b. Surface $\psi = \psi(p,q)$, if $\alpha = \lambda = 1$, $\gamma = 3/4$, $\mu = -1/4$, $\beta = -1$ and $(p,q) \in [1,4] \times [-2.9, 2.9]$.

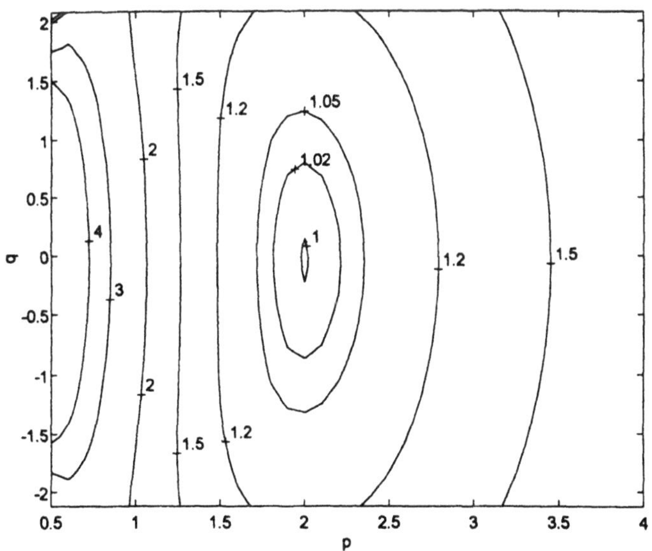

Fig. 126 a. Contour curves for $\varphi=\varphi(p,q)$, if $\alpha=\lambda=1, \gamma=3/4, \mu=-1/4, \delta=-9/8, \beta=-1$ and $(p,q)\in[0.5,4]\times[-2.12,2.12]$.

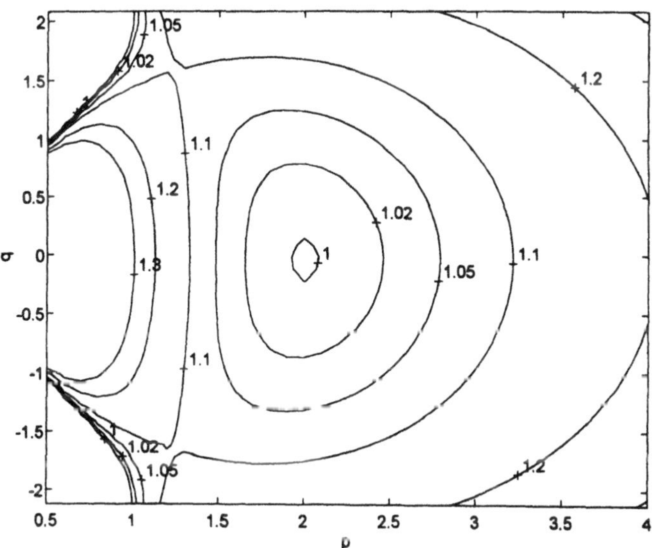

Fig. 126 b. Contour curves for $\psi=\psi(p,q)$, if $\alpha=\lambda=1, \gamma=3/4, \mu=-1/4, \delta=-9/8, \beta=-1$ and $(p,q)\in[0.5,4]\times[-2.12,2.12]$.

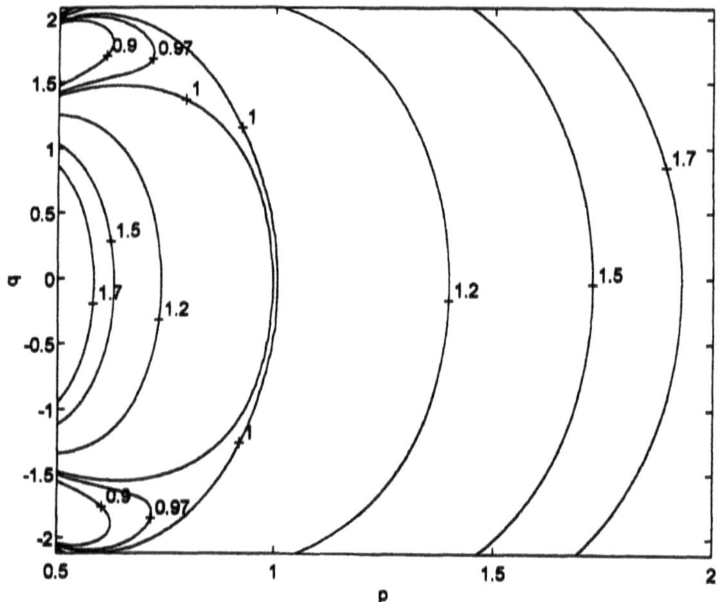

Fig. 127 a. Contour curves for $\varphi=\varphi(p,q)$, if $\alpha=\lambda=1$, $\gamma=3/4$, $\mu=-1/4$, $\delta=-9/8$, $\beta=-1/2$ and $(p,q)\in[0.5,2]\times[-2.12,2.12]$.

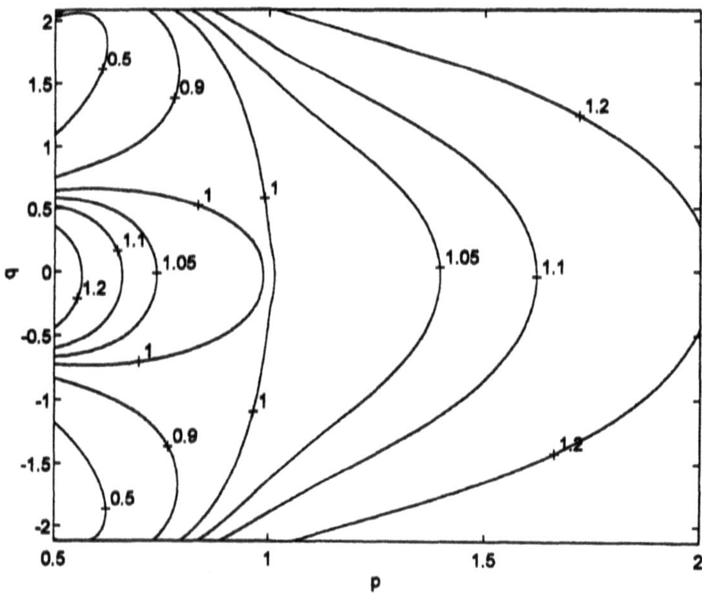

Fig. 127 b. Contour curves for $\psi=\psi(p,q)$, if $\alpha=\lambda=1$, $\gamma=3/4$, $\mu=-1/4$, $\delta=-9/8$, $\beta=-1/2$ and $(p,q)\in[0.5,2]\times[-2.12,2.12]$.

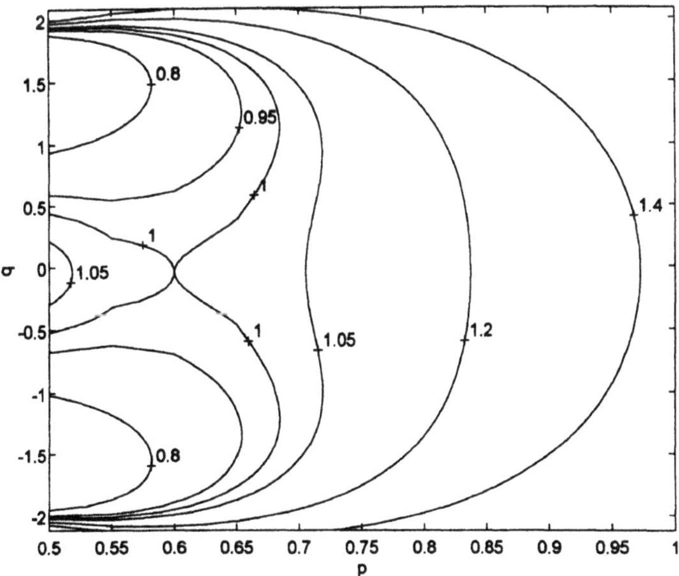

Fig. 128 a. Contour curves for $\varphi = \varphi(p,q)$, if $\alpha = \lambda = 1$, $\gamma = 3/4$, $\mu = -1/4$, $\delta = -9/8$, $\beta = -0.3$ and $(p,q) \in [0.5,1] \times [-2.12, 2.12]$.

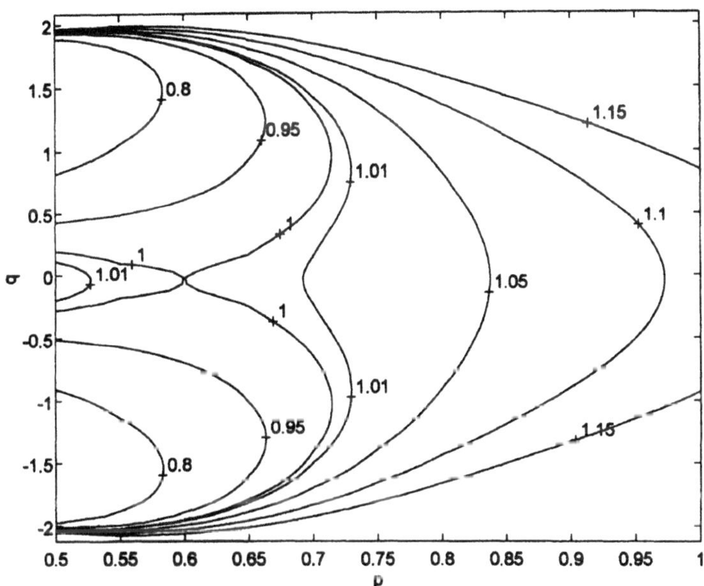

Fig. 128 b. Contour curves for $\psi = \psi(p,q)$, if $\alpha = \lambda = 1$, $\gamma = 3/4$, $\mu = -1/4$, $\delta = -9/8$, $\beta = -0.3$ and $(p,q) \in [0.5,1] \times [-2.12, 2.12]$.

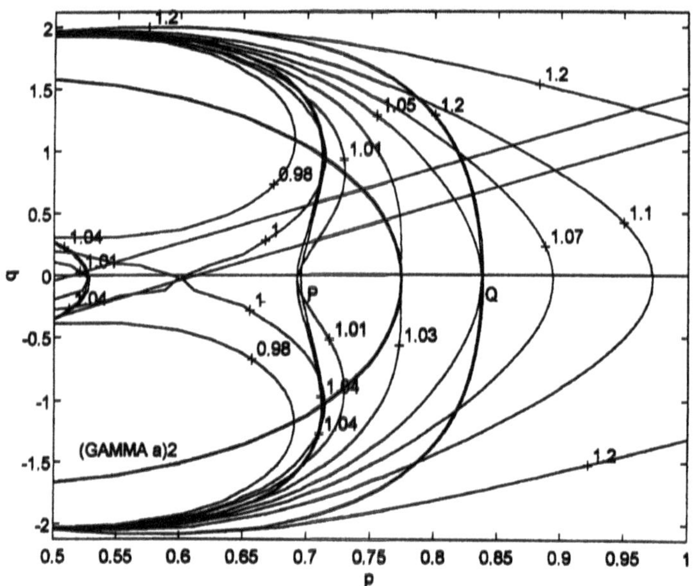

Fig.129. Curves $\varphi(p,q)=1.04$, $\varphi(p,q)=1.2$, $\psi(p,q)=$ k, k = 0.98; 1; 1.01; 1.05; 1.07; 1.1; 1.2 and curve (Γ_a) for β = - 0.3.

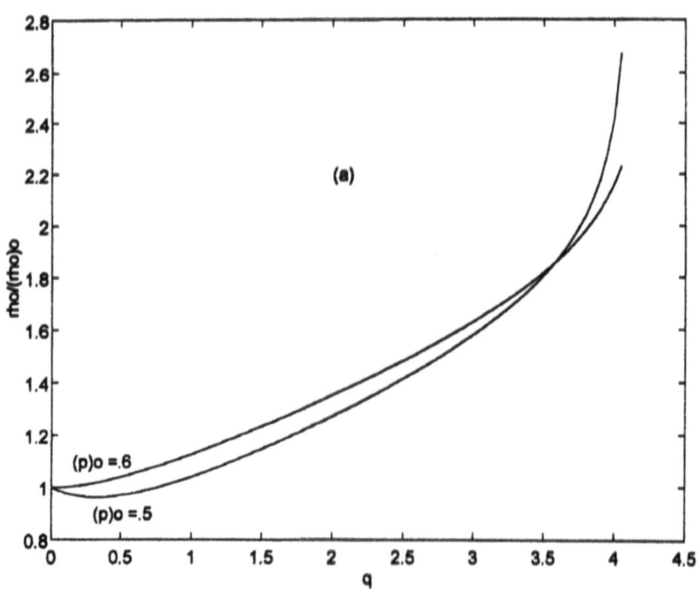

Fig.130 a. Deviatoric stress-mass density curves for $p=q/3+p_0$, $\beta=-0.3$;

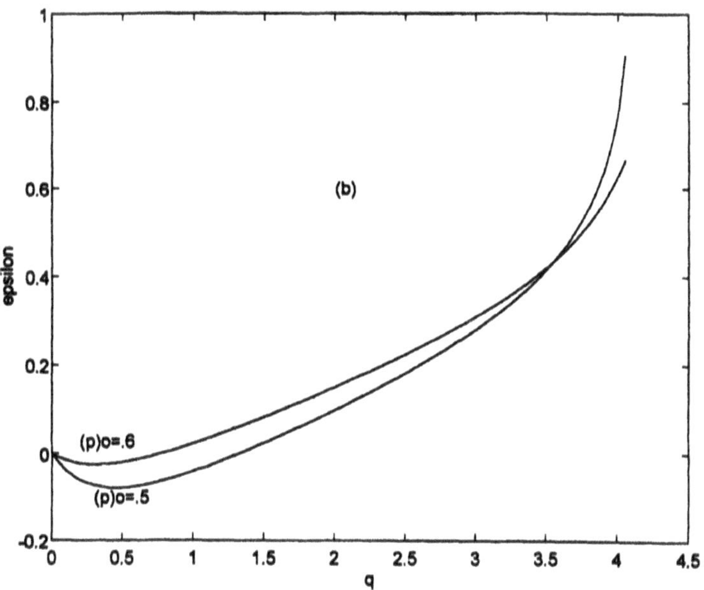

Fig. 130 b. Deviatoric stress-shear strain curves for $p=q/3+p_0$, $\beta=-0.3$;

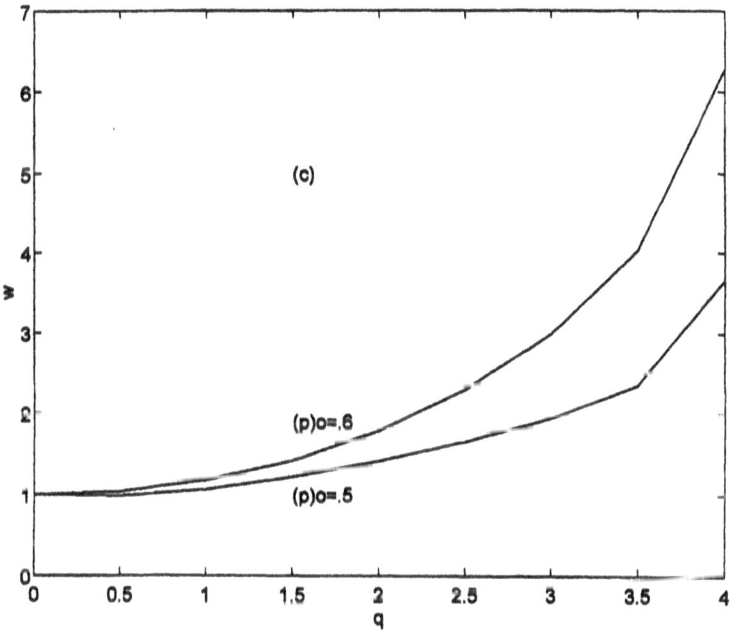

Fig. 130 c. Deviatoric stress-stress work curves for $p=q/3+p_0$, $\beta=-0.3$.

11.3. CONCLUSIONS

1. For the stability of granular compacted materials ($3\alpha_7 - \alpha_{15} > 0$), the consolidation pressure must be greater than its bifurcation value -2β.

2. On the accessibility curve, the curves ρ = const., w = const. have the same tangent.

3. For granular materials (soils, powders, ...) in loading, unloading and reloading, the different material constant values should be considered. The loading, unloading and reloading paths must be the accessible paths.

4. Some granular materials such as sand, salt,... have a dilation before failure. For those materials we get $3\alpha_7 - \alpha_{15} < 0$ and the surface $\varphi = \varphi(p,q)$ (see Fig.125a) have in $(-2\beta, 0)$ a maximum point, not a minimum point.

5. The materials with dilation have an interesting behavior for different values of the constitutive parameters. They become unstable before failure.

6. This mathematical model can explain the loss of volume stability (the appearance and disappearance of the dilation) and the total loss of stability.

In consequence, the mechanical behavior of a granular new material, obtained by combination of two granular materials, essentially depends on their constitutive parameters, the stress path, the place of the initial stress and the initial configuration. Because the material constant values experimentally deduced have a certain approximation degree, knowing the bifurcation conditions is absolutely necessary.

11.4. REFERENCES

[1] C. Truesdell, *J. Rat. Mech. Anal.* **4**, 83, 1019 (1955).

[2] L. Drăguşin, *Int. J. Engng. Sci.* **19**, 511 (1981).

[3] L. Drăguşin, *Rev. Roum. Sci. Techn.-Méc. Appl.* **34**, 323 (1989).

[4] L. Drăguşin, *Int. J. Engng. Sci.* **33**, 279 (1995).

[5] L. Drăguşin, *Int. J. Engng. Sci.* **33**, 1183 (1995).

[6] L. Drăguşin, *Int. J. Engng. Sci.* **36**, 1839 (1998).

[7] G.Ioos and D.D. Joseph, *Elementary Stability and Bifurcation Theory,* Springer-Verlag, Berlin (1980).

[8] C. Udrişte, *Linii de câmp*, Editura Tehnică, Bucureşti (1988).

[9] J. Hale and H. Kocak, *Dynamics and Bifurcations,* Springer-Verlag, Berlin (1991).

BIBLIOGRAPHY

1. V. Arnold, Ecuaţii diferenţiale ordinare, Bucureşti, Editura Ştiinţifică şi Enciclopedică, 1978.

2. V. Arnold, Metodele matematice ale mecanicii clasice, Bucureşti, Editura Ştiinţifică şi Enciclopedică, 1980.

3. V. Barbu, Ecuaţii diferenţiale, Iaşi, Editura Junimea, 1985.

4. Y. Bibikov, Local theory of nonlinear analytic ordinary differential equations, Berlin, Springer-Verlag, 1979.

5. S. Bobbio, Struttura topologica dei campi magnetici nelle esperienze di fusione termonucleare controllata, Notiziario della Unione Matematica Italiana, Cagliari, 1-3 Gugne 1987, 125-152.

6. S. Bobio, G. Marrucci, Classical thermodynamics formulated as a field theory in the representative space, Il Nuovo Cimento 13, 9 (1991), 1189-1196.

7. F. Brickell, R. Clark, Differential manifolds, London, Van Nostrand Reinhold Company, 1970.

8. V. Brînzănescu, O. Stănăşilă, Matematici speciale, Editura All, Bucureşti, 1994.

9. C. Caratheodory, Grundlagen der Termodinamik, Math. Ann. 67 (1909), 369.

10. J. Carr, Applications of centre manifold, Berlin, Springer-Verlag, 1981.

11. G. Cartianu et al., Semnale, circuite şi sisteme, Bucureşti, Editura Didactică şi Pedagogică, 1980.

12. G. Chilov, Analyse mathematique, Moscou, Mir, 1975.

13. A. Chorin, J.E. Marsden, A mathematical introduction to fluid mechanics, Berlin, Springer-Verlag, 1979.

14. I. Cornfeld et al., Ergodic theory, Berlin, Springer-Verlag, 245, 1982.

15. M. Craiu, M. Roşculeţ, Ecuaţii diferenţiale aplicative, Bucureşti, Editura Didactică şi Pedagogică, 1971.

16. T. Creţu, Fizică generală, Curs universitar, Bucureşti, Editura Tehnică, 1996.

17. Cursul de fizică Berkeley, I - V, Bucureşti, Editura Didactică şi Pedagogică, 1982-1983.

18. R. Devaney, Chaotic dynamical systems, Reading, MA, Addison-Wesley Publishing Company, Inc., 1989.

19. O. Dogaru, I. Ţevy, C. Udrişte, Extrema constrained by a family of curves and local extrema, Journal of Optimization Theory and Applications, 97, 3(1998), 605-621.

20. B. Dubrovin, and al., Modern Geometry, Methods and Applications, Berlin, Springer-Verlag, 1984.

21. E. Durand, Electrostatique, I - III, Paris, Masson et Cie, 1966.

22. D. Ebin, Completeness of Hamiltonian vector fields, Proc. Amer. Math. Soc. 26,4 (1970), 632-634.

23. L. Eisenhart, Continuous groups of transformations, New York, Dover Publications, Inc., 1961.

24. Gh. Gheorghiev, V.Oproiu, Varietăţi diferenţiabile finit şi infinit dimensionale, Bucureşti, Editura Academiei , 1976.

25. V. Gioncu, M. Ivan, Teoria comportării critice şi postcritice a structurilor elastice, Bucureşti, Editura Academiei R.S.R., 1984.

26. W. Gordon, On the completeness of Hamiltonian vector fields, Proc. Amer. Math. Soc. 26 (1970), 329-331.

27. A. Halanay, Teoria calitativă a ecuaţiilor diferenţiale, Bucureşti, Editura Academiei R.S.R., 1963.

28. P. Hartman, Ordinary differential equations, New York, John Wiley, 1965.

29. B. Hassard et al., Theory and applications of Hopf bifurcation, Cambridge, UK, Cambridge University Press, 1981.

30. S. Ianuş, Geometrie diferenţială, Bucureşti, Editura Academiei R.S.R., 1983.

31. D. V. Ionescu, Ecuaţii diferenţiale şi integrale, Bucureşti, Editura Didactică şi Pedagogică, 1972.

32. I. Gerard, J. Daniel, Elementary stability and bifurcation theory, Berlin, Springer-Verlag, 1980.

33. St. Ispas et al., Cosmosul, Laborator şi uzină pentru viitorul omenirii, Bucureşti, Editura Tehnică, 1984.

34. M. Krasnoselskii et al., Vektornîe polea na ploskosti, Moscova, Gosatomizdat, 1983.

35. M. Kubicek, Algorithm for evaluation of complex bifurcation points in ordinary differential equations, Siam, J. Appl. Math. 38 (1980), 103-107.

36. G. Leitmann, Optimization techniques with applications to aerospace systems, New York, Academic Press, 1962.

37. E. Lorenz, Deterministic nonperiodic flow, Journal of the atmospheric sciences, 20 (1963), 130-141.

38. J. Marsden, M. McCracken, The Hopf bifurcation and its applications, Berlin, Springer-Verlag, 1976.

39. S. Mirică, Ecuaţii diferenţiale, Litografia Universităţii Bucureşti, 1979.

40. R. Miron, Geometrizarea sistemelor Pfaff în spaţii riemanniene cu metrică nedefinită, St. Cerc. St. Acad. R.S.R., Iaşi (Matematică), 1, 1958.

41. R. Miron, M. Anastasiei, The geometry of Lagrange spaces; theory and applications, Fundamental Theories of Physics, 59, Dordrecht, Kluwer Academic Publishers, 1994.

42. R. Miron, The geometry of higher - order Lagrange spaces, Fundamental Theories of Physics, 82, Dordrecht, Kluwer Academic Publishers, 1996.

43. C. Mocanu, Teoria câmpului electromagnetic, Bucureşti, Editura Didactică şi Pedagogică, 1981.

44. L. Nicolescu, Lecţii de grupuri Lie, Litografia Universităţii Bucureşti, 1984.

45. V. Obădeanu, Mechanics (Newtonian formalism, Lagrangian formalism), Universitatea Timişoara, 1987.

46. V. Olariu, T. Stănăşilă, Probleme de ecuaţii diferenţiale şi cu derivate parţiale, Bucureşti, Editura Tehnică, 1982.

47. D. Opriş, I. Butulescu, Geometrical methods in the study of differential systems

of equations, Editura Mirton Timişoara, 1987.

48. E . Petrişor, Sisteme dinamice haotice, Universitatea din Timişoara, 1992.

49. E. Petrişor, The dynamics of a magnetic field around a heteroclinic structure, Seminarul de Mecanică, Universitatea din Timişoara, 48, 1995.

50. E. Petrişor, A study of the Rimmer bifurcation of symmetric fixed points of reversible diffeomorphisms,Balkan Journal of Geometry and Its Applications, 1,2(1996),87-95.

51. E. Petrişor, Heteroclinic conections in the dynamics of a reversible magnetic - type vector field, Physica D 112 (1998, 319 - 327).

52. L. Pontryaguin et al., Theorie mathematique des processus optimaux, Moscou, Mir, 1974.

53. W. Poor, Differential geometric structures, New York, Mc Graw-Hill Book Company, 1981.

54. M. Postnikov, Lectures in geometry, Moscou, Mir, 1982.

55. M. Puta, Hamiltonian mechanics and geometric quantization, Dordrecht, Kluwer Academic Publishers, 1993.

56. V. Radcenco, C. Udrişte, D. Udrişte, Thermodynamic systems and their interaction, Scientific Bulletin, Politechnic Institute of Bucharest, Electrical engineering, 53, 3-4 (1991), 285-294.

57. A. Ramsey, Newtonian attraction, Cambridge, UK, Cambridge University Press.

58. M. Săvescu et al., Metode de optimizare în analiza circuitelor electronice, Bucureşti, Editura Tehnică, 1982.

59. L. Segel, Mathematical models in molecular and cellular biology, Cembridge, UK, Cambridge University Press, 1980.

60. Gh. Silaş et al., Vibraţii mecanice, Bucureşti, Editura Tehnică, 1973.

61. I. Singer, J. Thorpe, Lectures notes on elementary topology and geometry, Chicago, lL, Scott, Foresman and Company, 1967.

62. S. Smale, The mathematics of time, Berlin, Springer-Verlag, 1980.

63 S. Ştefănescu, Lignes de champ magnetique d'une ramification de courants, Bull. Math. Phys. Pures et Appl., 1-9(1936).

64. S. Ştefănescu, Pour la prospection electrique du sous-sol, Note presentee a l'Academie Roumaine, 1927.

65. S. Ştefănescu, Pour la prospection electrique du sous-sol, etude du champ S normal, Note presentee a l'Academie Roumaine, 1928.

66. S. Ştefănescu, Lignes de champ magnetique d'un circuit filiforme, symetrique et plan, deux fois coude, Bull. Math. Phys. Pures et Appl., 1,2 (1935-1936), 19-20.

67. S. Ştefănescu, Un nouveau cas d'applications en electromagnetisme des fonctions cylindrique generales, Bull. Math. Phys. Pures et Appl., 1,2,2(1936-1937), 22, 23, 24.

68. S. Ştefănescu, Un cas particulier des lignes H algebrique, Bull. Math. Phys. Pures et Appl., 1,2,3 (1937-1938), 25, 26, 27, 1-7.

69. S. Ştefănescu, Liniile de câmp magnetic ale unui curent electric filiform şi plan de doua ori cotit, Comunicarile Academiei, 1(1951), 8, 769-774.

70. S. Ştefănescu, Liniile de câmp magnetic ale poligoanelor regulate de curenţi rectilinii (I), St., Cerc. Fiz., 5(1954), 1-2, 63-70.

71. S. Ştefănescu, Liniile de câmp magnetic ale poligoanelor regulate de curenţi

rectilinii (II), St., Cerc. Fiz., 6(1955), 1-2, 459-471.

72. S. Ştefănescu, Asupra unor linii de câmp magnetic definite prin transcedente elementare, St. Cerc. Fiz., 7,4 (1956), 519-530.

73. S. Ştefănescu, Les lignes e champ magnetique d'un triangle de courants rectilignes, Revue de Physique, 1(1956), 89-102.

74. S. Ştefănescu, Open magnetic field lines, St. Cerc. Fiz., 1, 9(1958), 151-166, Revue Roum. Phys, 3, 2(1958).

75. S. Ştefănescu, Liniile de câmp magnetic ale unui curent directiliniu strimb, St. Cerc. Fiz., 10, 3(1959), 387-396.

76. S. Ştefănescu, M. Nabighian, Magnetic field lines of two equal rectilinear electric currents, St. Cerc. Fiz., 3(1960), 563-583; Rev. Roum. Geo., Geophys. et Geogr., Geophysique, 31(1987), 95-112.

77. S. Ştefănescu, M. Nabighian, Asupra liniilor de câmp magnetic ale emitatorului AB, Probleme de Geofizică, 1(1961), 181-186.

78. S. Ştefănescu, Liniile de câmp magnetic imprejurul unei prize de pamânt intr-un teren cu stratificaţie paralela, Probleme de Geofizică, 2(1963), 135-145.

79. S. Ştefănescu, Liniile de câmp magnetic ale unui dreptunghi centrat de curenţi rectilinii egali, St. Cerc. Fiz., 21, 1(1969), 21-32.

80. S. Ştefănescu, Nouveaux exemples de lignes de champ magnetique ouvertes, Rev. Roum. Phys., 15 (1970), 1, 11-25.

81. S. Ştefănescu, Lignes de champ magnetique d'un parallelogramme centre de courants rectilignes egaux (I), Rev. Roum. Phys., 17(1972), 9, 1041-1052.

82. S. Ştefănescu, Lignes de champ magnetique d'un parallelogramme centre de courants rectilignes egaux (II), Rev. Roum. Phys., 18(1973), 9, 35-48.

83. S. Ştefănescu, Sur les lignes de champ magnetique d'un circuit electrique en forme de losange aplati, Rev. Roum. Phys., 21 (1976), 4, 421-430.

84. S. Ştefănescu, Sur les lignes de chmap magnetique d'une ligne electrique bifilaire, plane symmetriquement coudee, Rev. Roum. Phys., 22 (1977), 9, 911-921.

85. S. Ştefănescu, Open magnetic field lines (II), Rev. Roum. Phys., 31 (1986), 7, 701-721.

86. S. Ştefănescu, Addenda 1987 - Open magnetic field lines (III), Rev. Roum. Geol. Geophys., Geogr. - Geophysique, 31 (1987), 113-119.

87. S. Ştefănescu, Une hobby mathematique, Rev. Roum. Phys., 31(1987), 89-93.

88. S. Ştefănescu, Lignes H, circuits rectiligne coudes, manuscript notices, 1944-1992, unpublished.

89. S. Ştefănescu, C. Udrişte, Magnetic field lines around filiform electrical circuits of right angle type, Scientific Bulletin, Politehnica University of Bucharest, Applied Mathematics and Physics 55 (1993), 3-18.

90. Z. Stoian, Ecuaţii diferenţiale, Litografia Institutului Politehnic Bucureşti, 1982.

91. C. Teleman, Asupra sistemelor mecanice neolonome, Analele Univ. Bucureşti, 1957, p.43.

92. R. Thom, Structural stability and morphogenesis, Boston, MA, W.A. Benjamin, Inc., 1975.

93. J. Thorpe, Elementary topics in differential geometry, Berlin, Springer-Verlag, 1979.

94. L. Timothy, B. Bone, State space analysis, New York, Mc Graw-Hill Book Company.

95. N. Teodorescu, V. Olariu, Ecuaţii diferenţiale şi cu derivate parţiale, Bucureşti, Editura Tehnică, 1978-1980.

96. I. Teodorescu, S. Teodorescu, Culegere de probleme de geometrie superioară, Bucureşti, Editura Didactică şi Pedagogică, 1975.

97. A. Ţugulea, Al. Timotin, R. Răduleţ, Teoreme de unicitate pentru regimuri variabile ale câmpului electromagnetic, St. Cerc. Energetică, Electrotehnică, 21(1971),109-128.

98. A. Udrişte, C. Udrişte, Magnetic dynamics around electrical circuits, Ed. Gr. Tsagas, Global Analysis, Differential Geometry, Lie Algebras, BSG Proceedings 1, Geometry Balkan Press 1997, 109-122.

99. A. Udrişte, C. Udrişte, Dynamics induced by a magnetic field, Ed. J. Szenthe, New Developments in Differential Geometry, Budapest (1996), 429-442, Dordrecht, Kluwer Academic Publishers.

100. C. Udrişte, Independents vector fields on orientable hypersurfaces, Bucureşti, Editura Academiei , 1976, 163-164.

101. C. Udrişte, E. Tănăsescu, Minime şi maxime, Bucureşti, Editura Tehnică, 1980.

102. C. Udrişte, and al., Probleme de algebră, geometrie şi ecuaţii diferenţiale, Bucureşti, Editura Didactică şi Pedagogică, 1981.

103. C. Udrişte, and al., Algebră, geometrie şi ecuaţii diferenţiale, Bucureşti, Editura Didactică şi Pedagogică, 1982.

104. C. Udrişte, Linii de câmp, Editura Tehnică Bucureşti, 1988.

105. C.Udrişte, Extremum points of square lengths of some vector fields, Colocviul Naţional de Geometrie şi Topologie, Buşteni, 27-30 iunie 1981, Bull. Math. 30 (78), 4 (1986), 361-370.

106. C. Udrişte, Proprietăţi ale câmpurilor vectoriale afine şi proiective, St. Cerc. Mat. 36, 5 (1984), 444-452.

107. C. Udrişte, Properties of conformal vector fields, ICM, Warsaw, Poland, 16-24 august, 1983.

108. C. Udrişte, Properties of torse forming vector fields, Colocviul Naţional de Geometrie şi Topologie, Piatra Neamţ, 16-19 iunie 1983; Tensor, N.S. 42 (1985), 137-144.

109. C. Udrişte, C. Radu, A. Zlătescu, Completitudinea câmpurilor vectoriale hamiltoniene, Colocviul Naţional de Geometrie şi Topologie, Piatra Neamţ, 16-19 iunie 1983, Buletinul IPB, 46-47 (1984-1985), 15-20.

110. C. Udrişte, Properties of irrotational vector fields, Journal of Geometry and Physics, Pitagora Editrice Bologna, 2 (1985), 117-125.

111. C. Udrişte, Convex functions and optimization methods on Riemannian manifolds, Mathematics and Its Applications 297, Dordrecht, Kluwer Academic Publishers, 1994.

112. C. Udrişte, O. Dogaru, Extrema with nonholonomic constraints, Buletinul Institutului Politehnic Bucureşti, seria Energetică, 50 (1988), 3-8.

113. C. Udrişte, O. Dogaru, Mathematical programming problems with nonholonomic constraints, Seminarul de Mecanică, Universitatea din Timişoara, 14, 1988.

114. C. Udrişte, O. Dogaru, Extreme conditionate pe orbite, Buletinul Institutului Politehnic Bucureşti, Seria Mecanică, 51 (1989), 3-9.

115. C. Udrişte, O. Dogaru, Convex nonholonomic hypersurfaces, The Mathematical Heritage of C.F. Gauss, Edited by G.M. Rassias, Singapore, World Scientific Publishers, (1990), 769-784.

116. C. Udrişte, O. Dogaru, I. Ţevy, Sufficient conditions for extremum on differential manifolds, Scientific Bulletin, Politehnic Institute of Bucharest, Electrical Engineering 53, 3-4 (1991), 341-344.

117. C. Udrişte, Applications of algebra, geometry and differential equations, Bucuresti, Editura Didactică şi Pedagogică, 1993.

118. C. Udrişte, O. Dogaru, I. Ţevy, Extrema points associated to a Pfaff form, Tensor, N.S., 54 (1993), 115-121.

119. C. Udrişte, O. Dogaru, I. Ţevy, Open problems in extrema theory, Scientific Bulletin, Politehnica University of Bucharest, Applied Mathematics and Physics, 55, 3-4 (1993), 273-277.

120. C. Udrişte, M. Postolache, A. Udrişte, Acad. Sabba Ştefănescu, conjecture; Lines of magnetic field generated by filiform electrical circuits, Revue Roumaine Geophysique, Romanian Academy, 36 (1992), 17-25.

121. C. Udrişte, M. Postolache, A.Udrişte, Energy of magnetic field generated by filiform electrical circuits of right angle type, Tensor, N.S., 54 (1993), 185-195.

122. C. Udrişte, M. Postolache, A.Udrişte, Numerical simulation of dynamic magnetical systems, Scientific Bulletin, Politehnica University of Bucharest, Applied Mathematics and Physics, 55 (1993), 51-64.

123. C. Udrişte, C. Radu, C. Dumitrescu, A. Zlătescu, Biot-Savart-Laplace integral, Tensor, N.S., 54 (1993), 196-202.

124. C. Udrişte, A.Udrişte, Properties of magnetic lines and surfaces, Proceedings of 23-rd Conference on Geometry and Topology, Babeş-Bolyai University, Cluj-Napoca, Sept 27-29 (1993), 203-208.

125. C. Udrişte, A. Udrişte, V. Balan, M. Postolache, Magnetic dynamical systems, Eds. L.Tamassy, J.Szenthe, New Developments in Differential Geometry, Dordrecht, Kluwer Academic Publishers (1996), 407-414; Analele Stiintifice ale Univ. AL.I. Cuza Iaşi, Informatică (1995), 105-126.

126. C. Udrişte, A. Udrişte, V. Balan, M. Postolache, Phase portraits and critical elements of magnetic field generated by piecewise rectilinear electric circuits, Eds. P.Antonelli, R.Miron, Lagrange and Finsler Geometry, Dordrecht, Kluwer Academic Publishers, 1995, 177-187.

127. C. Udrişte, A. Udrişte, V. Balan, M. Postolache, Magnetic field generated by two coplanar electrical circuits of fixed angle type and its field lines, Proceedings of 24-th National Conference of Geometry and Topology, University of Timişoara, July 5-9, 1994, 285-301.

128. C. Udrişte, A. Udrişte, V. Balan, M. Postolache, Zeros of magnetic fields generated around filiform electrical circuits, Tensor, N.S., 57 (1996), 119-134.

129. C. Udrişte, A. Udrişte, C. Dumitrescu, T. Vasile, Geometry of magnetic flow,

Scientific Bulletin, Politehnica University of Bucharest, Applied Mathematics and Physics 55, 3-4 (1993), 279-283.

130. C. Udrişte, A. Udrişte, Electromagnetic dynamical systems, Balkan Journal of Geometry and Its Applications, 2,1 (1997), 129-140.

131. C. Udrişte, Differential Geometry, Differential Equations, Bucharest, Geometry Balkan Press, 1997.

132. C. Udrişte, Geometric Dynamics, Second Conference of Balkan Society of Geometers, Aristotle University of Thessaloniki, June 23 - 26, 1998.

133. C. Udrişte, S. Udrişte, Biot-Savart-Laplace dynamical systems, Balkan Journal of Geometry and Its Applications, 1,2 (1996), 125-136.

134. D. Udrişte, Dynamical systems of classical thermodynamics, Scientific Bulletin, Politehnica University of Bucharest, Applied Mathematics and Physics, 55, 3-4 (1993), 299-309.

135. S. Udrişte, Magnetic field generated by electrical circuits seated on a pair of coplanar isosceles triangle, Scientifc Bulletin, Politehnica University of Bucharest, Electrical Engineering, 55, 3-4 (1993), 69-74.

136. G. Vrănceanu, Lecţii de geometrie diferenţială, Bucureşti, Editura Didactică şi Pedagogică, 1962, 1964.

137. G. Vrănceanu, Opera matematică, Bucureşti, Editura Academiei , 1971-1975.

138. K. Yano, B. Chen, On the concurrent vector fields of immersed manifolds, Kodai Math. Sem. Rep. 23, 1971, 343-351.

139. J. Walker, Dynamical systems and evolution equations, New York, Plenum Press, 1980.

140. A. Weinstein, J.A. Marsden, A comparison theorem for Hamiltonian vector fields, Proc. Amer. Math. Soc. 26, 4 (1970), 629-631.

INDEX

GPSR Compliance
The European Union's (EU) General Product Safety Regulation (GPSR) is a set of rules that requires consumer products to be safe and our obligations to ensure this.

If you have any concerns about our products, you can contact us on

ProductSafety@springernature.com

In case Publisher is established outside the EU, the EU authorized representative is:

Springer Nature Customer Service Center GmbH
Europaplatz 3
69115 Heidelberg, Germany

www.ingramcontent.com/pod-product-compliance
Ingram Content Group UK Ltd.
Pitfield, Milton Keynes, MK11 3LW, UK
UKHW021858190726
13853UKWH00003B/1327

* 9 7 8 9 4 0 1 1 4 1 8 8 8 *